# SCHOOL
# HEALTH
# PROGRAM

*Health Education, Physical Education, and Recreation Series*

RUTH ABERNATHY, Ph.D.

EDITORIAL ADVISER
*Director, School of
Physical and Health Education
University of Washington, Seattle*

# SCHOOL HEALTH PROGRAM

## third edition

### JESSIE HELEN HAAG, Ed.D., F.R.S.H.

*Professor, Health Education,*
*Department of Physical and Health Education,*
*The University of Texas at Austin*

LEA & FEBIGER • *Philadelphia* • *1972*

ISBN 0-8121-0380-7

Library of Congress Catalog Card Number 70:175461

Published in Great Britain by Henry Kimpton Publishers, London

Printed in the United States of America

*To Edna and Sterling Harris*

# Preface

School and community personnel concerned with the health needs of the elementary or secondary school pupil are aware that sources of information to discover these health needs are often not known. Frequently, the pupil's health needs are ignored, although the pupil's physical and mental health status and his health practices, attitudes, interests, and knowledge can affect learning, either positively or negatively. Why sources of information to discover the pupil's health needs are not known has puzzled workers in school and community health for many years. Is it not possible to devise a total school health program from which these pupil health needs might be found? Or, have school health services developed independently of health education? Or, have the "why" and "what" of health education been lost in the multiplicity of methods and materials of instruction? Or, has healthful school living been taken for granted in this day of modern school facilities?

This text is written for teachers and prospective teachers and for those school and community personnel who would prefer the total school health program to be a means by which the pupil's health needs could be made known. These needs can become the *basis for the selection of subject matter in health education.* Satisfying these needs can justify some of the functions of school and community health personnel.

In the third edition, the text of *School Health Program* has been rewritten and reorganized. Four parts of the health program are presented: school health services, healthful school living, health education,
and organization and administration of the school health program. The implications of school health services and healthful school living for health education are stressed as well as the consideration of the *total* health program.

Among the objectives of the third edition of *School Health Program* are the following:

1. To reveal the teamwork needed by school and community personnel in the total school health program.
2. To disclose everyday situations arising within school health programs of elementary and secondary schools.
3. To identify the health problems of elementary school children and secondary school youth.
4. To reveal community resources which can be used in the total school health program.
5. To disclose the diversity and range of health education topics, for use from kindergarten through grade 12, which might be used to solve the health problems of elementary and secondary school students.
6. To indicate the in-depth subject matter of health education.
7. To reveal some of the health problems of school personnel and the procedures which might be taken to solve these problems.
8. To identify the functions of parents, school administrators, health education personnel, school nurses, family and school physicians, elementary school classroom teachers, physical educators, dentists, and dental hygienists, other school personnel, and

professional workers in local health departments and other health agencies.

9. To disclose some of the research which might be used to develop the school health program.

Some of the outstanding features of the third edition are discussions of common observable health problems; recent health appraisal techniques; health counseling and follow-through; diseases common to all school-age students including venereal diseases; dental diseases and defects; chronic health conditions including vision defects; tort liability in emergency care for the ill or injured pupil; and health problems of school personnel. Other topics covered are up-to-date improvements in the school environment; recent research studies in child nutrition; competencies and units of health education, K through 12; sources to discover the pupil's and community's health problems; health education curriculum; controversial topics; areas and units of health education; lessons within controversial units; conceptual approach and other methods of instruction; and community resources. In addition, there are discussions of the responsibilities of school and community personnel in the total school health program; school health council; and evaluation of health services, healthful school living, health education, and the total health program. Appendix A and Appendix B have been revised and Appendix C added.

Throughout the text, teamwork among teachers, school and community health service personnel, parents, and pupils is emphasized. Also, the pupil's health status, practices, attitudes, interests, and knowledge are stressed.

Many groups and personnel sharing the responsibility for the development of the school health program can use this text. Teacher education institutions preparing elementary and secondary school classroom teachers, physical educators, teachers of health education, special education teachers, and school counselors can use the text for the basic information concerning the school health program. School nurses, physicians, dentists, and dental hygienists will appreciate the numerous health problems among elementary and secondary school pupils and the procedures for solving these problems. Elementary and secondary school classroom teachers, principals, consultants, and superintendents of schools will find this text useful in any health education workshop. Community voluntary health agencies, local and state departments of health, and professional schools of medicine, nursing, and public health can use the text to extend their services. All of these groups can benefit from the References for Further Study at the end of each chapter and the footnotes in each chapter.

Permissions were granted to the author by the Joint Committee on Health Problems in Education of the National Education Association and the American Medical Association; Texas State Department of Health; and State Education Department, The University of the State of New York.

Austin, Texas                    JESSIE HELEN HAAG

# Contents

# Chapter 1

# *INTRODUCTION*

In a society where community health problems such as air pollution and noise are so prominent, the relation of the school health program to the *community health problems* is often disregarded. Without any doubt, community health problems affect the health of all school-age children both directly and indirectly. Every teacher is a team member of the school health program and is the vital link between the community and the elementary or secondary school students. No teacher can function in the school's environment without an awareness of the community's health problems. Because of the impact of the community's health problems upon the school health program, the teacher and other school personnel face the challenge of improving the *health* of not only the student but also those persons not enrolled in the elementary and secondary schools.

## AN INCIDENT

In discussing health problems of pupils with teachers, a school administrator uses these terms: "school health program," "school health services," "healthful school living," and "health education." Some teachers ask the administrator to explain the terms. Teachers should not only know what each term means but also understand how the school health program developed in the United States.

The modern school health program can provide the best justification for health education in the elementary and secondary schools. This justification is revealed when the adult accepts his responsibilities in promoting individual and community health. This acceptance of the adult's re-

sponsibilities is a result of elementary and secondary school health education and well-coordinated school health programs.

The school health program has been divided into three interrelated parts—school-health services, healthful school living, and health education.[1] *School health services* has been defined as

> school procedures carried out by physicians, nurses, dentists, social workers, teachers, and others to appraise, protect and promote the health of students and school personnel. Such procedures are designed (a) to appraise the health status of pupils and school personnel, (b) to counsel pupils, teachers, parents and others for the purpose of helping pupils obtain needed treatment or for arranging school programs in keeping with their abilities, (c) to help prevent and control communicable diseases, (d) to provide emergency care for injury or sudden illness, . . . (f) to protect and promote the health of school personnel.[2]

*Healthful school living*

> simply means living within a school where all environmental conditions, every social relationship, and every curriculum experience is carried on with due attention to health. None of these conditions or experiences should be allowed to endanger health or safety; they all should contribute to well-being.[3]

[1] Joint Committee on Health Problems in Education of the National Education Association and the American Medical Association: *Healthful School Environment.* Rev. ed. Washington, D.C.: National Education Association, 1969, p. 8.

[2] _____ : *Health Appraisal of School Children.* 4th ed. Washington, D.C.: National Education Association, 1969, p. 2.

[3] _____ : *Healthful School Environment, op. cit.,* p. 7.

*Health education* has been defined as

> the process of providing experiences for favorably influencing understandings, attitudes, and practices relating to individual, family and community health.[4]

The goal of health education is not directed at a high level of health simply for health's sake, but rather to help *each* individual view health as *a way of life* that will attain individual goals and utilize one's highest potential for the betterment of self, family, and community.[5]

The health professions readily endorse the school health program. The history of the American school health program reveals the dedicated efforts of educators, physicians, nurses, dentists, public health personnel, and professional leaders in the official and nonofficial health agencies.

## HISTORICAL DEVELOPMENT OF SCHOOL HEALTH SERVICES

In some ways, school health services in the United States were influenced by activities of physicians in European schools. During 1842 and 1843, physicians were ordered to visit public boys' and girls' schools in Paris. Each physician was requested both to inspect the school building and to examine the children's health. By 1898, certain German cities had a plan established for detecting communicable diseases in children. As the children entered school and as they entered the third, fifth, and eighth school years, they were examined by a physician.

The first public school medical officer in the United States was appointed in New York City in 1892. The Boston Board of Health, in 1894, initiated the first medical inspection of school children. During 1899, public school personnel of Connecticut were required to test the pupils' vision. The first school nurse was employed by the New York City schools in 1902. Other cities employing school nurses within a few years were Los Angeles, Philadelphia, Boston, and Pueblo, Colorado. In 1903, the first school dentist was appointed, in Reading,

Pennsylvania.[6] Massachusetts made state medical inspections compulsory in its public schools in 1906.[7] School dental services were financed in Cincinnati and New York City in 1910.[8] Dental hygienists were employed in the public schools of Bridgeport, Connecticut, in 1914.[9]

At the 1909 White House Conference on Care of Dependent Children, it was proposed that "every needy child should receive the best medical and surgical attention."[10] School health services were considered at the White House Conference on Child Welfare Standards in 1919. Vision and hearing testing, the compilation of health records, control of communicable diseases, and establishment of dental and nutrition clinics were recommended at this conference.[11] In 1925, the National Congress of Parents and Teachers promoted the Summer Round-Up Campaign. The purpose was to promote among parents a realization of their responsibility for sending children to school prepared through adequate medical attention.

The health of teachers was emphasized in a report by James Frederick Rogers in 1926. This was the first attempt to stress the importance of the teacher's health as a part of the school health program.[12] Later, in 1938 and 1957, the health of the teacher was the main topic in the publication *Fit to Teach*. The health of teachers and other school personnel was also considered at the 1940 White House Conference. In 1964, the Joint Committee on Health Problems in Education of the National Education Association (NEA) and the American Medical Association (AMA) published *Health of School Personnel*.

The American Association of School Physicians was established in 1927; in 1938 this society became the American School Health Association, which publishes *The Journal*

[4]Health education terminology. *J. Health, Physical Education and Recreation 33* (November, 1962) :27.
[5]School Health Education Study: *Health Education: A Conceptual Approach to Curriculum Design.* Washington, D.C.: 3M Education Press and the Study, 1967, p. 11.
[6]Charles H. Keene: Development of school health services. *J. School Health 23* (January, 1953) :23.
[7]Richard Means: *A History of Health Education in the United States.* Philadelphia: Lea & Febiger, 1962, p. 268.
[8]Charles H. Keene: School health services—second section. *J. School Health 23* (February, 1953) :51.
[9]Kenneth Veselak: Historical steps in the development of the modern school health program. *J. School Health 39* (September, 1959):268.
[10]Means, *op. cit.*, p. 90.
[11]*Ibid.*, p. 134.
[12]*Ibid.*, pp. 212-213.

*of School Health.* Delegates to the 1930 White House Conference on Child Health and Protection gave detailed suggestions for school health services. Daily health inspections, dental care, weighing, immunization, and follow-through activities of the nurse were some of the phases of school health services mentioned.[13] The 1940 White House Conference on Children and Youth recognized the deficiencies in school health services. The delegates proposed that adequate school health services include examination of the teeth, immunizations, early detection of diseases, thorough medical examinations, vision and hearing tests, medical examination of athletes, and complete follow-through activities.[14]

In 1947, the AMA inaugurated the series of Conferences on Physicians and Schools. The Mid-Century White House Conference on Children and Youth advocated that all school personnel work closely with school health services. This conference focused attention on the handicapped child. In 1953 and 1957, two publications of the Joint Committee on Health Problems in Education of the NEA and the AMA had considerable impact on school health services. The two publications were *School Health Services* and *Health Appraisal of School Children.* The 1960 White House Conference on Children and Youth dealt extensively with school health services. Some of the problems considered by the delegates were hearing and vision screening, dental and medical examinations, tuberculin testing, prevention and control of diseases, health records, immunization, the handicapped child, and health service facilities.[15]

The American Academy of Pediatrics published the outstanding *Report of the Committee on School Health* in 1966. In the same year and in 1969, the Joint Committee on Health Problems in Education of the NEA and the AMA published the fourth editions of *Suggested School Health Policies* and *Health Appraisal of School Children.*

During the sixties, school nurses, encouraged by the growth of school health services, established standards for the functions and preparation of school

nurses.[16],[17] In addition, a National Conference on School Nurse Leadership was held in 1968 sponsored by the National Council for School Nurses, American Association for Health, Physical Education and Recreation. In 1967, the Study Committee on School Physicians of the American School Health Association published a pamphlet, "Manual for School Physicians."[18] Evidence of continuing growth of dental health care in school health services was found in the 1968 Report of the Study Committee on Dental Health of the American School Health Association.[19] Involvement of other health personnel in the school health services was disclosed in *The Journal of School Health* from 1960 to 1971.

## HISTORICAL DEVELOPMENT OF HEALTHFUL SCHOOL LIVING

As early as 1829, the importance of improving school buildings was recognized by William A. Alcott in his *Essay on the Construction of Schoolhouses.* In 1837, school hygiene was discussed by Horace Mann in his first report to the Massachusetts Board of Education. The Los Angeles Board of Education, in 1880, requested school personnel to be aware of classroom ventilation and temperatures.[20] The 1919 White House Conference on Child Welfare Standards issued significant statements concerning healthful school living.[21] The 1930 White House Conference on Child Health and Protection indicated that healthful school living was the most important phase of education and made recommendations regarding environmental factors and the school day. Adequate lighting, heating and ventilation, water supply, and toilet and shower room facilities were some of the items considered necessary to healthful school environment. Planning activities, ar-

[13]*Ibid.*, pp. 260-261.
[14]*Ibid.*, pp. 328-329.
[15]*Ibid.*, pp. 330-332.

[16]American Nurses' Association: *School Nursing Practice: A Guide for Evaluating, Implementing and Improving the Functions of School Nurses.* New York: The Association, 1961.
[17]Report of the School Nursing Committee on proposed guidelines for qualifications of school nurse supervisors. *J. School Health 36* (June, 1966) :262.
[18]Annual Report of the Study Committee on School Physicians. *J. School Health 39* (March, 1969) :190.
[19]Report to the Governing Council of the Study Committee on Dental Health. *J. School Health 39* (June, 1969) :418.
[20]Veselak, *loc. cit.*
[21]Means, *op. cit.*, p. 134.

rangement of the curriculum, and discipline were some of the items mentioned in their recommendations for the school day.[22] "Hygiene of the environment" and "school hygiene" were replaced by the term "healthful school living" in 1934. Differences in desirable and actual conditions of healthful school living were presented at the 1940 White House Conference on Children in a Democracy. More comprehensive statements about healthful school living were made at the 1940 Conference than at previous White House Conferences. The quality of daily school meals were stressed for both educational and dietary values. The Mid-Century White House Conference on Children and Youth discussed healthful school living in detail, involving environmental factors, school nutrition, and the school day. The 1960 White House Conference provided optimum standards for lighting, heating, ventilation, cooling, and other environmental factors; school nutrition; and factors related to school day.[23]

Many professional societies and governmental agencies have assisted in promoting healthful school living. Since 1948, the Illuminating Engineering Society has published the *American Standard Guide for School Lighting*. The American Society of Heating, Refrigerating, and Air-Conditioning Engineers have published standards biennially. The American Association of School Administrators and the Council of Educational Facility Planners have promoted the need for construction of safe, efficient, modern school buildings. The United States Public Health Service, the American Public Health Association, and the American Society of Mechanical Engineers have provided standards for water supply, plumbing, and waste disposal. The National Safety Council and the United States Department of Labor have established safety standards for schools. The United States Department of Agriculture, the United States Office of Education, the United States Public Health Service, and the National Sanitation Foundation have published guidelines for school nutrition. In 1957, *Healthful School Living* was published by the Joint Committee on Health Problems in Education of the NEA and the

AMA. In 1962, the Joint Committee published *Health Aspects of the School Lunch Program* and, in 1969, *Healthful School Environment*.

## HISTORICAL DEVELOPMENT OF HEALTH EDUCATION

The historical development of health education reveals the efforts of leaders in education, medicine, and official and nonofficial health agencies. In 1843, Horace Mann emphasized the need for the study of hygiene and physiology as parts of the elementary and secondary school curriculum. Seven years later, Massachusetts became the first state to require hygiene and physiology as compulsory subjects in the public schools. Previously, in 1845, a course consisting of hygiene, physiology, and first aid was offered in the Boys' High School of Philadelphia.[24]

During the period between 1850 and 1900, developments in public health, education, and the temperance movement stimulated progress of health education. Lemuel Shattuck's "Report of the Sanitary Commission of Massachusetts," in 1850, focused attention not only on the public health field but also on school health education. The American Public Health Association was organized in 1872, and the American Association for the Advancement of Physical Education, now the American Association for Health, Physical Education and Recreation, was established in 1885. These two societies were influential in the development of health education of that period. The national movement of the Women's Christian Temperance Union, from 1880 to 1890, succeeded not only in having legislation passed concerning the teaching of the effects of alcohol, tobacco, and narcotics but also in focusing national attention on hygiene and physiology as important parts of the curriculum. By 1890, 38 of our states and territories had passed legislation requiring the teaching of hygiene and physiology in the public schools.[25] At the National Education Association's meeting in 1896 two significant recommendations were made. First, support was given to hygiene teaching in elementary and secondary schools. Second, instruction in hygiene was

[22]*Ibid.*, p. 261.
[23]*Ibid.*, pp. 328-332.
[24]*Ibid.*, pp. 33-36.
[25]*Ibid.*, pp. 50-56.

to be included in the preparation of the teacher. However, a year earlier Edward M. Hartwell had revealed the nonexistence of teachers prepared to teach hygiene in the United States. In 1898, Hartwell indicated that school hygienists were being prepared in Europe but not in the United States.

New concepts of health education appeared from 1900 to 1915. Open-air classrooms demonstrated practical health education. The White House Conference on the Care of Dependent Children stressed that every child should receive health instruction. The Joint Committee on Health Problems in Education of the NEA and the AMA was established in 1911. The early publications of this committee received attention because of its greater emphasis on health education than that found in previous publications. From 1911 to 1938, the committee's chairman was Thomas D. Wood, who formulated the modern school health program and health education. During this period, preparation of teachers of health education received more attention than previously.

From 1915 to 1920, rapid growth occurred in school health education. The Modern Health Crusade of the National Tuberculosis Association emerged with 100,000 children receiving health information and developing health habits. The Child Health Organization of America, founded in 1918, changed the concepts of health education. "Hygiene" was replaced by the term "health education." The organization stressed a positive approach to health rather than traditional practices. The American School Hygiene and the American Child Hygiene Association were established at the same time that the National Society for the Prevention of Blindness and the National Dairy Council were founded. Each of these groups assisted in the promotion of health education. At the White House Conference on Child Welfare specific reference was made to the content areas of health education and to compulsory courses in health education in public schools. During this period, the Child Health Organization stimulated interest among teachers in health education as a teaching field.

The third decade of the twentieth century disclosed that health education had gained some acceptance as a subject-matter field. In 1921, the Malden Study showed that health education was practical, could change children's health habits, and could influence the child's growth. Other studies were the Child Health School, health education survey of the 48 states by the National Tuberculosis Association, health survey of 86 cities by the American Child Health Association, and the School Health Study. The first issue of *Health Bulletin for Teachers* was published by the Metropolitan Life Insurance Company in April 1929. Many conferences were held to promote the acceptance of health education. The 1924 publication *Health Education* did more than any other publication of the period to promote health education. In 1927, delegates to the Fourth Health Education Conference of the American Child Health Association recommended specific health education courses in the secondary schools. Safety education emerged during the early 1920s and developed quickly.[26] The Joint Committee on Health Problems in Education of the NEA and the AMA made this statement in 1924:

Every prospective teacher when not specializing in Health Education should be required to take one course where the health program as a whole is considered, synthesis indicated, and methods of securing the standardized desired results are discussed.[27]

Health education, from 1930 to 1940, as a subject-matter field had difficulty, owing to the emphasis on the traditional fields. The Cattaraugus County studies, the National Survey of Secondary Education, the Joint Committee on Health Problems in Education's study, and studies in rural New York communities revealed significant findings about the importance of health education. In 1938, the *Journal of School Health* was first published, and it has continued throughout the years to be a leading influence in the development of school health education. The 1930 White House Conference urged not only the necessity of health education and total school health programs but also the importance of the

[26]*Ibid.*, pp. 154-237.
[27]Joint Committee on Health Problems in Education of the National Education Association and the American Medical Association: *Health Education—A Program for Public Schools and Teacher Training Institutions.* New York: The Committee, 1924, p. 76.

preparation of qualified teachers of health education. Personal, home, and community health; safety; and mental and sex hygiene were listed as areas of health education. Practical learning was stressed in methods of health education, and the provision of a time allotment for health education received more attention. Studies of this decade indicated that some progress had been made on the inclusion of health education in the preparation of teachers. The Joint Committee on Health Problems in Education's 1930 publication *Health Education* stressed motivation, facts and procedures in strengthening health practices, and establishment of permanent desirable health attitudes and habits.[28]

During the forties, fifties, and sixties of the twentieth century health education as a single subject-matter field won recognition as an essential part of the modern school curriculum. In the forties, these research studies were among the many studies of that decade: Kellogg Foundation Health Projects, Astoria Study, New York City Study, and the Denver Study *Health Interests of Children*. Conferences dealt with undergraduate and graduate preparation of teachers of health education, functions of school administrators in health programs, and health in colleges. The 1940 White House Conference on Children in a Democracy stressed mental health and the need for health education in elementary and secondary schools. The Mid-Century White House Conference recommended that teaching of health ought to be given more time in the curriculum and teachers of health ought to be better prepared. The 1960 White House Conference mentioned specific areas of health education: mental health, alcoholism, tobacco, safety education, nutrition, accident prevention, family life education, dental health and fluoridation, and community health. Many statements of the 1960 White House Conference made specific reference to health education in elementary and secondary schools.

Many outstanding publications appeared in these decades. Some of these publications were *Suggested School Health Policies* (1946) of the National Conference for Cooperation in Health Education; *Health in Schools* (1942 and 1951), Twentieth Yearbook

of the American Association of School Administrators; and *Health Education* (1941, 1948, and 1961) of the Joint Committee on Health Problems in Education.

Among the many noteworthy developments during the sixties was the School Health Education Study. Conducted on a nationwide basis through the combined efforts of the National Education Association, the American Medical Association, the United States Office of Education, the United States Public Health Service, and the National Congress of Parents and Teachers, the Study was financed by the Samuel Bronfman Foundation of New York City. Questionnaires were sent to school administrators, teachers, and students in 38 states. Health behavior questionnaires were submitted to 6th, 9th, and 12th grade students in 1,101 individual elementary schools and 359 secondary schools. The replies to the questionnaires revealed answers to three broad questions: (1) What is health education like in the public schools of the United States? (2) What do students appear to know and understand about health education? (3) What strengths and weaknesses are disclosed by the findings that can provide a basis for the development of future health education?[29] The findings and recommendations of the School Health Education Study precipitated a nationwide interest in health education and the development of new curriculum materials in health education. Within a few years after the School Health Education Study, educational leaders in various state departments of education sought mandatory requirements for health education in the elementary and secondary schools with accompanying regulations concerning the preparation of teachers of health education in the secondary schools. With the growth of health education in the elementary and secondary schools, two professional societies provided outstanding leadership: the American School Health Association and the School Health Division of the American Association for Health, Physical Education and Recreation. National conferences were held concerning the health education curriculum (K through 12th grade), prepara-

---

[28]Means, *op. cit.*, pp. 238-290.

[29]School Health Education Study: *Summary Report of a Nationwide Study of Health Instruction in the Public Schools*. Washington, D.C.: The Study, 1964.

tion of teachers of health education for secondary schools, graduate programs in school health education, research promoting health education, and future plans for the development of health education. The fifties and sixties have witnessed the publication of a wealth of literature on school health education by independent authors. Some of these authorities, by their school health experiences and preparation, have provided a scholarly depth to the school health program not found in the literature of the third, fourth, and fifth decades of the twentieth century.

## SYNTHESIS

At the beginning of this chapter, the school health program was divided into three interrelated parts—school health services, healthful school living, and health education. In this text, *four* parts of the school health program will be presented: Part I—School Health Services; Part II—Healthful School Living; Part III—Health Education; and Part IV—Organization and Administration of the School Health Program. Throughout the text, the relations existing among school health services, healthful school living, and health education are emphasized. However, the final synthesis of the total school health pro-

gram occurs in Part IV—Organization and Administration of the School Health Program, so that pupil and community health problems can be discovered and solved. Thus, this text attempts to fulfill the recommendations of the Joint Committee on Health Problems in Education of the NEA and the AMA in that the total school health program is presented and the parts of the program are interrelated.

## References for Further Study

Anderson, C. L.: *School Health Practice*. 5th ed. St. Louis: The C. V. Mosby Company, 1972.

Cornacchia, H. J., Staton, W. M., and Irwin, L. W.: *Health in Elementary Schools*. 3rd ed. St. Louis: The C. V. Mosby Company, 1970.

Hamburg, M., and Hamburg, M. V.: *Health and Social Problems in the School*. Philadelphia: Lea & Febiger, 1968.

Kilander, H. F.: *School Health Education*. 2nd ed. New York: The Macmillan Company, 1968.

Nemir, A.: *The School Health Program*. 3rd ed. Philadelphia: W. B. Saunders Company, 1970.

Smolensky, J., and Bonvechio, L. R.: *Principles of School Health*. Boston: D. C. Heath and Company, 1966.

Turner, C. E., Randall, H. B., and Smith, S. L.: *School Health and Health Education*. 6th ed. St. Louis: The C. V. Mosby Company, 1970.

Willgoose, C. E.: *Health Education in the Elementary School*. 3rd ed. Philadelphia: W. B. Saunders Company, 1969.

# Part I
## *SCHOOL HEALTH SERVICES*

# Chapter 2

## *APPRAISAL OF THE PUPIL'S HEALTH STATUS*

## AN INCIDENT

The school nurse and the special education teacher have informed teachers that some pupils will have vision and hearing screening. The teachers have asked their principals whether the pupils could have other types of health appraisals in addition to vision and hearing screening. The principals have asked the teachers to explain other types of health appraisal and the reasons for these appraisals.

At the beginning of the twentieth century, the prevention of diseases among school children was the main objective of school health services. State medical inspections were compulsory in Massachusetts' public schools in 1906. School nurses were employed in the public schools of New York City, Los Angeles, Philadelphia, Boston, and Pueblo, Colorado, by 1910.

Today, though prevention of diseases remains an objective, there are many other varied and complex objectives of school health services. *School health services* was defined in Chapter 1. With this definition in mind, Part I of this textbook will include discussion of each of the facets of school health services.

## PURPOSES OF HEALTH APPRAISAL

Many procedures are utilized in determining the pupil's health status. After a medical examination of the pupil, the family physician can present information that is vital in assessing the pupil's health status. Using full-mouth x-rays and dental examinations revealing dental diseases and defects, the family dentist can assist health appraisal. The teacher, nurse, and parent also can observe changes in the pupil's behavior and appearance. Posture and nutritional screening, tuberculin tests, and screening of vision and hearing can disclose data. Parent-teacher, parent-nurse, and teacher-nurse conferences can add information to the student's health history. Emergency care records show the incidence of illness and injury. Immunization records often indicate reasons for school absenteeism; some children have not had the necessary childhood immunizations. Physical performance tests and psychological and psychometric tests can provide valuable data to physicians at the time of the medical examination.

Why is the health appraisal important? *First,* the health appraisal indicates the presence of hidden and known diseases. It reveals unsuspected chronic health conditions, some of which can be corrected. It discloses types of emotional illnesses. Health appraisal may show the need for medical care of injuries. It can indicate dental diseases and defects. In addition, the health appraisal can broaden the pupil's understanding of his health status. *Second,* the health appraisal can reveal the pupil's health practices and attitudes and, to some extent, his fund of health information. *Third,* the health practices, attitudes, and knowledge can disclose the content (subject matter) of the health education needed to improve the pupil's existing health status. *Fourth,* the health appraisal can reveal adjustments in the school's activities and curriculum necessary to assist the pupil with health problems. *Fifth,* the health appraisal is necessary so that a classification for physical education can be had. This classification results from the physician's assessment of the pupil's health status after the completion of the medical examination. *Sixth*, when the appraisal of school health services can be related to health education and healthful school living, the total school health program becomes meaningful to pupils, parents, and school and community personnel.

## PARENTAL RESPONSIBILITIES

The pupil's health is primarily a parental responsibility, one that does not end with the entrance of the teenager into the secondary school. Rather, the responsibility shifts from the parent to the adolescent, with parental guidance. *One* of the parental functions in school health services is to supply information concerning a pupil's illnesses, injuries, operations, possible physical health difficulties, health habits, and emotional health problems. This information should be placed in the pupil's health history record.

A *second* function of parents in school health services is to develop close working relations with physicians and dentists. These relations result from the interchange of health information between parents and physicians and dentists, through health guidance sought by parents, and parental willingness to carry out the physician's and the dentist's requests. The physician and the dentist rely on the day-to-day observations of parents to supplement their examinations.

A *third* function of parents in school health services is to accept their responsibilities in seeking correction of the child's remediable health problems. Too often, elementary and secondary schools have not emphasized to parents that, while school personnel may observe certain health conditions, it is the parents' responsibility to seek correction of the child's remediable problems. Occasionally, parents assume that school personnel will correct the pupil's health difficulty. The school or public health nurse acquaints the parent with medical and dental services needed to correct the difficulty, but the parent must seek and obtain the needed care. Local health departments can assist the personnel of school health services and administrative personnel when parents are unable, or refuse, to seek and obtain care for their child.

The *fourth* function of parents in school health services is to secure early immunization of their child. Local boards of education may require certain immunizations for pupil entrance into local public schools, but again it is a parental responsibility to comply.

A *fifth* function of parents in school health services pertains to parents of elementary school children. The parents should be present at medical and dental examinations performed in the offices of the physician and dentist. The parents' cooperation will add to the success of the examination. Questions can be asked by or directed to the parents. The elementary school pupil should realize the value of these examinations. As he becomes older, he should accept the responsibility for his own medical and dental checkups.

A *sixth* function of parents is to cooperate with the instructional personnel, the school nurse, and the school administrator in school health services. This cooperation begins during the readiness-for-school medical examination and continues with parental compliance with the school's procedures for emergency care and prevention of disease, with parental insistence that medical and dental examination be a definite part of family living, and with parental interest in the total school health program. To strengthen parental cooperation, the personnel of school health services might provide parents with information about general observable signs that might indicate diseases, chronic health conditions, or injuries occurring to their son or daughter.

The *seventh* function of parents in school health services is to become aware of the many agencies within the community to promote the child and teenager's health. Parents with low incomes and parents of children with unusual health problems should be assured that some medical and dental assistance may be available in their communities. In one study, medical and dental examinations were given to 618 teenagers from families whose income was low enough to qualify for programs of financial assistance from local, state, or national agencies. Those teenagers having medical and dental care available, without cost, had less severe untreated dental disease and fewer medical abnormalities than the teenagers not receiving medical and dental care.[1]

## HEALTH RECORD

The essential information on the cumulative health record should be clearly stated, legibly written, and comprehensive. Also, school personnel should understand the privileged nature of the information and how the information can help the pupil.[2]

Results of any appraisal should be recorded on a cumulative pupil health record. Eight sections can comprise the health record.

1. Pupil identification and teacher observations
2. Pupil health history (detachable)
3. Medical examination (detachable)
4. Physician's report to the school on significant findings of the medical examination (detachable)
5. Follow-through and hearing and vision screening (detachable)
6. Dental examination with recommendations for further dental care (detachable)
7. Height Weight Interpretation Folder (detachable)
8. Posture screening and summary of health data to be used by the teacher in the instructional program

A sample health record including these sections is given in Appendix A. Six of these sections are detachable. Physicians and dentists can retain in their files confidential data resulting from their examinations. Detachable sections allow physicians and dentists to send to the schools significant pupil information. With a detachable section for the follow-through, the nurse can record pertinent information needed by teachers.

The health record (Appendix A) was designed to assist school personnel in accumulating pupil data resulting from many types of health appraisals. The front cover of the record contains information needed

during emergency care of the ill or injured pupil. The health record can be used during the pupil's 12 years of school life, even when he changes residence. A summary of the health data can be utilized in planning health instruction. The six sections can be separated from the main sections, mailed, and returned to the complete record.

The health record (Appendix A) resulted from suggestions of nurses, family physicians and dentists, state departments of health and education, city and rural schoolteachers, and school administrators. Most state departments of health and education have sample health records to assist school personnel in developing their own health records.

### Accessibility of Health Records

Most teachers of elementary pupils are responsible for informing the parents of any continuously observed signs of health problems, physical education activities, and health education. To complete these responsibilities, teachers should have access to the pupil's health record, which might well be kept in the pupil's cumulative folder. A copy of the health record should be sent to the new school if the pupil transfers.

The health record of the secondary school student should be filed in his cumulative folder, usually kept in the administrative offices. Many members of the school personnel will use the health record: the school health educator can discover problems to be considered in health instruction; the health coordinator can obtain information necessary for developing the total school health program; the school nurse can use the health data for pupil conferences; the physical educator can discover the pupil's health grade classification; counselors can use data for teacher-counselor conferences; and the classroom teachers can refer to the health record as they observe changes in the student's behavior and appearance.

Stennett and others have noted significant by-products or applications of the magnetic-tape, master student health record file. Computerized records can reduce the nurse's time spent on clerical tasks, and they have several other possible applications. One of these applications is to obtain

[1] Arthur Salisbury and Robert B. Berg: Health defects and need for treatment of adolescents in low income families. *Public Health Reports 84* (August, 1969): 705.
[2] Harriett B. Randall: Strengths and limitations of the cumulative health record. *J. School Health 37* (February, 1967) :861.

lists of students with special health problems.[3]

In the 1967-1969 school years, the Denver Public Schools' Department of Health Services had a trial of IBM cards for health data processing in one high school. In the 1969-70 school year, health data collection was accomplished by a school nurse in interviews with newly enrolled pupils. Also, the processing included annual or semi-annual updating of the data.[4]

## Implications for Health Education

The information on the pupil's health record can reveal to the teacher units of health education that should be taught. Units are divisions of areas of health education and are a series of lessons built around a central topic. On the pupil's health history (Section 2 of the health record), the teacher may discover that a large number of pupils have not received immunization for rubeola, rubella, mumps, and tetanus. One of the areas of health education (Chapter 4) is "The Prevention and Control of Diseases" and a unit might be "Measles, mumps, and tetanus and the immunizations for these diseases."

In Section 5 of the health record is found the results of hearing and vision screening. A teacher may find that many pupils have failed the hearing and vision screening. Another area of health education is "The Care of All Parts of the Human Body" and a unit could be "Eyeglasses, contact lenses, and hearing aids." Many other units of health education will be suggested to the imaginative teacher who studies the information on the health records of her pupils.

## TEACHERS' AND NURSES' OBSERVATIONS

Continuous and systematic observations by the teacher and nurse can reveal a wealth of health data regarding the pupil. The teacher should be aware of many signs indicating changes in his behavior and appearance. During the preservice teacher preparation, the teacher should become acquainted with these signs. Projected slides depicting health problems common

to the elementary and secondary school pupil can be shown. Descriptive photographs of these problems can be used.

What are some characteristics of a *healthy* elementary school child or a secondary school youth? He gets along well with himself and other persons. He has an abundance of vitality. He is happy and smiles easily, showing clean, straight teeth. His skin is clear, and his hair is lustrous. He has good muscle tone and body mechanics that provide satisfactory standing, sitting, and walking postures. He participates in many types of physical activity and is developing leisure-time activities. He has safety skills that prevent unnecessary injuries. His eyes are bright and clear, and his hearing is acute. He gets sufficient sleep, has daily periods of rest, has a hearty appetite, and gains weight and height as his growth patterns change. He has developed daily habits and control of elimination. He has no illnesses and has had his remediable health difficulties corrected. When he has a chronic health condition, he has made adjustments in daily living. He has a wholesome outlook on life and is willing to seek assistance when emotional health problems arise.

The teacher and nurse observations are not limited to morning inspections but are continuous throughout the school day. Nor can these observations be confined to signs of communicable diseases, but must include every phase of the whole child—mental and physical health, social characteristics, intellectual capacities, and achievements.

A word of caution might be added. Because many persons will be appraising the pupil, the term "normal" should be avoided. This term will be interpreted differently by each person appraising the pupil's physical and mental health status. A physician may not agree with the results of nutrition screening. The medical diagnosis may consider physiological factors that are not included in the nutrition screening. Also, elementary and secondary teachers should be aware that signs indicating changes in the pupil's appearance and behavior can be altered within a short interval of time.

As the teacher and nurse observe many signs of health problems, they should compile their data so that differences among pupils can be compared. Bodily growth

[3]R. G. Stennett, D. M. Cram, Dorothy Gibson, and Kathryn Dukacz: Exploring the possibilities of computerized health records. *J. School Health 41* (February, 1971) :59.

[4]Department of Health Services, Denver Public Schools: *Forty-fourth Annual Report, 1968-1969.* Denver, Colorado: Public Schools, 1969, p. 5.

skin conditions, posture habits, fatigue and energy levels, appetites, visual and hearing difficulties, dental health problems, bodily cleanliness, and emotional health problems of two girls of the same age will reveal distinct variations in observable signs. These observations should be continued over a reasonable period of time so that deviations can be detected.

Before listing signs of possible diseases and defects, school personnel should be acquainted with conditions relative to these signs. *First*, there may be signs of health problems that are repeated regardless of the disease or defect. *Fatigue, irritability, listlessness, failure to achieve capacity of work, apathy, loss of appetite, and slumped posture may be common to many health problems. Second*, there are specific signs that identify each health problem. *Third*, health problems may be interrelated. For example, hearing difficulty may be one of the causes of an emotional health problem. *Fourth*, the signs of diseases and defects given in this textbook, are only *some* of the signs observable to nonmedically prepared persons. *Fifth*, only physicians and dentists make the diagnosis of the disease, defect, injury, and emotional illness. *Sixth*, diseases are caused by bacteria, viruses, fungi, protozoa, metazoa or helminths, and rickettsiae. Defects are due to malfunctioning of one or more parts of the human body.

## Some Signs of Possible Communicable Diseases

Unusual pallor or flushing of the face
Inflammation (redness, soreness, heat, pain) of the mucous membranes of the nose, throat, and mouth
Inflamed and watery eyes
"Runny nose"
Sneezing, coughing, sniffling
Swelling or tenderness of the glands of the neck
Faintness, nausea, or vomiting
Fever or chills
Headache
"Runny ear"
Upset stomach
Stiff neck
Backache
Noisy breathing
Blueness of lips

Signs designating characteristics of diseases such as measles (spots appearing on face, neck, chest, arms of child), chicken pox, mumps, scarlet fever, and the like.

Many of the signs of a possible cold may actually be the symptoms of other communicable diseases.

## Some Signs of Possible Visual Difficulties

Rubbing of the eyes
Continual frowning
Blinking more than usual
Holding of a book for reading either too close or too far away
Sensitivity to light
Red-rimmed and watery eyes
Swollen eyelids
Repeated sties
Complaints of dizziness
Stumbling and tripping over objects
Shutting or covering of one eye when reading
Tendency to reverse words or syllables
Excessive head movements while reading
Body rigid while looking at close objects
Complaints of headaches
Difficulty in distinguishing colors
Requests to have writing on chalkboard repeated orally
Dislike of assignments requiring close work
Drawings described in a confused manner
Difficulty in reading (especially undue hesitancy and frequent loss of place)
Screwing up of face when reading
Poor hand-eye coordination
Poor score on accuracy tests, such as target throwing
Complaints of double vision
Head turned to one side when reading or writing
Unnatural position of the head in an attempt to avoid glare
Squinting
Voluntary changes in seating to see better
Crusted eyelids
Inability to distinguish symbols nearly similar in appearance, such as *a* and *o*, *e* and *c*, *m* and *n*, *n* and *r*, *f* and *t*, *8* and *6*, *7* and *1*, *3* and *8*
Crossed eyes
Erratic eye movements
Body tenseness during class work
Loss of peripheral vision
Head thrust forward

## Some Signs of Possible Hearing Difficulties

Requests for repetition of what has been said
Complaints of earaches
"Runny ear"
Swollen glands

Complaints of noises in the head, such as ringing, buzzing, or hissing

Breathing through mouth

Peculiar-sounding voice (pitch too high, too low, too loud)

Complaints of heaviness, stuffiness, or fullness in the ear

Cocking of an ear toward the speaker

Repeatedly answering questions incorrectly

Sensitivity

Suspiciousness

Aloofness

Failure to locate source of sound

Watching other children before beginning to work or copying from other pupils

Bewildered facial expression

Use of his hands in making known his wants

A look of "watchful waiting"

Close attachment to the teacher during group activities—"shadowing" of the teacher

Poor sense of balance

Monotonous speaking and singing

Faulty articulation

Tendency to lip-read

Hand held to ear

Observing other pupils during teachers' directions

Interrupting conversations of other pupils

## Some Signs of Possible Emotional Health Problems

Undue restlessness such as facial grimacing, nail biting, lip sucking, twisting or pulling the hair, pulling the ear, playing with hands not attributable to any observable physical cause

Excessive daydreaming

Extreme sensitivity

Crying easily

Overtimidity, seclusiveness, extreme docility, withdrawal

Overaggressiveness, extreme "showing off"

Resistance to authority

Complaints of being "picked on," not being treated fairly, or being discriminated against

Antagonism

Poor sportsmanship

Difficulty in reading or reciting not caused by any observable physical cause

Chronic absence

Continual lying

Lack of cooperation (negative attitude)

Frequent bullying

Continual selfishness

Unacceptable sexual conduct

Temper tantrums

Destructiveness

Cruelty

Uncontrollable emotions

Overstudiousness

Domineering attitude

Depression and unhappiness

Lack of respect for the property of others

Obstinacy

Stealing, cheating

## Some Signs of Possible Nutritional Deficiencies

Failure to show a steady gain in weight

Avoidance of normal play activities

Poor posture habits

Complaints of pains on sitting and standing

Chronic diarrhea or constipation

Repeated respiratory infections

Persistent cracking and slight redness at the corners of the mouth

Small or flabby muscles

Excessive thinness

Excessive fat or poor distribution of fat on body surfaces

Strained, worried look

Poor dental health

Pallor

Continual hunger

Abnormalities of bone growth (bowlegs, pigeon breast)

Rough, scaly skin

Dry, coarse, brittle, lusterless hair

Inflammation of margins of eyelids

Headaches

Eye fatigue and sensitivity to light

Tender, swollen, bleeding, or spongy gums

Easily bruised skin

Sore joints

Pains in the musculature

Sore, beefy tongue

Spindly arms and legs, flat chest

Chronic indigestion

Abnormal discharge of tears

Weakness and loss of strength

Skin abrasions slow to heal

Brittle nails

Burning and prickling of skin

Burning or itching of eyes

## Some Signs of Possible Posture Conditions

*Standing Posture*

Round shoulders

Sway-back

One shoulder higher than other

One hip prominent

Markedly inclined head

Markedly depressed or deformed chest

Knock-knees or knees extended back

Bowlegs

Flat feet

Protruding shoulder blades

Protruding and sagging abdomen

Toes pointed outward, ankles turned in

ward, body weight on inner side of feet
General body appearance—slumping
Weight on one foot
Uneven walking gait

*Sitting Posture*

Sitting on the end of the spine—slumping
Hunching over
Leaning to one side because chair arm is too high
Curling one foot under the body
Not placing feet on the floor

## COMMON OBSERVABLE HEALTH PROBLEMS

In addition to the signs of certain health difficulties, there are health problems easily observable to teachers and nurses. The descriptions of these problems are given in general terms and do not include descriptions used in medical diagnosis. To acquaint teachers with these health problems, descriptive photographs and projected slides can be used. These health problems are as follows:

### Ears, Nose, and Throat

*Adenitis*—Inflammation of lymph nodes in the neck. Adenitis is often called "swollen glands."

*Chronic otitis media*—Chronic inflammation of the middle ear.

*Conduction deafness*—Caused by obstruction of sound vibration. Obstruction may be the result of dirt and wax in the outer ear, adhesions, scar tissue, perforations of the eardrum, an abscess in the middle ear, or congestion of the eustachian tube.

*Earache*—Pain in the outer, middle, or inner ear due to infection or other cause.

*Enlarged adenoids*—Collection of lymphoid tissue in posterior nasopharynx which obstructs nasal breathing.

*Impacted wax*—Unusual amount of waxlike secretion lodged in the outer ear canal.

*Mastoiditis*—Extensive inflammation of the mastoid process. Complaints of pain and tenderness in back of the ear may be signs of mastoiditis.

*Nosebleed*

*Obstruction of nasal breathing*—Obstruction may be due to enlarged adenoids, congestion of the mucous membranes covering nasal bones, acute infection from common colds or other disease, allergies, presence of foreign bodies such as beans, fracture of nasal bones, or polyps (small benign grapelike growths).

*Perception deafness*—Caused by some injury or disease in the inner part of the ear, resulting in destruction of segments or all of the auditory nerve.

*"Runny ear"*—Drainage from an infected ear.

*Sinusitis*—Inflammation of the mucous membranes lining sinuses. Acute or chronic forms are characterized by aching in the cheeks and over the eyes.

*Tonsillitis*—Inflammation of the tonsils.

### Eyes

*Accommodation difficulties*—Lack of ability of the eyeball to alter the size of its lens properly in order to change the focus of the eye for near seeing and for distance.

*Amblyopia*—Dimness of vision from disuse or nonuse of an eye. Often called "lazy eyes." Muscle imbalance prevents focusing both eyes on an object, and the child learns to see with the stronger eye.

*Ametropia*—Images are not brought to a proper focus on the retina because of an imperfection in the refractive process of an eye.

*Astigmatism*—A condition caused by an irregularly shaped eyeball so that the refractive surfaces are distorted, and light rays are not in sharp focus on the retina.

*Blepharitis*—Inflammation of the margin of the eyelids.

*Cataract*—Cloudy or opaque lens.

*Color blindness*—An inability to distinguish certain differences in color.

*Conjunctivitis*—Inflammation of the mucous membranes of the eyelid and exposed surface of the eyeball. Often called "pinkeye."

*Diplopia*—Double vision.

*Ectropion*—Edge of the eyelids turns out.

*Entropion*—Eyelids roll in.

*Esotropia*—One eyeball is observed to turn inward.

*Glaucoma*—Intense intraocular pressure of the eyeball. Cupping of the optic disc.

*Hyperopia*—Eyeball is too short from front to back so that light rays focus *beyond* the retina instead of *on* the retina. Often called "farsightedness." Near distance is blurred, but far distance is clear.

*Inflammation of eye*—Redness in appearance often accompanied by pain, excessive tearing, or vision difficulty.

*Myopia*—Eyeball is too long from front to back so that light rays focus *in front of* the retina instead of *on* the retina. Often called "nearsightedness." Near distance is clear, but far distance is blurred.

*Nystagmus*—Eyeballs involuntarily move rapidly from side to side, up and down, or in rotary motion.

*Occlusion*—Forcing the use of one eye by obscuring the vision of the other eye.

*Phoria*—A tendency toward deviation from the normal axis, causing focusing and fusion problems.

*Ptosis*—Lack of muscular control which results in a drooping of the upper eyelid.

*Refractive error*—Light rays not focusing exactly on the retina because of a defect in the eyeball.

*Scotoma*—A blind spot, or area of poor perception, in the field of vision.

*Strabismus*—Deviation of the eyes when external eye muscles do not function correctly in focusing both eyes on an object at the same time. Commonly called "cross-eyes," "squint," or "wall-eyes," depending on the direction of the deviation.

*Sty*—Infection of the glands surrounding the roots of eyelashes.

*Trachoma*—Viral disease of the conjunctiva and cornea which may produce loss of vision. A usual sign is abnormal sensitivity to light.

## Posture

*Lordosis*—Deviation of anterior-posterior posture with an extreme curvature in the lumbar region (sway-back).

*Kyphosis*—Deviation of anterior-posterior posture with an exaggerated curvature in the thoracic region (round shoulders).

*Rickets*—Nutritional deficiency due to the lack of vitamin D. Normal process of bone formation is disturbed. Knock-knees, bowlegs, and pigeon breast are possible signs.

*Scoliosis*—Lateral curvature of the spine. *Functional* scoliosis is caused by poor walking, standing, and sitting posture. *Structural* scoliosis may be caused by rickets, polio, or osteomalacia (nutritional deficiency which results when bones are deprived of sufficient calcium, phosphorus, and vitamin D). Effects may include C-shaped left-total curve, S-shaped combined curve, and right lumbar curvature.

## Skin, Hair, and Nails

*Acne*—Skin condition with blemishes, blackheads, and pimples.

*Birthmark*—Abnormal condition of the surface blood vessels creating discoloration or pigmentation of the skin.

*Blackheads*—Hard, black plugs found in skin pores. Plugs are collections of oil and dirt which clog and enlarge the pores.

*Boils*—Inflammation of the skin. Bacteria enter the skin through hair follicles or sweat glands.

*Carbuncles*—Many-headed boils.

*Eczema*—Itchy, inflamed skin. Small blisters form, and watery discharge appears. Discharge dries into scales or crusts.

*Favus*—Fungal infection marked by cup-shaped yellowish crusts found over hair follicles. Favus is usually located on the scalp and results in loss of hair.

*Hangnails*—Drying or cracking of cuticle around nail. Because cuticle is poorly oiled and cracks easily, it is often picked or bitten off.

*Hives*—Small pink and white skin elevations of various sizes resulting from an allergen within or outside the body. Intense itching accompanies elevations.

*Impetigo*—Highly contagious disease consisting of sores arising on inflamed skin areas. Sores ooze a thick, sticky yellow or brown liquid. Scabs or crusts are built around liquid. Sores create intense itching. Crusts are shed and the exposed dermis looks red and "weepy." Direct or indirect contact can spread impetigo.

*Infectious dandruff*—Excessive scaling of the scalp. Large flakes hang loosely in the hair. Sometimes flakes are oily and yellow. Itching accompanies dandruff.

*Lacerations*—Wounds made by tearing.

*Moles*—Densely packed skin cells pigmented either brown or black.

*Pediculosis*—Skin disease caused by lice. Head lice create irritation to the scalp. Lice lay their eggs, or nits, in glistening lumps connected to hair and at a short distance from the scalp. Severe itching occurs.

*Pimple*—Small, solid elevation which forms a head. Obstruction of normal functioning of sebaceous glands.

*Plant toxins*—Severe inflammation can occur from a mere trace of toxins from certain plants such as poison ivy, oak, or sumac. Small, swollen, red, itchy spots and blisters form.

*Psoriasis*—Silvery-scaled red patches on exposed surfaces such as the scalp, knees, and elbows.

*Ringworm*—A fungal growth occurring on the skin and at the margin of the nails. Round, elevated, irregular, reddish patches spreading from red edges while healing in the center. Itching accompanies scaling. It can be transferred from one part to other parts of the body or from one person to another.

*Ringworm of the groin and crotch*—Inflamed skin patches with intense itching. Infected areas become raw from scratching, and severe bleeding occurs.

*Ringworm of the scalp*—Round, grayish, scaly, slightly elevated patches covered by stubs of broken hairs. The broken hairs become dull and brittle and snap off near the root, leaving bald spots. Gray scaly patches appear and itching occurs at bald spot.

*Scabies*—Irritation caused by a mite burrowing molelike under the skin. The itch mite produces a minute, slightly elevated black trail. The trail is found on the inner side of the fingers and thighs, on the wrists and backs of hands, at the armpits, and on the abdomen. Intense itching accompanies scabies.

*Seborrheic dermatitis*—Severe extension of dandruff. Red, irritated patches which may ooze fluid appear on the scalp.

*Shingles*—Painful viral disease of the nerve endings in which blisters erupt on the skin in a band or over a large area of the skin.

*"Threadbare skin"*—Skin disease having bright red patches covered with silvery scales. These scales are shed, leaving outer skin "threadbare" in spots.

*Warts*—Cauliflowerlike overgrowths of epidermal cells.

*Wheals*—Localized white or pinkish elevations or ridges on the skin, such as those caused by hives or insect bites.

## Miscellaneous

*Accelerated maturation and growth*—Too rapid a change into adolescence or adulthood.

*Allergy*—Hypersensitivity to a particular allergen (may be a protein or a nonprotein). Foods, dust and pollens, animal hair, and drugs are among common allergens.

*Anemia*—Condition in which the red corpuscle count or the hemoglobin content of the blood is low or both deficiencies are present. Lack of vitality and endurance result.

*Appendicitis*—Inflammation of appendix causing abdominal pain. Nausea or vomiting may or may not accompany pain.

*Chorea* (St. Vitus' dance)—Jerky, involuntary movements. Definite sign of rheumatic fever.

*Delayed maturation and growth*—Too slow a change into adolescence or adulthood.

*Gastroenteritis*—Inflammation of the stomach and intestines. Accompanied by nausea, vomiting, diarrhea, abdominal pains, and bodily discomfort.

*Hypertension*—High blood pressure.

*Hyperthyroidism*—Excessive functional activity of the thyroid gland. Increased basal metabolism. Child may be highly excitable.

*Hypothyroidism*—Deficiency of thyroid activity. Child may fatigue easily, perspire very little, have slow reaction time, and sleep heavily.

*Hysteria*—Lack of control over acts and emotions, explosive conduct, absence of sensation. Child may become unconscious or semiconscious.

*Low vitality*—General sluggishness.

*Pinworms*—Small white worms found in the upper part of the large intestine, occasionally in the female reproductive organs and bladder, and in the rectum of children. Itching accompanies pinworms.

*Polyarthritis*—Discomfort in joints of ankles, hips, knees, wrists, elbows, and shoulders. Discomfort may spread from joint to joint, may last a day or longer, and may show swelling. Accompanies rheumatic fever.

*Obesity*—Excessive accumulation of body fat.

*Overweight*—Weight in excess of normal range.

## Implications for Health Education

Having observed some signs of possible health problems among students, how can the teacher use this information? The teacher should be aware that there are applicable areas of health education: "Care of All Parts of the Human Body," "Prevention of Diseases To All Parts of the Human Body," "Chronic Health Conditions," "American Red Cross First Aid," "Mental Health," and "Nutrition." These areas are divided into units which are series of lessons built around a central topic.

Many suggested units can result from the teacher's observations. Each unit is taught so that the student understands the health problem; how he can prevent the problem in the future; and what he can do for the problem.

Some suggestions follow:

| Observable health problem | Area of health education | Suggested unit |
| --- | --- | --- |
| Visual difficulties | Care of All Parts of the Human Body | Visual defects and their care |
| Hearing difficulties | Care of All Parts of the Human Body | Injuries to the ear and hearing loss |
| Emotional health problems | Mental Health | Self-control and self-discipline |
| Nutritional deficiencies | Nutrition | Obesity |
| Posture conditions | Care of All Parts of the Human Body | Scoliosis |
| "Runny ear" | Prevention of Diseases | Ear infections and their prevention |
| Sty | Prevention of Diseases | Eye infections and their prevention |
| Impetigo | Prevention of Diseases | Skin problems and their prevention |
| Lacerations | American Red Cross First Aid | Wounds and their care |
| Allergy | Chronic Health Conditions | Allergies |

## MEDICAL EXAMINATIONS

The National Committee on School Health Policies of the NEA and the AMA has suggested that physicians giving medical examinations

be sufficiently painstaking and comprehensive to command medical respect, sufficiently informative to guide school personnel in the proper counseling of the pupil and sufficiently personalized to provide a desirable educational experience.[5]

The final decision regarding possible sources for the medical examination rests with the superintendent of schools and the local medical society. Some pupils may be examined by their own physicians in the physicians' offices, but pupils who are not examined by their own physicians perhaps can be examined by a physician at a clinic of the local health department, or the outpatient department of a local hospital. The decision must be made before any planning of the procedures for medical examination can be done. As soon as the decision is made, the local or county medical society should be informed.

The school health committee of the local or county medical society can assist in the cooperative planning of the medical examination. One of the duties of this committee will be to submit to the schools a list of physicians who are available to examine pupils having no family physician. Another duty will be to advise individual physicians upon the desired extent of each medical examination. Local medical practices will partially determine the extent of the medical examination. If school physicians are employed by boards of education, they will usually determine the extent of the medical examination. In some localities the school health committee of the local or county medical society establishes the procedures for schools and physicians. These procedures should be followed, and conflicts arising from the procedures should be resolved as soon as possible. Among the potential difficulties in the procedures are requirements about the date of examination for each pupil, payment for services rendered by physicians, availability of the

[5]National Conference for Cooperation in Health Education: *Suggested School Health Policies.* 3rd ed. Washington, D.C.: National Education Association, 1956, pp. 17-18.

school health record to the examining physician, pupil excuses from school in order to be examined, accessibility of the physician's recommendations to the schools, and exchange of information between the school and physician following the examination.

The Joint Committee on Health Problems in Education of the NEA and the AMA has indicated that the medical examination by a pupil's own physician in his private office has become increasingly common. The physician can discuss any health problem that arises, can prescribe therapy, has the equipment and the facilities to do special tests, has records of the pupil's previous examinations, can give immunizations, and can be assured of privacy. Also, a medical examination in the physician's office provides an opportunity for the physician to explain the necessity for medical care and to encourage the pupil to seek medical advice from the physician when it is required.[6]

## What Is the Medical Examination?

The extent of the medical examination that is desirable will depend upon information given in the health history indicating the need for medical exploration. Also, the extent of the examination will depend upon whether the physician is the student's personal physician or a physician with whom the student has had no previous contact. The physician will examine all areas of the body, although not all areas should be exposed throughout the examination. Older girls should be provided with a slipover or other covering, and girls should be examined in the presence of a nurse or another adult female. The genital organs of boys and girls should be covered except for the brief time required for their examination. Since shoes and hose are removed, protection for the feet should be provided.[7]

The medical examination should include all of the following:[8]

[6]Joint Committee on Health Problems in Education of the National Education Association and the American Medical Association: *Health Appraisal of School Children.* 4th ed. Washington, D.C.: National Education Association, 1969, pp. 18-19.
[7]*Ibid.*, p. 20.
[8]Committee on School Health of the American Academy of Pediatrics: *Report of the Committee.* Evanston, Ill.: The Committee, 1966, p. 13.

skin
external eye structures, distant visual acuity, and muscle coordination of the eyeballs
nasal passages
ear canals, membranes of the ears, and hearing acuity
tooth structure and occlusion
mouth and pharynx
thyroid gland
bones of the thoracic area
breasts
lungs
heart
abdomen
external reproductive organs
function and structure of bones and muscles
lymph nodes
height
weight
blood pressure
pulse
detection of organic heart disease

A medical examination by the pupil's own physician may include other procedures such as urinalysis and serologic tests. Boys might be examined for possible hernia. Toes might be inspected for fungal growth. The rectum of a younger boy or girl might be examined if the parent has reported that the child complains of itching.

Following the medical examination, the physician gives recommendations to be entered on the health record used by school personnel. Such recommendations call attention to remediable health defects and to the importance of immediate medical care. To the teacher, the physician suggests modifications in school work. He may indicate whether the pupil can or cannot climb stairs, needs special seating placement, should have supplementary school feeding, or has chronic health problems. The physician classifies the student for physical education activities. (See Health Record— Appendix A)

## Frequency of Examinations

The frequency of medical examinations for the school-age pupil has been a subject for debate for many years. In some states, the frequency of the routine medical examination is set by law. The American Academy of Pediatrics recommends three routine medical examinations: before entrance to kindergarten or grade 1, either at grade 6 or grade 7 (early adolescence), and at or near grade 11 (adolescence). In addition, there should be more frequent medical examinations of a child having specific health problems which produce academic difficulties.[9] The Joint Committee on Health Problems in Education of the NEA and the AMA recommends four periodic medical examinations during the pupil's school years: at the time of entrance into school, at grade 4, at grade 7, and at grade 10.[10]

In the suggested frequency of medical examinations, there may not be any medical examination at the time of the student's entrance into the junior or senior high school. Not all young people reach adolescence at the same time. Thus physical education teachers, depending on the physician's classification of the student for physical education activities, may not have a valid health grade for the student. One of the purposes of the medical examination is to classify the student for physical education. Therefore, students entering the junior or senior high school should have a medical examination so that they are properly classified for physical education.

### Readiness-for-school Medical Examinations

There are four general types of medical examination: readiness-for-school, routine, special, and referral. Readiness-for-school examinations can be given to entering first-graders and new students. Routine examinations might be given when the child enters sixth grade and ninth grade. Special examinations are given to the pupil with a physical handicap, the student fulfilling requirements for after-school employment, and the athlete competing in interscholastic and intramural sports. Referral examinations take place after the teacher detects unusual signs in the pupil's appearance and behavior, when emergency care of a sick or injured pupil is needed, or when screening procedures are carried out.

In planning the readiness-for-school examinations, many school personnel and Parent-Teacher Association members will be involved. The superintendent of schools has a census of potential kindergarten or first-grade children a year before their entrance. The health coordinator, school nurses, and designated PTA members select a preregistration date in late April. The preregistration meeting will acquaint parents with the necessity for medical and dental examinations and immunizations previous to the child's entrance into kindergarten or first grade. Principals, first-grade teachers, health coordinators, school nurses, and PTA members plan this preregistration meeting. Invitations are sent to parents of children entering kindergarten or first grade and of new pupils in elementary schools. Enrollment cards and health records are distributed and explained at the preregistration meeting. During June, members of the PTA telephone parents on the invitation list to follow up and remind them of the necessity for medical and dental examinations and immunizations. Parents should be encouraged to have the child's health difficulties corrected before he enters school. On the opening day of school in September, the first-grade teachers or school nurses check whether the children have had medical and dental examinations and the required immunizations. This information is recorded on the pupils' health records. In home visits, school nurses or social workers interview the parents of children who have not fulfilled the requirements. At this time they can arrange for examinations and immunizations of indigent children.

### Routine Medical Examinations

Meyerstein "has compiled evidence about the abolition of a required *annual* medical examination for every pupil. State laws requiring annual medical examinations of every pupil should be repealed. Modified medical examinations should replace the annual examinations. These modified examinations should be at less frequent intervals; however, greater emphasis should be placed upon the comprehensiveness and quality of the medical examinations."[11]

Routine examinations do not take the place of yearly examinations given by the family physician. Parents should be encouraged to continue yearly medical examinations even though the schools may de-

[9]*Ibid.*, p. 11.
[10]Joint Committee on Health Problems in Education of the National Education Association and the American Medical Association, *op. cit.*, p. 20.

[11]Albert Meyerstein: The value of periodic school health examinations. *Amer. J. Public Health* 59 (October, 1969):1910-1926.

sire less frequent routine examinations.

Routine medical examinations may be given as the pupil enters the sixth and ninth grades. They are used to classify students for required physical education and are given by school or family physicians.

Required physical education refers to regularly scheduled class periods of physical education and does not include interscholastic or intramural sports. The examining physician should understand (1) the importance of the medical examination to physical education; (2) the physical education program, staff, and facilities; and (3) the implications of the classifications that he (the physician) will give.

The physician should be aware that the physical educator discovers the student's physical capacities through motor ability tests, physical fitness indices, and athletic ability tests. With this battery of information and with knowledge of students' interests in physical education, the physical education activities are planned to meet the student's capacities, needs, and interests. At the secondary level, the physical education activities are designed to prepare the young adult for recreational activities used in later life. At the elementary level, the basic physical education fundamentals and skills are taught. In the modern program of physical education, the physiological capacities of each student must be known. The physical educator realizes that there are individual pupil differences in body build and physiological conditions. He is aware that some of his students cannot participate in strenuous activities. The medical examination will provide data on the health status of the individual pupil and will determine the extent of the pupil's participation in physical education. In the elementary school, the classroom teacher who teaches physical education needs this classification by the physician as does the physical education teacher.

The physician should understand the types of pupil classification for physical education. In Section 4 of the health record (Appendix A), there is a subdivision called "Classification for Physical Education." There are three possible classifications:

A. Unlimited physical education activity, including interscholastic and intramural sports.

B. Moderate physical activity, limited to physical education classes and excluding interscholastic sports and more strenuous activities.

C. Adapted physical education or physical education for the handicapped.

Also provided is space for the physician to make recommendations for activities for students classified "B" and "C." Using these three classifications, the physician has no reason to issue a "blanket" medical excuse from physical education.

Physical educators occasionally ask how a medical examination can be given when there are no routine medical examinations or when students have no family physicians. In most localities there are county medical societies from which physical educators can seek medical assistance in the classification of students for physical education. When the county medical society has a school health committee, the society may recommend a panel of physicians to give the medical examinations.

Routine medical examinations are also used by family physicians to check the pupil whose personal health needs constant surveillance. This child may be recovering from prolonged illness or a serious operation or the child may have a chronic condition such as diabetes or asthma. These routine medical examinations not only check the pupil's health status but also enable the physician to recommend proper care including the amount of rest and relaxation needed, food intake, health habits, school and home activities, and adjustments to emotional health problems. The pupil may or may not need physical education for the handicapped. He may attend adapted physical education classes for several weeks and then return to regular physical education activities after recovery. Whenever possible, the pupil with a chronic condition should be encouraged to participate in regular physical education activities.

## Special Medical Examinations

In addition to the readiness-for-school and routine medical examinations, there is a definite need in school health services for special medical examinations. These examinations can include those for the handicapped pupil, for the athlete participating in interscholastic and intramural sports, and for the student complying with regulations for an employment certificate. The American Academy of Pediatrics defines a handicapped child as one

> with a physical, mental, or emotional problem that interferes with normal growth and development. From the standpoint of the school, children with handicaps are those who require special attention beyond that given to other children.[12]

Handicapped students include those with many remediable and chronic health problems. Such students may have hearing or visual impairments, severe posture conditions, nutritional deficiencies, or major disabling conditions resulting from tuberculosis, heart disease, poliomyelitis, traumatic injuries, epilepsy, cerebral palsy, or neurological problems. Some students may be mentally retarded while others may be emotionally disturbed. Students may be overweight; some may have delayed or accelerated maturation and growth; and others have signs of polyarthritis, hyperthyroidism, or hypothyroidism. An anemic child might be placed in physical education for the handicapped.

*Adapted physical education* has been defined as

> a diversified program of development activities, games, sports, and rhythms suited to the interests, capacities, and limitations of students with disabilities who may not safely or successfully engage in unrestricted activities of the general physical education program.[13]

Some of the objectives of adapted physical education are as follows:

1. To acquaint students with their capacities for exercise and at the same time to encourage awareness that exercise does not aggravate their handicaps.
2. To have students develop physiological benefits from exercise within the limits of their handicaps.
3. To provide students with opportunities for social development.
4. To assist students with permanent handicaps to adjust to those handicaps.

5. To provide students with activities which will assist learning to function more effectively.
6. To assist students in developing pride in their success in overcoming or adjusting to their handicaps.[14]

Some public school systems provide special education teachers for these children. Successful programs for exceptional children depend partially on special medical examinations that can be given by the family physician, a medical specialist such as an ophthalmologist, or a panel of cooperating local physicians. Special medical examinations occur more frequently than routine examinations and differ in diagnostic medical procedures. Health information can be brought to the attention of special education and classroom teachers as a result of special medical examinations.

Physical education for the handicapped can be provided when there is medical supervision and a physical educator qualified to teach physical education for the handicapped. The medical supervision begins with the student's first routine medical examination. If the student is classified "C," the physician makes recommendations for the handicapped student's physical education. The written recommendations by the physician are the result of conferences between the physical educator and the physician regarding the activities offered in physical education program for the handicapped.

The personal physician will continue special medical examinations of the student and will have overall periodic medical responsibility for the student's physical education. A student with a severe posture condition not only will be classified for physical education for the handicapped but also will have medical recommendations for posture exercises and physical education activities to remedy the problem. From time to time during the school year, the physician should visit the student during the physical education class. The physician should suggest changes or modifications in activities. The physical educator in charge of the handicapped student's physical education must change and modify activities according to the physician's suggestions. The physical educator should seek the phy-

[12]Committee on School Health of the American Academy of Pediatrics, *op. cit.*, p. 35.
[13]Adapted physical Education. *J. Health, Physical Education and Recreation 40* (May, 1969):45.
[14]*Ibid.*, p. 46.

sician's advice about the handicapped student's progress. In physical education for the handicapped, the physical educator cannot assume any medical responsibility but must follow the recommendations of the physician. If the physical educator has specialized preparation in physical education for the handicapped, he can choose physical education activities to the handicapped student's capacities and satisfy medical recommendations.

Special medical examinations are vital in determining the health status of the athlete participating in interscholastic and intramural sports because of the physiological demands on the body in such sports. Before the athlete is allowed to participate in these sports, he should have a medical examination. The Joint Committee on Health Problems in Education of the NEA and the AMA has suggested that medical examinations for athletes enable the physician: (1) to determine the health status of the athlete before competition; (2) to initiate prompt treatment for remediable conditions of athletes and arrange for further examinations; (3) to counsel the athlete in order to have him participate in those sports which provide the best activity for him; and (4) to restrict those athletes who have physical limitations causing undue risk. The Joint Committee further suggests that one annual medical examination for athletes is sufficient. More than one medical examination should be given the athlete when he (1) has had a significant injury or illness since the last examination or (2) has been urged to have a medical examination after successful surgery and/or treatment.[15]

The elementary or secondary school student participating in intramural sports should have a special medical examination at frequent intervals. Most schools do not require these students to have special medical examinations, but school administrators who are aware of the physiological demands placed on the student and the probable lack of physical conditioning insist on special medical examinations.

Many industrial corporations and businesses insist upon medical examinations for new employees. In some instances, physicians who are retained by the employer give the medical examination. In other instances the prospective employee may have the medical examination given by his family physician who will usually answer a questionnaire submitted by the employer.

## Referral Medical Examinations

Referral medical examinations can also provide information for physicians and school personnel. These examinations can result from teachers' and nurses' observations; emergency care for the ill or injured pupil; screening procedures for vision, hearing, nutritional status, heart disease, and posture; psychological testing; health counseling; tuberculin testing; and home visits by the nurse. The family physician and medical specialist responsible for these examinations will utilize many diagnostic procedures and will often rely on health information given by parents and school personnel.

Questions have been raised as to the ways in which parents can be encouraged to seek medical care for their children's health problems. Two studies by Cauffman and others have revealed that there are factors which influence the outcome of referral from personnel in school health services. Several notifications describing the child's health problem were found to be significantly more successful than a single written notice. Parents receiving two notifications were more likely to seek medical care than parents receiving only one notification. Follow-through by school personnel is therefore very important.[16,17]

## Implications for Health Education

The importance of medical examination should be stressed as a unit of health education in the area "Care of All Parts of the Human Body." Children in the intermediate grades of the elementary school should be aware of some of the diagnostic techniques used by the physician during a medical examination, such as inspection, palpation,

[16]Joy C. Cauffman, Eleanora Peterson, and John Emrick: Medical care of school children: factors influencing outcome of referral from a school health program. *Amer. J. Public Health* 57 (January, 1967): 60-73.

[17]Joy C. Cauffman, Edward Warburton, and Carl S. Shultz: Health care of school children: effective referral patterns. *Amer. J. Public Health* 59 (January, 1969):86-91.

[15]Joint Committee on Health Problems in Education of the National Education Association and the American Medical Association, *op. cit.*, p. 21.

auscultation, and percussion. In the high school, the unit on the medical examination can include instruction about the laboratory tests such as the urinalysis, blood chemistry and serologic tests, examination of fecal material, sputum tests, and cytology tests; chest x-rays; and electrocardiogram, in addition to the diagnostic techniques used by the physician during the medical examination. The need for pelvic examination, Papanicolaou's smear ("Pap" test), and examination of the female breasts can be taught in this unit along with the need for rectal examination of men. The teacher needs to stress that students are wise to develop physician-patient relations that will carry over into the post-school years.

## DENTAL EXAMINATIONS

Dental caries, malocclusion (irregularities of tooth position), and periodontal diseases (diseases of the gums and supporting structures of the teeth) are considered the most prevalent school health problems. Examinations by dentists to reveal these problems are important in the pupil's total health appraisal. Because of the frequency of such dental health problems among school children and young persons, an entire chapter is devoted to dental health. In Chapter 4, dental examinations and other phases of dental health will be discussed.

## SCREENING PROCEDURES

A part of health appraisal, screening procedures are preliminary evaluations of the pupil's health status. These procedures do not take the place of the physician's medical examination. Instead, they designate which children need more intensive medical examinations and diagnosis.

Several questions should be raised concerning these procedures. How do they affect school health services, teacher and nurse observations, medical examinations, functions of school personnel following appraisal, and the nurse's home visit? When there are screening procedures, how are the results used to improve the school's lighting, seating, acoustics, and other environmental conditions? Do elementary and secondary teachers use the results of screening to alter the school day so that the pupil's total health will be benefited? How do the results of screening influence instructional methods and materials? Are

school personnel prepared to carry out these screening procedures? How frequently shall these procedures be required? What role does the special education teacher have in the procedures? To what extent should there be administrative control of these procedures?

The Joint Committee on Health Problems in Education of the NEA and the AMA has raised these questions. (1) Is the screening applicable to the health problems of elementary and secondary school students? Some health problems detected by screening procedures have a low incidence among school-age children. (2) Is the screening medically sound? The procedures should be medically acceptable. Physicians are aware of the possibility of overreferral, the number of missed cases, and faulty interpretation of the results of screening. (3) Is the screening educationally sound? (4) Is the cost of the screening feasible? The equipment needed, the technical personnel to perform and interpret the results of the screening, and the types of screening procedures will affect the cost. (5) Is the screening acceptable to public relations? Many persons will be affected by the screening procedures such as family physicians, parents, local health departments, optometrists, children receiving the screening, and school personnel.[18]

### Vision

Vision screening devices will indicate some of the pupil's visual difficulties, but school personnel should realize that vision screening procedures do not reveal diseases of the eye. An ophthalmologist must diagnose eye diseases and malfunctionings. To assist school systems in deciding the types of screening devices to use, the American Medical Association, the National Society for the Prevention of Blindness, state departments of health and education, and local ophthalmologists and optometrists can give suggestions.

The Joint Committee on Health Problems in Education of the NEA and the AMA has indicated that the common vision screening procedures are the Snellen test, the plus sphere test for ability to accommodate, the Maddox rod test or some other screening

[18]Joint Committee on Health Problems in Education of the National Education Association and the American Medical Association, op. cit., pp. 8-9.

procedure for muscle imbalance, and a screening for color discrimination performed once during the school years.[19]

Vision screening should be done at the beginning of the school year so that needed medical care can be obtained before visual difficulties interfere with school progress. In the elementary school, the vision screening should be done annually. However, if a child wears glasses and is known to be under the continuous supervision of an ophthalmologist, he does not need to be tested. In the secondary school, vision screening might be limited to students referred by teachers and to students having had previous possibilities of visual difficulties.

Pupils need to understand the purpose and the procedures of screening. With pre-school children and first-graders, a demonstration of vision screening should precede the screening.

One of the common visual difficulties of school children is amblyopia; it can be prevented or if it begins, it can be quickly and easily detected; it is never learned. The image from one eye is blurred because of some other eye defect such as astigmatism. The child does not see well because he tries to fuse the image of the weak eye with the image of the good eye. Later, the child reduces the blurry image of the weak eye. The vision of the weak eye can be corrected by glasses, minor surgery, or eye exercises. Time is an important factor as the child must have the vision of the weak eye corrected by the age of six or seven since his visual development ends at those ages. If the amblyopia is not detected, the child will never have depth perception.[20] In a study by Flom and Neumaier, there was an analysis of previous studies of the prevalence of amblyopia. In 1561 children in kindergarten and 1201 children in grades 1 through 6, 1% of the children had amblyopia of 20/40-or-worse visual acuity. Assuming that some of the children had had amblyopia prevented or eliminated before the study was made, the prevalence of amblyopia was estimated at 1.8%. No significant difference was reported in the preva-

lence of amblyopia in the different age groups.[21]

*The Snellen Test*

The Snellen test has several advantages. It is inexpensive, requires no mechanical equipment, is easy to administer, and can be given within one minute to each pupil. It requires the reading of letters, numbers, or symbols (test objects) from a distance of 20 feet. The test objects are of graduated sizes on a chart. A person with normal visual acuity should be able to identify each size at a standard distance. Each size is numbered to indicate this standard distance. Thus, if the student can read the 20-foot line at a distance of 20 feet, the student is said to have 20/20 vision. The numerator indicates the distance of the student from the chart, and the denominator the smallest line read correctly. A young child, however, may not have 20/20 vision even though his vision is normal for his stage of development.

The Snellen chart is hung on a wall of a room. The pupil can sit or stand 20 feet away. The chart is artificially illuminated, and daylight is excluded from the room. The lights illuminating the chart should not shine in the pupil's face.

The pupil should be familiarized with the screening procedures before he is tested. Both eyes are kept open during the test, and the eye not being tested is covered with a small card resting obliquely across the nose. If a child wears glasses, the child reads the Snellen chart with his glasses *and then* without his glasses.

1. Test the right eye, the left eye, and then both eyes together.
2. Begin with the 30-foot line on the chart, and follow with the 20-foot line. If the pupil fails to read the 30-foot line correctly, proceed to the 20-foot line.
3. Use cards with circular cutouts to expose one letter at a time so that unused parts of the chart are covered.
4. Move from one symbol to another at a speed with which the pupil can keep pace.

[19]*Ibid.*, p. 9.

[20]Patricia and Ron Deutsch: The hidden threat to children's eyes. *Today's Health 43* (August, 1965): 29-32, 64-65.

[21]Merton C. Flom and Richard W. Neumaier: Prevalence of amblyopia. *Public Health Reports 81* (April, 1966):329-341.

5. If the pupil reads correctly three of four symbols on a line, he is considered to have read the line satisfactorily.

6. Record results so that the numerator represents the distance from the chart and the denominator the smallest line read correctly.

After the Snellen test, the parents of pupils needing eye examinations should be notified. These pupils are (1) those who have been observed to have signs of visual difficulties, regardless of the results of the Snellen test; (2) older children who have a visual acuity of 20/30 or less in either eye; and (3) younger children (7 years or less) who have 20/40 or less in either eye.

## Other Vision Tests

Screening for farsightedness and the student's ability to accommodate for close work can be accomplished by the use of suitable convex lenses. The pupil wears convex lenses (+2.25 diopter strength for grades 1 through 3 and +1.75 diopter strength for grade 4 and above). The pupil reads the 20-foot line of a Snellen chart with both eyes open and uncovered. If the pupil can read the 20-foot line, he *fails* the test. This test for accommodative ability is given only to those students who pass the Snellen test.

Vertical heterophoria (failure of both eyes to maintain alignment on the same level) can be screened by reliable tests. Screening for lateral heterophoria does not clearly differentiate between physiological conditions not requiring treatment and significant eye problems. Thus, the value of screening "muscle balance" is limited.

Opinions of the value of using stereoscopic devices vary. These devices may be employed if they are based on the physiological principles of central acuity as in the Snellen test, convex lens test, and distance muscle imbalance tests. Stereoscopic devices use test targets viewed through a binocular device which tests central visual acuity, color vision, and muscle balance.

Tests for identification of colors should be given to students before the sixth or seventh grade. Tests do not need to be repeated as the ability to perceive color correctly does not change.[22]

The National Society for the Prevention of Blindness suggests additional tests. First, there may be a test of accommodative ability to determine the student's ability to accommodate for close work while wearing a pair of convex or plus lenses. Second, there may be a test of muscle balance or the ability of both eyes to work together. Third, there may be tests for depth perception or visual perception of three-dimensional space.[23]

Lampe has reported the results of color vision tests with more than 3400 five- and six-year-old children in the Denver Public Schools. One approach to color vision testing employed color matching and another approach included recognition of symbols of the test color different from other colors. Some conclusions were that (1) with experienced examiners, the color vision tests take only two minutes per child; (2) color vision tests were practical with five- and six-year-old children; (3) color deficiency was 3 to 3.5% for boys and .5% for girls; and (4) the color symbol test was more definitive than the color matching test.[24]

## Hearing

At least 3 to 4% of school-age children or about three million children in the United States have a measurable hearing loss, although very few children are totally deaf. The hearing of pupils in the elementary and secondary schools is not checked early enough.[25] Often the hearing difficulty is not suspected by the child, the parents, or the teacher. Thus, hearing screening should be done annually in the elementary school and at least every three years in the secondary school.

The audiometer should meet the specifications established by American Standards Association for identification audiometry. Audiologists must know the calibration of their audiometers.

A good testing environment is necessary to obtain valid measurement of hearing loss. A quiet room, acoustically treated and with a quiet ventilating and heating sys-

[22]Joint Committee on Health Problems in Education of the National Education Association and the American Medical Association, *op. cit.*, pp. 26-27.

[23]National Society for the Prevention of Blindness: *Vision Screening of Children.* New York: The Society, 1969, p. 4.

[24]John M. Lampe: An evaluative study of color-vision tests for kindergarten and first grade pupils. *J. School Health 39* (May, 1969):311-313.

[25]Statements on deafness today. *J. School Health 37* (March, 1967):150-151.

tem, is advantageous for audiometric screening. The health service unit with a standard "soundproof" booth which can guarantee at least 40-decibel attentuation is recommended. The screening room should be removed from sounds of traffic, music and typewriter rooms, shops, and cafeteria.

The five frequencies recommended for identification audiometry are 500, 1000, 2000, 4000, and 6000 cycles per second. The established procedure is to test many frequencies until definitive data are available to justify testing one or two frequencies.

*Sweep Test*

This test is called the "sweep test" because the audiologist or tester can sweep through all of the frequencies in rapid order. Frequencies of 1000, 2000, and 6000 cps are tested at the 10-db level, and 4000 cps are tested at the 20-db level. The tester must be sure that the pupil can detect the presence of the tone of the audiometer. The interrupter key can be used for this purpose. Both ears of the pupil can be tested in about two minutes.

The pupil will fail the sweep test and be a candidate for the threshold test if he cannot hear all of the tones tested in either ear. The sweep test thus identifies pupils whose hearing at one or more frequencies is outside the range of normal hearing. About 5 to 10% of students fail the sweep test.

*Threshold Test*

An audiogram chart, as found in Section 5 of the Health Record (Appendix A), should be used to record the thresholds at each of the test frequencies to which the pupil fails to respond. The better ear should be tested first if there is a difference in the hearing acuity between the pupil's ears. The threshold test starts at 1000 cps. If the pupil hears a tone, the pupil may raise a finger, push a button that operates a signal light, or say yes. If the pupil hears no tone, the pupil may lower the finger, release the button that operates a signal light, or say no. The tester searches for the minimum intensity level at which the pupil responds at least 50% of the time. Several trials are required so that the tester is satisfied that the pupil is consistent. The frequency selector is moved to other frequencies when the threshold has been determined at 1000

cps. A repeat threshold measurement is made at 1000 cps after all other frequencies have been measured so that there is another check upon the consistency of the pupil's responses. The pupil is not consistent if at the second test of 1000 cps the threshold measurement is not ±5 db of the first measurement.

After the tester has charted the audiogram for the first ear, the same procedures are followed for obtaining the threshold measurements at all test frequencies for the other ear. In some pupils, there may be differences in acuity between the two ears of 40 or more db at some or all frequencies. These pupils may be responding to the tone in the better ear even though the other ear is being tested.

The pupil is referred to an otologist when there is a loss in either ear of 20 db or more at two or more frequencies or a loss of 30 db or more at any single frequency. A loss of this magnitude is usually considered medically significant, although some physicians consider that a loss measurable only at 4000 cps is not.[26]

Harrelson and others have reported their findings in comparing hearing screening methods of 603 elementary school children of the Tacoma, Washington, public schools. The three hearing screening methods were the individual pure-tone sweep check, group pure-tone test, and individual three-tone sweep check. Some of the conclusions were (1) the three screening methods differed significantly in ability to detect hearing loss; (2) the three-tone screening method was superior to the other two methods; and (3) the three-tone screening method required the least time per pupil, was cheaper in cost, was more reliable, and had less than 1% misdiagnosis.[27]

A five-year hearing screening project involving 35,435 school-age children in Kansas has been reported by Gendel. These children had their screening by the sweep test in a mobile testing unit by two audiologists and a public health nurse. At least 1404 children were referred for medical care. The ages of the children having the

[26]Joint Committee on Health Problems in Education of the National Education Association and the American Medical Association: *op. cit.*, pp. 27-30.

[27]Orvis A. Harrelson, Donna G. Ferguson, G. Paul Killian, and Irving Zimmer: Comparison of hearing screening methods. *J. School Health 39* (March, 1969): 161-165.

highest rates of medical referral were 7 years—9.7%; 13 years—9.6%; 14 years—9.0%; 8 years—8.6%; and 17 years—7.9%. Thirty-four percent of the parents of the 1404 children expressed indifference to providing their children with follow-up medical examinations. The study clearly showed the need for widespread hearing screening.[28]

Hollien and others have reported on the Hollien-Thompson group screening test of hearing designed to survey the hearing acuity of large numbers of school children quickly for the purpose of identifying medically significant hearing problems. The test consists of controlled signals that reach the pupil through earphones connected to the audiometer. Each pupil indicates on his answer sheet the number of signals he heard through his earphones. Nearly 5000 elementary school students have been involved in the research for development of the Hollien-Thompson test so that the validity, reliability, and efficiency of the test could be established.[29]

Hodgson has presented a study of the misdiagnosis of children with hearing loss for the purpose of classifying the types of hearing loss that have been mistaken for other problems. In the first group, the children were uncooperative and difficult to test. When auditory thresholds could not be established, some testers concluded that the child was retarded, was too mentally disturbed, or had some auditory problem. In the second group, the children had mild hearing losses but had learned to use their hearing well enough to respond to sounds in their environments. In the third group, the children had high frequency loss but responded to many sounds around them. These children understood only a part of what was said to them so their responses were considered inappropriate.[30]

## Heart Disease

Mass screening tests for detection of heart disease in children have been conducted since 1959. This screening has been facilitated by the use of the Phono-Cardio Scan, a portable computer which can detect marked right axis deviation, bradycardia (abnormal slowness of the heart beat), tachycardia (excessive rapidity in the action of the heart), and arrhythmia (absence of rhythm, or variation from normal rhythm of the heart). Cayler and others have reported on the mass screening of 3518 fourth-grade children for heart disease in the Sacramento City Unified School District, California. Definite organic heart lesions were detected in 18 children, and 24 children had suspected heart disease. Following the screening, electrocardiograms and chest x-rays were given in addition to pediatric cardiology consultation. Of the 42 children, twenty children had organic heart lesions, and seven children were considered to have suspected heart disease. Of the 27 children, sixteen had histories of murmurs or heart disease, and eleven had heart conditions not previously found. The cost of the mass screening for heart disease was $.52 per child or about $166 per unknown case detected.[31]

Physicians may indicate that a child has a heart murmur. Sounds produced by the passage of blood through the chambers and valves of the heart are heart murmurs. Most heart murmurs detected in children are "functional" and disappear during adolescence. An "organic" heart murmur indicates that there is a disease or defect of the heart. In detection of heart disease by a heart screening device, the physician may find it necessary to re-examine the child periodically. Physicians may check the functioning of the heart through x-ray or fluoroscope, with an electrocardiograph, or by laboratory tests of blood samples to discover whether infection or anemia is causing the murmur.

## Nutritional Status

Measurements of height and weight can indicate factors relative to the pupil's nutritional status. Platform beam-type scales and a yardstick or measuring tape are commonly used measuring devices.

[28]Evalyn S. Gendel: Hearing conservation of children—a special five-year project in Kansas. *Amer. J. Public Health* 58 (March, 1968):499-505.

[29]Harry Hollien, Joseph M. Wepman, and Carl L. Thompson: A group screening test of auditory acuity. *J. School Health* 39 (October, 1969):583-589.

[30]William R. Hodgson: Misdiagnosis of children with hearing loss. *J. School Health* 39 (October, 1969): 570-576.

[31]Glen G. Cayler, Gordon Mannerstedt, Michael W. Adams, Grace Tanner, Harold S. Hunt, and Wilma Bujack: Mass screening of school children for heart disease. *Public Health Reports* 84 (June, 1969):479-483.

The elementary and secondary pupil should be weighed and measured at the beginning and close of every school year. The procedures of weighing and measuring should be performed accurately. Before weighing the child, the teacher should place all weights at the zero marks, check to be sure that the scales are balanced, adjust scales when they are not balanced, and require each child to remove his shoes and sweater or jacket before stepping on the scales. Each child should stand in the center of the scales. The child's weight can be measured to the nearest half-pound.

A yardstick or measuring tape can be fastened either to a special board or directly to a smooth wall. The headpiece can be a wooden object having two faces at right angles. The child should stand with his heels, the lower part of his back, his shoulders, and the rear of his head touching the yardstick or measuring tape. The child's heels should be nearly together on the floor but not touching. His arms should hang at the sides. His face should be straight forward. As soon as the child is in position, one face of the headpiece can be placed against the yardstick or tape measure. The other face of the headpiece, held in a horizontal position, should be in contact with the top of the child's head. The child's height can be measured to the nearest 1/4-inch.

Figures 1 and 2 show height/weight interpretation for boys and girls. Don Jones weighs 75 pounds, is 55 inches in height, and is just past his tenth birthday.

## Recording Height

1. Find age 10 along the bottom of the chart in Figure 1.
2. Locate 55 inches along the upper left-hand margin.
3. Place a dot at the intersection of the two lines.
4. Below this dot write "55."

## Recording Weight

1. Find age 10 along the bottom of the chart.
2. Locate 75 pounds along the lower right-hand margin.
3. Place a dot at the intersection of the two lines.
4. Above this dot write "75."

Over the years, Don's progress in height can be shown by drawing lines connecting the various dots on the height chart. Lines connecting the various dots on the weight chart will show Don's progress in weight. Don's height and weight falls in the "average zone." In the event that Don's height and weight do not fall in corresponding zones, he should have medical attention. The child's progression in height and weight should run about parallel with the lines on the chart. Also, the child should be in corresponding zones at each age level.[32]

Wear has reported on the use of combining height and weight data into two-way classification tables for group evaluation and an analysis of the resulting data. The heights and weights were taken from boys in four age groups—12, 13, 14, and 15 years. A total of 1200 boys were involved in the study. The average of the heights and weights of the 1200 boys was higher than that of the boys of the same age groups measured to calculate the figures on which the 1963 Height Weight Interpretation for Boys was based. Wear suggested that the Height Weight Interpretation for Boys be revised periodically, every 10 or 15 years. He also suggested that these Height Weight Interpretation charts be used as a screening device to detect sudden or gradual changes in height and weight.[33]

## Posture Screening

The true validity of posture screening rests with the skill of the examiner, who in all likelihood will be a physical educator. Posture screening is classified into four categories: (1) static anterior-posterior posture tests; (2) functional appraisal methods; (3) observation; and (4) refined posture appraisal. Static anterior-posterior posture tests may be divided into two groups. The first group, used to determine lateral standing posture, consists of silhouettes or shadow prints. The second group, used to determine certain body landmarks, are

[32]Height weight interpretation for boys, 1963 revision. Prepared for the Joint Committee on Health Problems in Education of the National Education Association and the American Medical Association by Howard V. Meredith and Virginia B. Knott. Chicago: American Medical Association, 1967.
[33]Carl L. Wear: An analysis of height-weight relationships of Midwestern boys. *Research Quarterly* 40 (October, 1969):607-613.

# HEIGHT WEIGHT INTERPRETATION FOR BOYS

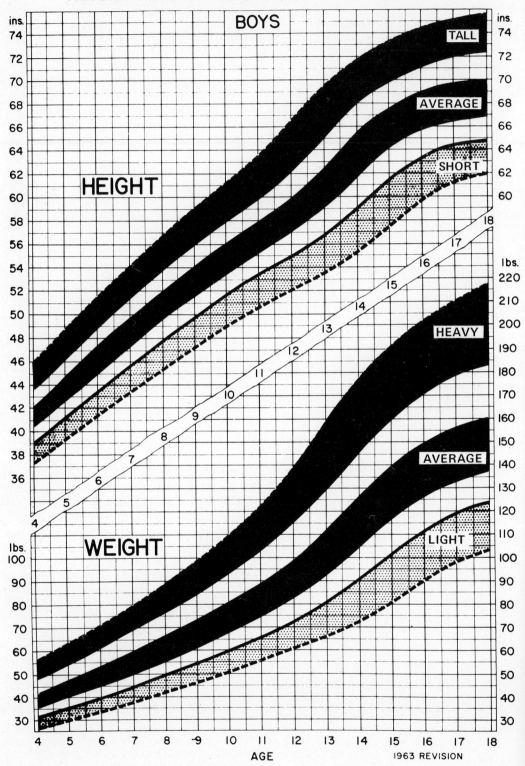

Figure 1

# HEIGHT WEIGHT INTERPRETATION FOR GIRLS

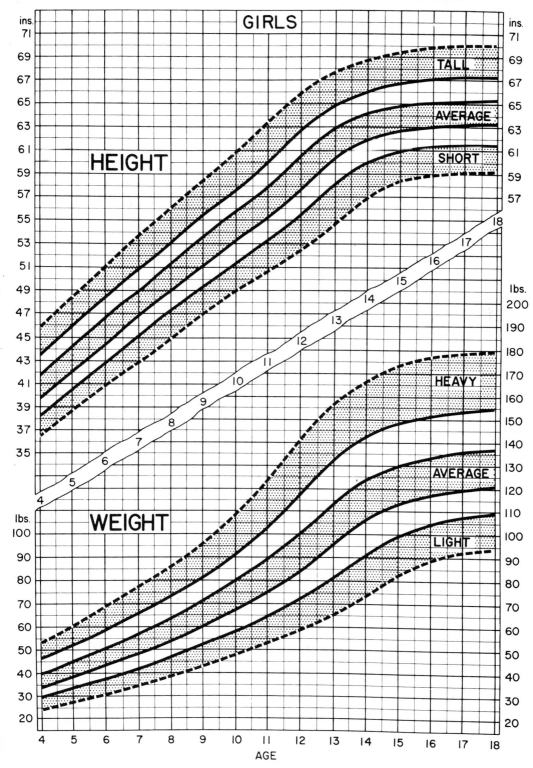

Figure 2

based on photographs. Calipers and other specially designed instruments are used in the objective anterior-posterior posture tests. Two of these specially designed instruments are the conformateur and spinograph. The pupil stands with his back to the conformateur. Rods, extending from the conformateur, touch the spinous processes of the pupil's vertebrae. The pupil's spinous processes are traced by a pointer of the spinograph, thus making a record of the pupil's spinal contour on a blackboard. The Massey posture test measures standing anterior-posterior posture. The Howland Alignometer indicates structural balance of the pupil's body trunk while standing. The center of gravity test reveals that there is a distance in front of the line coordinating the center of gravity at the pelvis with the ankle bone. The functional appraisal methods and observation include the Washington State University test and observation of walking gaits. The Washington State University test includes anterior-posterior posture, and lateral balance, and alignment of legs and feet in a standing position. The student's efficiency of walking gait is observed from side, front, and back positions. Another appraisal method is functional posture screening.[34]

In Section 8 of the health record (Appendix A) there is a score card for posture screening. The card consists of a check list for evaluating posture in a static and dynamic status. The evaluation takes about four minutes per pupil and consists of the following procedures:

Functional Posture Screening

1. The pupil is standing. The examiner, from a side view, looks for shoulder overhang, forward head, round back (kyphosis), hollow back (lordosis), hyperextended knees, and pronated foot.
2. The pupil makes a quarter turn. The examiner checks lateral balance: shoulder height for left and right shoulders.
3. The pupil walks to a chair and is seated. The examiner checks that the pupil keeps the body weight over the rear foot as the pupil is seated.

[34]Donald K. Mathews: *Measurement in Physical Education.* 3rd ed. Philadelphia: W. B. Saunders Co., 1968, pp. 258-270.

The hands and arms of the pupil are relaxed, and one foot is to the rear of the other foot.

4. The pupil stands up. The examiner checks how the pupil transfers his body weight from the rear foot to the forward foot.
5. The pupil walks the length of the room. The examiner observes the pupil from the rear. The examiner checks whether the pupil has proper heel-to-toe movement and whether the pupil thrusts his weight to the inside of his foot.
6. The pupil turns to his right as he nears the end of the room. The pupil walks three-quarters of the width of the room. From the side of the pupil, the examiner checks the walking position and the anterior-posterior posture.
7. At three-quarters of the width of the room, the pupil is asked to stop walking and to reach upward toward the ceiling. The examiner watches to see if the pupil can reach upward and slightly forward with mechanical efficiency.
8. The pupil continues walking across the room and is seated. Again the examiner checks the transfer of body weight and body position as in numbers 3 and 4.
9. The pupil rises from the chair and walks toward the examiner. The examiner checks the foot and leg functions in walking, head tilt, and erectness of body position.
10. The pupil climbs and descends three steps. The examiner checks the transfer of body weight and alignment of the different parts of the pupil's body. The pupil repeats climbing and descending the three steps. The examiner checks the pupil from the side, front, and back view. As the pupil ascends, the examiner checks to see that the ball of the pupil's foot makes the first contact and then is followed by the heel. As the pupil descends, the examiner notes whether the pupil bends the leg supporting the body weight as the toe of the opposite leg is lowered.
11. The pupil lowers a weight of 5 to 8

pounds from a shelf above his head to the floor and returns the weight to the shelf. (A series of shelves arranged from the floor is necessary.) The examiner watches the manner in which the pupil's legs are used when the pupil moves the weight. The examiner checks how the pupil holds the weight to his gravity line.

12. The pupil skips rope. The examiner checks the coordination and control the pupil has as the pupil skips rope and as the pupil lands.[35]

The refined posture appraisal tests include the Kraus-Weber refined test which provides objective evidence to assist the physical educator in planning posture exercises.[36]

In posture screening, the physical educator may wish to evaluate the student's feet. One method of evaluating feet uses a pedograph to record the footprint. The Clarke footprint angle may be used, as well as the pedorule which measures the position of the foot in relation to the leg. The Truslow foot ratio determines the functional efficiency of the foot by the ratio of

the height of the arch to the length of the foot.[37]

## Tuberculin Testing

Tuberculin tests can be indicators of the pupil's health status and are considered by most physicians to be specific and reliable measures of susceptibility to tuberculosis. Chapter 6 has a section on tuberculosis in which tuberculin testing will be discussed.

## Implications for Health Education

Screening for vision, hearing, heart disease, nutritional status, and posture can be the subject of many units of health education. The area in which these units should be taught is the "Care of All Parts of the Human Body."

Not only should these units acquaint students with the procedures involved but they should also familiarize students with the purposes of the screening. Since these screening procedures precede medical diagnosis, students need to understand that the screening procedures are intended to identify those persons with health problems which may be medically significant.

| Type of screening | Suggested unit of health education |
|---|---|
| Vision | Snellen test and other vision screening procedures |
| Hearing | Sweep test and threshold test |
| Heart disease | Heart disease and how detected |
| Nutritional status | Height Weight Interpretation for Boys and Height Weight Interpretation for Girls |
| Posture | Procedures for posture screening |

## References for Further Study

Anderson, C. L.: *School Health Practice*. 5th ed. St. Louis: The C. V. Mosby Company, 1972.

Ballantyne, J.: *Deafness*. Boston: Little, Brown and Company, 1960.

Breckenridge, M. E., and Vincent, E. L.: *Child Development*. 5th ed. Philadelphia: W. B. Saunders Company, 1966.

Daniels, A., and Davies, E.: *Adapted Physical Education*. 2nd ed. New York: Harper and Row, 1965.

Davies, E. A.: *The Elementary School Child and His Posture Problems*. New York: Appleton-Century-Crofts, 1958.

Dun, L., ed.: *Exceptional Children in Schools*. New York: Holt, Rinehart and Winston, 1963.

Ellis, R. B.: *Child Health and Development*. New York: Grune & Stratton, Inc., 1966.

Eye Health Committee, American School Health Association: *Teaching About Vision*. New York: National Society for the Prevention of Blindness, 1969.

Fait, H.: *Special Physical Education*. 3rd ed. Philadelphia: W. B. Saunders Company, 1971.

Falkner, F., ed.: *Human Development*. Philadelphia: W. B. Saunders Company, 1966.

Fortier, E. G.: *Eye Muscle Problems in Children*. Roselle, Ill.: Roselle Publishing Company, 1962.

Gallagher, R., and Harris, H.: *Emotional Problems of Adolescents*. rev. ed. New York: Oxford University Press, 1964.

Joint Committee on Health Problems in Education of the National Education Association and the American Medical Association: *School Health Services*.

[35]*Ibid.*, pp. 270-274.
[36]*Ibid.*, pp. 274-277.

[37]*Ibid.*, pp. 278-283.

2nd ed. Washington, D.C.: National Education Association, 1964.

———': *Answers to Health Questions in Physical Education*. Washington, D.C.: National Education Association, 1970.

Kaplan, S. A.: *Growth Disorders in Children and Adolescents*. Springfield, Ill.: Charles C Thomas, 1964.

Krugman, S., and Ward, R.: *Infectious Diseases of Children*. 4th ed. St. Louis: The C. V. Mosby Company, 1968.

Lindsey, R., Jones, B. J., and Whitley, A. V.: *Body Mechanics*. Dubuque, Iowa: Wm. C. Brown Book Company, 1968.

Mawson, S. R.: *Diseases of the Ear*. Baltimore: The Williams & Wilkins Company, 1963.

Mayer, J.: *Overweight*. Englewood Cliffs, N.J.: Prentice-Hall, Inc., 1968.

National Committee on School Health Policies of the National Education Association and the American Medical Association: *Suggested School Health Policies*. 4th ed. Chicago: American Medical Association, 1966.

National Society for Prevention of Blindness, Inc.: *Vision Screening of Children*. New York: The Society, 1969.

Rathbone, J., and Hunt, V. V.: *Corrective Physical Education*. 7th ed. Philadelphia: W. B. Saunders Company, 1965.

Sauer, G.: *Teen Skin*. Springfield, Ill.: Charles C Thomas, 1965.

Silverthorne, N. H., Anglin, C. S., and Schusterman, M.: *Principal Infections and Diseases of Children*. 2nd ed. Springfield, Ill.: Charles C Thomas, 1966.

Sussman, M.: *Growth and Development*. 2nd ed. Englewood Cliffs, N.J.: Prentice-Hall, Inc., 1964.

Wheatley, G., and Hallock, G. T.: *Health Observation of School Children*. 3rd ed. New York: McGraw-Hill Book Company, 1965.

Wheeler, R., and Hooley, A.: *Physical Education for the Handicapped*. Philadelphia: Lea & Febiger, 1969.

# Chapter 3

# FOLLOWING APPRAISAL OF THE PUPIL'S HEALTH STATUS, WHAT CAN SCHOOL PERSONNEL DO?

## AN INCIDENT

Elementary school classroom teachers, aware of some signs of possible visual difficulties, have asked what they can do to help children with these difficulties. Junior high or middle school teachers, familiar with some signs of possible hearing difficulties, have asked how they can assist students with these hearing difficulties. Senior high school teachers, recognizing some signs of possible skin infections and other communicable diseases, have asked what they should do concerning those students who have communicable diseases.

When the appraisal of the pupil's health status is complete and the results indicate certain health problems, what can be done? The Joint Committee on Health Problems in Education of the NEA and the AMA suggests that school health personnel "counsel pupils, teachers, parents and others for the purpose of helping pupils obtain needed treatment or for arranging school programs in keeping with their abilities."[1]

School personnel can be informed of their duties following appraisal only if continuous in-service health education is made imperative. The in-service health education for teachers should stress (1) the ease by which these procedures can be followed without requiring the teacher to neglect other responsibilities, (2) the limitations of these procedures, and (3) the relation of

the procedures to the total school health program.

## PROCEDURES COMMON TO ALL HEALTH PROBLEMS

The teacher should be familiar with the procedures in her school system for *referral medical examinations* (Chapter 2). School systems vary in their methods of reporting suspected health problems to the family or the school physician. The signs observed by the teacher should, however, be a part of any report as they assist the physician in determining the extent and nature of the health problem.

At the same time, *parents should be informed* of the results of the appraisal. Here, too, school systems do not agree entirely on how the results of the appraisal should reach the parents. In some communities, a letter summarizing the results of the appraisal is sent to the parents. In other communities, a parent-teacher conference is held, at which time the teacher informs the parents of the results of the appraisal. Often the public health nurse or school nurse approaches the parents directly, as will be discussed under *"follow-through."*

At some point school personnel *should encourage parents to seek medical or dental care* for their son's or daughter's health problems. Parents should understand and accept that this is primarily their responsibility and *not* the responsibility of school personnel. It may be necessary for the public health nurse or school nurse to inform parents of this fact.

When the student reaches the secondary school, he can be encouraged to assume some of this responsibility for seeking and acquiring his own medical or dental care.

[1] Joint Committee on Health Problems in Education of the National Education Association and the American Medical Association: *Health Appraisal of School Children.* 4th ed. Washington, D.C.: National Education Association, 1969, p. 2.

He should no longer be entirely dependent on his parents for caring for his health.

The *results of health appraisal* can be discussed with the student or parent at a teacher-pupil, nurse-pupil, teacher-parent, or nurse-parent *conference*. Whether the student or the parent is involved, the aims of health counseling should be considered.

## Health Counseling

The Joint Committee on Health Problems in Education of the NEA and the AMA has indicated that health counseling is a vital step toward obtaining the necessary medical and dental care for a student with a health problem. Health counseling takes place at a face-to-face conference between the teacher, nurse, or other member of the school health staff and the student or his parents. Health counseling has eight purposes. (1) The student is to be provided with information about the results of the appraisal of his health status. (2) Significant health problems are to be explained to parents, and the parents are encouraged to obtain medical and dental care for these problems. (3) Parents and students are motivated to seek medical and dental care and to accept changes in the school program which would help the students. (4) Each student is encouraged to accept responsibility for his own health, depending upon his age. (5) Students and parents are urged to seek and use available medical and dental resources. (6) School personnel recognize the need for establishment or enlargement of medical or dental treatment facilities for those students who are disadvantaged. (7) School personnel contribute to health education of students and parents during health counseling. (8) Educational programs for exceptional pupils are adapted to the pupil's abilities and needs.[2]

A teacher, nurse, or health educator might be assigned to act as the person to compile all information concerning a particular pupil. The parent will receive this information concerning his child's health problems during one visit to the school. As the information is being compiled, the records for all pupils having severe health problems (who need immediate medical or dental care, who require assistance from community agencies, or who are assigned to services of the school counselor) should be separated from those of students not having health problems necessitating these procedures.

Usually, when health problems are not severe, a single teacher-parent or teacher-pupil conference will be sufficient counseling. Teachers must be aware that during these conferences their tasks are to inform, interpret, explain, encourage, and motivate parents and pupils to seek correction of the health difficulty. Before teacher-parent conferences, the health coordinator or nurse must provide in-service education to acquaint teachers with the types of information to be given to parents, how this information is to be interpreted, and how health counseling is to proceed.

To ensure satisfactory health counseling, certain procedures should be followed. Before the conference, all information concerning the student should be reviewed by the teacher or nurse. At the beginning of the conference, a friendly conversation helps to establish rapport between the parent and teacher or nurse. The parent should recognize and analyze the son or daughter's health problems and indicate his observations about these health problems. The parent is encouraged to ask questions so that the significance of the problem is clearly understood. The parent compares different courses of action to solve the problem. Finally, the parent chooses a particular course of action to solve the student's health problem. If the parent chooses a poor course of action, the teacher or nurse can encourage the parent to review the reasons for the decision. The teacher or nurse tries to have the parent think through his son or daughter's health problems, stimulates the parent's thinking, serves as a sounding board for the parent's ideas, and is a source of information. Often, the teacher or nurse volunteers information helpful to the parent.[3] These same procedures are used with high school students themselves rather than with their parents.

Hochbaum suggests that to influence health behavior of another person, there

[2]———— : *School Health Services.* 2nd ed. Washington, D.C.: National Education Association. 1964, pp. 111-112.

[3]*Ibid.*, pp. 116-121.

must be attention focused upon the person himself. What kind of a person is he? What is important to him? How does he think and feel? What are his goals and values? Also, health personnel must *listen* to the person with whom they are dealing. Often, the person feels freer to discuss his problem within his own environment rather than in a school office.[4]

There are limitations in health counseling. Because many students and parents are reluctant to discuss their problems, school personnel may misinterpret the problems. If the health information is not sufficiently explained by the school personnel, it may have disturbing effects. The teacher doing health counseling must be fully informed about the pupil's mental and physical health in order to answer questions that arise during health counseling.

Privacy is a requisite for the conference. Following the conference, a written summary should be made. The summary of the teacher-pupil conference or teacher-parent conference should be accessible to other school personnel. To have effective health counseling, school administrators must allow teachers to have time during the school day to schedule conferences, to gather data needed for health counseling, to record the results of conferences, and to confer with other school personnel about their pupils.

After the secondary school student or the parent has received health counseling, the public health or school nurse is consulted; she completes the follow-through *or* checks that medical or dental care has been received.

## Follow-through by the Nurse

Guidelines for the school nurse have been prepared by the School Nursing Committee of the American School Health Association. These guidelines are responsibilities of the nurse in the school health program, the nurse as an educator, the nurse as a counselor, and factors influencing the pupil load of the nurse.[5]

One of the most important functions of the nurse in school health services is the follow-through. The nurse will come into contact with teachers, parents, pupils, community physicians and dentists, personnel of community agencies, school and administrative personnel, and the health coordinator and school health educator.

Some pupils take priority in the follow-through. These are the pupils who have several health problems, as indicated from medical and dental examinations, screening procedures, and teacher observations. Such pupils may have been excluded from school because of communicable disease or may have received emergency care for sudden illness or injury. Also, pupils not receiving proper immunizations might be included in a priority list, as well as new students not having readiness-for-school medical and dental examinations.

The nurse may place each pupil's name on a 3x5 card, together with the dates for nurse-pupil and nurse-parent conferences. The pupil's card is filed according to the dates of the next planned conference. At school, the nurse confers with the pupil to determine whether a home visit can be made; then she makes an appointment. High school students, however, usually prefer to be advised directly about their health needs. They can accept the responsibility for seeking medical and dental care without involving their parents. In schools having a school nurse, the follow-through takes the form of a series of nurse-student conferences within the school rather than at the home. These individual student-nurse conferences are useful in encouraging the adolescent to take the initiative in solving his own health problems.

Before the home visit, the nurse reviews the pupil's cumulative health record and anecdotal records, meets with the teacher and principal to obtain further information concerning the pupil, checks to see whether there are other home visits in the pupil's neighborhood, and telephones for an appointment. Letters, telephone calls, notes, and visits by parents to the school can be used in the follow-through, but the home visit is usually the best procedure.

The nurse must be well prepared for a home visit. She may use forms in duplicate, with space for notes or a notebook or she may sometimes take the cumulative health records with her. Whatever the method

Godfrey Hochbaum: Effecting health behavior: the professional and lay side of the coin. *Int. J. Health Education 10* (October-December, 1967):178.

School Nursing Committee, American School Health Association: The nurse in the school health program. *J. School Health 37* (February, 1967): # 2a.

she uses, she must have all pertinent data with her.

The nurse completing the follow-through supplements the health counseling of the teacher. She will inform, interpret, explain, encourage, and motivate parents to seek assistance for their child's health problem. Parents react in various ways to these home visits. Some will have no apparent interest in their child's health problems. Some, because of ignorance or religion, may even refuse to take action. When advising the parent to seek medical or dental care, the nurse should suggest that the parent consult the family physician or dentist. When a medical or dental specialist is needed, the family physician or dentist makes the recommendation. Some families have neither a family physician nor a dentist. The nurse might then suggest sources of names of physicians or dentists such as lists prepared by the local medical or dental societies.

If, because of the parents' low economic status, it is necessary for the nurse to contact a community health or welfare agency, the school principal should be informed.

The first home visit by the school nurse is usually followed by several others. The nurse will have to decide the degree of urgency of each pupil's problem, as well as the need for subsequent visits. When the pupil has an irremediable health problem, the nurse may have to explain the nature of the problem to the parents, assist them in accepting their child's difficulty, suggest ways of altering family living so that the child can adjust better, and help the child in these adjustments. When parents are not well informed about communicable diseases and their transmission to other family members, the nurse may have to acquaint parents with the signs of communicable diseases, the means of preventing their spread, the necessity for medical care of family members with communicable diseases, and the methods of caring for the ill child.

Encouraging parents to seek medical and dental attention is one of the nurse's most difficult tasks. Parents may not accept the importance of medical or dental services if they have been unduly influenced by the advertising of nostrums, charlatans, and quick cures. The fear of medical or dental treatment and its cost discourage many parents.

After the home visit, the nurse may wish to record her observations of the pupil, her recommendations for further medical care, and suggestions she gave to the parents for the care of the child. The nurse's observations and recommendations might be placed on a referral form or a written report to be sent to the physician handling the case. When parents have no family physician and their child needs medical care, the nurse may refer the parents to a panel of cooperating physicians or a clinic, together with her observations and recommendations.

The follow-through influences the total school health program, depending on the working relations existing between the nurse and the instructional staff. Following the home visit, the nurse should see the pupil's teacher. The nurse can supply the teacher with information for promoting the pupil's health during the school day. However, the utilization of this information by the teacher depends on the teacher's understanding of the total school health program, the in-service health education given by the health coordinator, and the rapport between the nurse and the teacher. The teacher can supply the nurse with data about the pupil's health status and practices, achievement, social tendencies, and possible capacities for schoolwork. To the school health educator and health coordinator, the follow-through can supply data for health teaching, school health council, in-service health education, and evaluation of school health services.

The nurse should be familiar with each community health agency and its means of assisting families with particular health problems. When the nurse wishes to refer a family to an agency, the family's permission and help must be secured so that the nurse can supply the agency with background information. The nurse should encourage the parents to request assistance from appropriate community agencies rather than to rely on her to obtain the assistance. Occasionally, several community agencies may be aiding one family. The nurse might suggest that representatives of these agencies meet together to discuss present methods of family assistance, to eliminate unnecessary agency efforts, and to foresee possible future problems.

The public relations program of a school should be well understood by the nurse because she must make effective contacts with parents, physicians, dentists, local health departments, hospitals, and community official and nonofficial health agencies. The school administrator should acquaint the nurse with the school system's public relations program, policies, and procedures. The administrator may be unaware of the many community contacts the nurse makes during the school day. A misinterpretation by the nurse of the school's philosophy, curriculum development, administrative and supervisory practices, and the total school health program can damage the efforts of the school's public relations program.

The school nurse should clearly understand her role in follow-through, in school health services, and in the total school health program. There has been a considerable body of literature written by nurses on the importance of school nursing, but there has been little opportunity for parents, school administrative officials, instructional personnel, and health coordinators to evaluate the effectiveness of school nursing.

Forbes[6] has revealed the teacher's expectations of the nurse's role and functions in schools. The study sample of 115 teachers in elementary and secondary schools suggested that

1. Teachers perceive that the nurse's main functions are health appraisal, follow-through, health protection, and safety.
2. Elementary school classroom teachers perceive more functions of the nurse than secondary school teachers.
3. The role of the nurse is, in large part, determined by the amount of time she is in the school providing school nursing services.
4. Teachers rated twenty selected school nursing services in the same way as did school nurses in a previous study.

## WHAT CAN ALL SCHOOL PERSONNEL DO FOLLOWING APPRAISAL OF THE PUPIL'S HEALTH STATUS?

Teachers, as well as the nurse, should be continually alert for signs of possible health difficulties (Chapter 2). There is a chance that other signs of the same health problem previously observed may occur. Or signs of a different health problem may be observed. A health problem that has received medical or dental care can recur.

In assisting the pupil with a health problem, teachers should be aware that environmental factors, the teacher's health, adjustments within the school day, and health education must be taken into consideration. Thus two of the parts of the total health program can be related to school health services: healthful school living and health education. In the following section, environmental factors, the teacher's health, adjustment within the school day, and direct health instruction will be emphasized.

## VISUAL DIFFICULTIES AND ADDITIONAL WAYS TO ASSIST THE PUPIL

Light and color in the classroom, arrangement of seating, and promotion of eye health by environmental factors can assist the pupil. Some of the ways to promote eye health are as follows:[7]

1. Check that no student works in his shadow.
2. Never seat a student with the sunlight in his direct line of vision.
3. Keep the upper portion of windows unshaded except when the sun shines on these window surfaces.
4. Use multiple seating arrangements.
5. Check condition of interior daylight controls, such as shades.
6. Keep chalkboards clean and free from accumulating chalk dust.
7. Be aware of direct glare on black slateboard surfaces.
8. Have all defective incandescent bulbs and fluorescent tubes replaced immediately.
9. Check height of desk-chair combinations so that the student receives the optimum light on the working surfaces.
10. Provide library or other special-purpose areas of classroom with ample brightness levels.

In addition, the teacher can use printed materials in clear type and in black ink, on dull-finished white paper with adequate

Orcilia Forbes: The role and functions of the school nurse as perceived by 115 public school teachers from three selected counties. *J. School Health* 37 February, 1967):101-106.

[7]Glare, brightness, and multiple seating arrangements will be discussed in Chapter 9.

spacing between words and lines and with generous margins. The teacher should be aware of the size of type on printed pages and choose the size of type to suit the pupil's needs. Eye injuries should be prevented by promoting safety skills in different teaching environments and activities. Emergency care procedures (Chapter 7) for eye injuries should be known to all school personnel.

The teacher's own eye health should be of vital concern, and there should be regular examinations by an ophthalmologist. Pupils soon become aware of the teacher who does or does not promote eye health. The teacher's actions in reading, writing on the chalkboard, playing a game, or giving a demonstration can reveal the teacher's own visual difficulties to pupils.

Daily activities can be modified so that the student with visual difficulties can remain a member of the class and have a sense of belonging. Targets used in accuracy tests can be made bigger. Printing or writing on the chalkboard by the teacher can be larger and more legible. The pupil should be allowed to change his seat so that he can see better. Discussion periods should alternate with reading sessions. Small objects on the floor should be picked up so that the pupil does not stumble over them. These are some of the ways in which the daily activities can be modified.

Elementary teachers and school health educators can include, among the units of direct health instruction, "care of the eyes" and "prevention of diseases and injuries to the eyes." An outline of the subject matter of these topics is found in Chapter 14. Since 30 out of every 100 pupils in elementary and secondary schools have poor vision, we certainly need to stress the care of the eyes, prevention of eye injuries and diseases, and understanding of early detection of eye defects.

## HEARING DIFFICULTIES AND ADDITIONAL WAYS TO ASSIST THE PUPIL

The teacher should be acquainted with the ways to control unnecessary classroom noise as well as the use of acoustical materials in the structure of the classroom. Seating arrangements can often assist the pupil with a hearing difficulty. If the pupil is placed so that the ear with better hearing acuity is toward the teacher, he has a better chance to hear the teacher's statements.

Loss of the teacher's hearing is not unusual. When the teacher often asks pupils to repeat what they said or repeatedly answers pupils' questions incorrectly, the pupils become aware of the teacher's loss of hearing. As the hearing loss progresses, the teacher may speak louder or fail to locate the source of sound. Teachers should be aware that their failure to recognize loss of their own hearing does *not* assist the pupil with a hearing difficulty.

Teachers can assist the pupil with a hearing difficulty throughout the school day by:

1. Being certain the pupil can see the teacher's lips when speaking.
2. Standing so that sunlight does not shine into the pupil's eyes and thus prevent him from watching the teacher's lips.
3. Keeping hands and pencils away from the face when speaking.
4. Standing still when speaking.
5. Repeating key words and assignments.
6. Speaking clearly without exaggerations.
7. Avoiding gestures.
8. Using a key vocabulary on the chalkboard when new subject matter is presented.
9. Encouraging the pupil to read ahead of his classmates.
10. Assigning a "big brother" to him.
11. Being certain that the pupil is looking at the teacher when the teacher speaks to the pupil.
12. Using homonyms like *meat* and *meet* in sentences to indicate which word is meant.
13. Having the attention of all classmates when the student is giving an oral report.
14. Encouraging older students to discover units to be studied *next*.
15. Encouraging students to understand pronunciation marks.

Elementary teachers and school health educators can include, in direct health instruction, "the care of the ears" and "the prevention of diseases and injuries to the ears." Such topics as "infections of the middle ear," "hearing aids," "screening hearing," and other health problems related to loss of hearing can be included within units of direct health instruction specifically concerned with the ears.

## EMOTIONAL HEALTH PROBLEMS AND ADDITIONAL WAYS TO ASSIST THE PUPIL

Of all health problems, emotional health problems are probably the least understood and accepted. No parent or pupil delights in being told of emotional health problems. Thus the teacher should be aware of the counseling services offered by the school system *before* informing the parent or pupil of the observed signs of emotional health problems. The counseling services can confirm the observed signs of emotional health problems and work with the teachers during assistance to the pupil. Most school systems will have established procedures for counselor-pupil conferences and psychological testing by counselors, as well as for exchange of pupil information among counselors, physicians, and teachers. Approved community child guidance clinics might be used, depending on the school system's referral system.

Teachers have obligations to evaluate their emotional health and its effect on pupils. Most teachers are aware that their emotional stability influences the pupil's mental health. A teacher with a clear understanding of his capacities can have a stabilizing effect on pupils. If the teacher shows evidence of self-confidence, pupils develop a sense of security. The teacher free from personal problems and pressures feels more secure. The teacher's sense of humor, courtesy, tact, kindness, patience, understanding, and honesty reveal some of the characteristics of emotional stability. Other characteristics include:

1. Accepting responsibilities.
2. Striving to do the best job one is capable of doing and gaining satisfaction from it.
3. Having self-respect.
4. Planning ahead and not fearing the future.
5. Setting realistic goals.
6. Accepting disappointments and shortcomings.
7. Doing one's own thinking and making one's own decisions.
8. Having personal relations that are lasting and satisfying.
9. Not permitting emotions such as guilt, worry, fear, anger, love, or jealousy to take precedence over teaching.
10. Being a part of a group.

In direct health instruction there are many units within the area of mental health. Some of these units are "getting along with others," "learning to understand oneself and others," "gaining self-confidence," "being honest," and "accepting tolerance." Thus the teacher not only promotes mental health during relations with pupils but also includes mental health units in direct instruction.

## NUTRITIONAL DEFICIENCIES AND ADDITIONAL WAYS TO ASSIST THE PUPIL

A recent national nutritional survey involving ten states revealed the extent of nutritional deficiencies among people in the lowest quarter of the four income groups. In the dietary assessment, there was a large number of persons, ten to 16 years old, who consumed 50% (or less) of the amounts of iron, vitamin A, vitamin C, and calories considered adequate. Over 60% of the young children had a low intake of iron. Among adolescents, almost 40% consumed less than half the desired amount of vitamin A. Biochemical measurements revealed that 16% of the persons studied had serum protein levels that were less than acceptable, 17% had unacceptable levels of serum albumin, and 9 to 19% had unacceptable levels of riboflavin and thiamine.[8]

The supervision, preparation, and serving of the school lunch will be discussed in Chapter 10. School personnel should encourage students to fulfill the following responsibilities:

1. Students should develop sound dietary habits and table etiquette.
2. They should maintain a quiet and clean lunchroom or cafeteria.
3. They should keep plate scrapings to a minimum.
4. They should only occasionally include candy and sweetened soft drinks in their noonday meal.

[8]Arnold E. Schaefer: Malnutrition in the U.S.A.? *Nutrition News 32* (December, 1969):1,4.

5. They should actively participate in school lunch committees.
6. They should hold campaigns to reduce food waste in the lunchroom or cafeteria.
7. They should try new foods on school menus and have an eagerness to eat their lunch in the cafeteria or lunchroom.
8. They should observe the rules of desirable social behavior.

Daily practice of two health habits should accompany the snack period and the noonday school meal. One of these habits is hand washing before entering and after leaving the cafeteria or lunchroom. Most elementary schools provide hand washing facilities at the entrance to the lunchroom, but hand washing facilities may not be available in every secondary school. The other health habit is tooth brushing. The toothbrush can be carried to the lunchroom or cafeteria, and when the pupil leaves, he can wash his hands, brush his teeth, and carry the toothbrush back to his classroom. In elementary schools having self-contained classrooms with boys' and girls' toilet rooms, children can use these toilet rooms for hand washing and tooth brushing. These toilet rooms are provided with sinks and have shelves on which toothbrushes can be placed or from which the brushes can be hung. Health instruction becomes meaningful when hand washing and tooth brushing accompany snacks and noonday meals.

Many units, from the area of nutrition, can be used in direct health instruction. Some of these units are "the essential four food groups," "carbohydrates," "proteins," "vitamins," "mineral elements," "obesity," "underweight," "influences on our dietary habits," "food fads and fallacies," "misuse of stimulants," "milk," and "food allergies." These and other units from the area of nutrition are found in Chapter 14.

## POSTURE CONDITIONS AND ADDITIONAL WAYS TO ASSIST THE PUPIL

Teachers should be aware of the relation of light and seating to posture and body mechanics. Desk-chair combinations can be adjusted to the pupil's body build. Students can become familiar with the adjustments for desk-chair combinations. Different varieties of classroom furniture can be used. Classroom activities can be alternated to eliminate long periods of sitting. Desk tops with glossy finishes should be avoided. In schools where students change rooms and seats throughout the day or in classrooms where traditional furniture is used, students should be aware of the different sizes of seats and the different heights of desks in each room. In classrooms having tablet-arm chairs, a few left-handed tablet-arm chairs should be provided. Additional information concerning school furniture will be presented in Chapter 9.

Students are influenced by the teacher's posture when standing, walking, and sitting. If he has reasonably acceptable posture, students follow his example. In fact, the control of the class may be dependent on his posture. If the teacher is observed to slump, carry one shoulder higher than the other, incline the head forward, stand with the weight on one foot, or point the toes outward, students are quick to notice.

Depending on the pupils' health needs and the age level, many lessons can be included in a posture unit. Some of the lessons teach proper walking posture, sitting posture, standing posture, deviations of bone growth because of poor posture, kyphosis, lordosis, structural and functional scoliosis, and the relation of seating and light to posture.

## COMMUNICABLE DISEASES AND ADDITIONAL WAYS TO ASSIST THE PUPIL

The teacher should be acquainted with procedures for isolation and the exclusion of pupils with communicable diseases. These procedures will be discussed in Chapter 4. At the same time, the teacher should be familiar with pupil readmission procedures following the pupil's recovery from communicable diseases (Chapter 4).

Proper sanitation in the school's facilities is a prime factor in controlling diseases. Disinfectants should be used in cleaning to destroy pathogenic bacteria. Urinals, toilets, washbasins, floors of toilet rooms, shower and locker rooms, lunchrooms, and health service units need disinfectants. The water supply should be purified so that water-borne diseases such as typhoid fever, enteritis, and amebic dysentery are prevented. Sewage, waste, and garbage dis posal systems should be adequate. When there is poor sewage treatment, the following sewage-borne diseases may occur: typhoid fever, amebic dysentery, and infectious hepatitis. When there is inadequate disposal of waste and garbage, breeding places multiply for insects, rodents and other animals. Sanitary procedures are needed in classrooms, corridors, and teaching laboratories as well as at all drinking fountains.

A teacher should have sick leave so that he will not spread any communicable disease he has to pupils and other school personnel. Sick leave provides the teacher with a length of time when he may be absent from his job because of a communicable disease, with partial or no loss in salary. Usually, on return to the school, the teacher is asked to submit a physician's certificate indicating he has fully recovered.

There are many units within the area of the prevention of diseases that can be presented in direct health instruction. These units can be used to instruct students about common diseases, such as colds, streptococcal infections, tuberculosis, rheumatic fever, rubella and rubeola, mumps and scarlet fever, poliomyelitis, chicken pox and whooping cough, tetanus, influenza and pneumonia, infectious mononucleosis, and typhoid fever. In the secondary school, a unit on venereal diseases must be included because of the incidence of venereal diseases among young persons. Among the units should be "the causative agents of communicable diseases and their transmission," and "the immunization procedures protecting the individual." In addition, units dealing with skin infections, such as ringworm, impetigo, and boils, should not be omitted from units on the prevention and control of diseases. Infections of the eyes, such as conjunctivitis and sties, should not be overlooked.

## References for Further Study

American Nurses' Association: *Functions and Qualifications for School Nurses.* New York: The Association, 1966.

Anderson, C. L.: *School Health Practice.* 5th ed. St. Louis: The C. V. Mosby Company, 1972.

Byrd, O.: *School Health Administration.* Philadelphia: W. B. Saunders Company, 1964.

*Conference Report on the Educational Preparation of the Nurse for School Health Work.* New York: Teachers College, Columbia University, 1967.

Joint Committee on Health Problems in Education of the National Education Association and the American Medical Association: *Health Appraisal of School Children.* 4th ed. Washington, D.C.: National Education Association, 1969.

———— : *Suggested School Health Policies.* 4th ed. Chicago: American Medical Association, 1966.

Mayshark, C., and Shaw, D. D.: *Administration of School Health Programs.* St. Louis: The C. V. Mosby Company, 1967.

Oberteuffer, D., Harrelson, O., and Pollock, M.: *School Health Education.* 5th ed. New York: Harper & Row, 1972.

Turner, C. E., Randall, H., and Smith, S. L.: *School Health and Health Education.* 6th ed. St. Louis: The C. V. Mosby Company, 1970.

# Chapter 4

## *PREVENTION AND CONTROL OF DISEASES*

### AN INCIDENT

A kindergarten teacher has sent home numerous children with colds, sore throats, and chicken pox. A fourth-grade teacher has many children absent with measles, whooping cough, and mumps. A junior high or middle school teacher has students absent because of infectious hepatitis, rheumatic fever, and infectious mononucleosis. A high school teacher of health education has received reports of gonorrhea and syphilis among the students while others are absent because of influenza. Previously, these teachers asked their principals about exclusion and readmission procedures.

### EXCLUSION OF THE PUPIL WITH COMMUNICABLE DISEASE

A school's exclusion procedures can succeed if school personnel and parents understand the purposes of the procedures. Exclusion of the pupil ill with a communicable disease protects other pupils and school personnel from contagion and hastens the recovery of the excluded pupil. Schools that stress perfect attendance at the cost of the pupil's health will not be able to carry out these purposes. The pupil with a severe "strep throat" who remains in school spreads streptococci to other children and school personnel. When he is at home in bed, his body has a chance to fight the infection, and he does not transmit the streptococci to others.

School personnel should follow standard procedures regarding the exclusion of pupils with such communicable diseases as measles, colds, impetigo, conjunctivitis, pediculosis, ringworm, and other infectious diseases. When the signs of a possible communicable disease are observed by a teacher, the pupil should be separated from his classmates immediately and sent to the school nurse. When there is no school nurse, the pupil should be sent to the school principal for permission to be excluded from the class. The parents must be notified, the pupil sent home, and the parents encouraged to seek medical attention. In secondary schools, the student is excused from school. The teenager, however, should be encouraged to feel that it is his responsibility to seek medical attention for himself. The practice of isolation and exclusion of sick pupils should be carried out consistently by all school personnel.

The ill pupil should never leave school alone or arrive at an empty home. Usually a parent comes to the school and takes the pupil home. When the parents cannot be reached, the health record of the pupil should be consulted for the names and telephone numbers of relatives or the family physician. If this information is not given on the health record, a cooperating local physician might be called. In severe emergencies, local hospitals can be used in accordance with the procedures for emergency care. The importance of notification of parents, of the pupil's safe transportation to his home, and the encouragement to seek medical attention cannot be over emphasized. In her follow-through, the nurse will check whether the parents did obtain medical care for the excluded pupil.

The personnel of local school health services should submit to the local board of education written policies and procedures for the exclusion of the pupil with communicable diseases. The policies and procedures should include provisions for the pupil to be legally excused from school

46

when he shows signs of a communicable disease during the school day. The written policies and procedures should include provision for notification of parents by health services' personnel or by teachers, medical care, pupil transportation, follow-through, American Red Cross First Aid or hospitalization in emergencies, and record of the care given to the pupil by school personnel.

Parents should realize the necessity for cooperating with the school's exclusion procedures. Health bulletins, PTA programs, and community-wide health action can inform parents about exclusion procedures. The pupil excluded from school because of illness should be isolated from other children and remain at home under medical care. Too often he is allowed to play with the neighborhood children or returns to school for the afternoon session.

Known cases of communicable diseases among pupils should be reported to the local health department. Little can be done to prevent the spread of disease within a community when the health department has not been informed about ill students excluded from the schools. The reporting to the health department can be done by the school nurse or principal immediately following teacher observation of possible signs of communicable diseases. Other members of the pupil's family are usually scrutinized for signs of the disease by public health nurses. When brothers and sisters of the excluded pupil are in other school buildings, school nurses cooperate with the local health officials in reporting signs of communicable diseases among these other members of the family. The local health department should continuously inform school administrative officials and school nurses of reported cases of communicable diseases within the community. In this way, school personnel can keep close observation upon students from stricken community areas.

The control of communicable diseases is joint project of the schools and the local health department. The effectiveness of the project depends on the consistency of early recognition of signs of communicable diseases, exclusion of pupils with communicable diseases, notification of the parents, parents' willingness to seek medical care, and notification of the local health depart-

ment. Surveys show that many local boards of education have not developed adequate policies and procedures for the exclusion of pupils with communicable diseases.

## READMISSION OF THE PUPIL RECOVERED FROM A COMMUNICABLE DISEASE

School readmission procedures should adhere to regulations established by public health officials and state and local health laws and ordinances. To readmit a pupil into the school during the period when he should be excluded would be flagrant disregard for pupil health.

The family physician will indicate when the pupil ill with a communicable disease can return to school. A certificate bearing the physician's signature might be used to indicate that the pupil has fully recovered from the disease. If pupils have no family physician, a certificate signed by a physician of the local or county health department might serve the same purpose. If possible, the physician who treated the pupil during the illness should be the one to determine when the pupil is fully recovered from the disease and can return to school.

In addition to the physician's certificate, some schools require that the returning pupil report to the school nurse. The nurse checks the pupil's temperature, observes his appearance and behavior, and is alert for any sign indicative of a recurrence of the disease. These procedures can be completed in the school's health service unit.

## CAUSATIVE AGENTS OF DISEASES

Communicable diseases have specific causative agents, which are minute microorganisms. In most instances, each disease has a specific agent, enabling the physician to identify and destroy the causative agent and thus to treat the person who is ill with the disease. These causative agents are classified as bacteria, viruses, protozoa, helminths, fungi, and rickettsiae.

*Bacteria* are one-celled organisms and can be *pathogenic* or *disease-producing*. Bacteria may be of three shapes. Rod-shaped bacteria are called *bacilli*. Round or spherical-shaped bacteria are *cocci*. Diseases such as streptococcal sore throat, pneumonia, gonorrhea, and boils related to staphylococci are caused by cocci. The coiled variety of bacteria are *spirilla*. Bacteria live on, between, and around human cells. Bacteria harm man when they produce poisonous substances called toxins. There are two groups of toxins: (1) endotoxins which are held inside the bacterial cells and are released after the death of the bacterial cells; and (2) exotoxins which wander out of the bacterial cells into surrounding human tissues. Within these two groups, toxins of some bacteria have a localized effect—killing and dissolving human cells near the site of the bacterial infection. Toxins of other bacteria are produced at one place within the human body, are carried by the blood to another part of the human body, and act upon cells in that distant part of the human body.

*Viruses* come in many shapes: rods, filaments, spheres, hexagons, and "tails." A virus is a core of nucleic acid, either ribonucleic acid (RNA) or deoxyribonucleic acid (DNA), wrapped in protein. Viruses must penetrate human body cells since they must live and reproduce within the living cell. The protein overcoat tries to find a site on a human cell wall which the virus can penetrate. The protein overcoat remains outside the living cell. When the nucleic acids penetrate the cell, changes occur in the cell, bringing about viral infections. Some of the diseases caused by viruses are colds, chicken pox, German measles, influenza, and mumps.

*Protozoa* are one-celled organisms and vary in size. Some are as small as the most minute bacterium, whereas others exceed the largest bacterium by many times. Only a few protozoa cause infectious diseases. Three diseases occurring in man which are caused by protozoa are malaria, African sleeping sickness, and amebic dysentery.

*Helminths* include many-celled animals of higher organization, such as flukes, hookworms, trichinae, tapeworms, lice and itch mites. The *flukes* include hair, lung, gastrointestinal, and blood flukes.

*Hookworms* live in the small intestine and can cause anemia and retarded mental and physical development. The hookworm pierces the human skin usually between the toes and finds its way to the lymphatics, circulatory system, respiratory tract, and small intestine. Hookworm disease is an international disease prevalent where there is inadequate sewage treatment and water purification.

*Trichinae*, causing trichinosis, are found in the meat of infected swine. These small roundworms are acquired when man eats infested pork not cooked sufficiently to kill the trichinae. Medical diagnosis of trichinosis is difficult. Often the larvae of the trichinae reach the circulatory system and heart before medical diagnosis of trichinosis has been made.

*Tapeworms* in man can be caused by the adult beef tapeworm or by larvae of pork tapeworms. Both beef and pork tapeworms are acquired by man when he eats raw or partially cooked beef or pork that is infested. In beef tapeworm disease, the flesh of infested beef contains larvae of the tapeworms. Specific treatment is available. In pork tapeworm disease, the eggs of the pork tapeworm are swallowed by man when eating raw or slightly cooked pork. The eggs hatch in the small intestine. The larvae develop in tissues beneath the skin, striated muscles, and other regions of the body. Persons having pork tapeworm disease need immediate medical care. There is no specific treatment.

*Head lice* are often found in children. The eggs or nits are firmly attached to the hair, near the scalp. Head lice are spread by personal contact, brushes, and hats. If the body louse bites a person with a rickettsial disease such as typhus and feeds on his blood, it will acquire the rickettsiae, the disease-causing agent, of typhus fever. The rickettsiae can then be passed to another person in three ways: the body louse may be crushed into the wound made by its bite; it may be crushed into a skin abrasion; or fecal material of the body louse may be rubbed into the wound that it caused by its bites.

*Itch mites* burrow under the superficial layer of the skin. They lay their eggs in the burrows and produce intense itching. The burrows become filled with dirt and create fine lines or black trails on the inner side of fingers and thighs, or wrists and back of hands, at armpits, and upon the abdomen. Scabies is highly contagious and spreads by actual contact or infected clothing.

*Pathogenic fungi*, which attack man, are microscopic. Athlete's foot and ringworm of the scalp are two common fungal infections. Ringworm of the foot (tinea pedis) appears as a lesion with a vesicle or veicles on the soles of the feet and between the toes; ringworm of the body (tinea corporis) appears on the hands and other parts of the human body other than the scalp. The lesion is ring-shaped, irregular, and reddish, and spreads from red edges while healing in center. All ages are susceptible, and males acquire the infection more often than females.[1] Sterilization of towels and general cleanliness in showers, dressing rooms, and floors can reduce the spread of the fungi. Ringworm can be prevented by thorough washing and drying of the skin. When the lesions become infected, the family physician should be consulted.

*Rickettsiae* are barely visible under the microscope and range in size between bacteria and viruses. They are transmitted by lice, fleas, and ticks. Two diseases caused by rickettsiae are typhus and Rocky Mountain spotted fever.

## IMMUNIZATION AS A MEANS OF PROTECTION

Twenty-eight states, the District of Columbia, Puerto Rico, and the Virgin Islands require immunizations for specific diseases before entry to school. The diseases for which immunization is most often required are smallpox, measles, poliomyelitis, diphtheria, pertussis, and tetanus. Penalties for noncompliance are not stated in the statutes. In October 1970, the Center for Disease Control indicated that 22 states had no mandatory school entry immunization requirements (Table 1).[2]

Immunization raises the human body's resistance to the effects of the causative agents of diseases as these agents enter the body. When bacteria enter the human body, poisons from these bacteria, called "toxins," create unusual disturbances in the body tissues. To combat the disturbances, antibodies are formed.

Antibodies may dissolve, neutralize, or take the toxin out of solution; clump the toxin together; or ingest the toxin. Antibodies are assisted by antibiotics, such as streptomycin or penicillin, which inhibit the multiplication of or kill pathogenic bacteria. It is possible for a person to have antibodies for a specific infectious disease after recovery from the acute disease or through the injection of an antigen stimulating the formation of antibodies for the specific disease.

Immunization affords protection against the results of infectious diseases within the human body. Each infectious disease creates damage to internal structures. The visual acuity of a child may be affected. Internal organs such as the kidneys may not perform their tasks as efficiently as before the disease struck. Thus immunization protects the person from the effects of infectious disease.

There are two kinds of immunity: natural and acquired. *Natural* immunity may result from the inheritance of specific antibodies to a particular disease. *Acquired* immunity is of two types: active and passive. *Active* acquired immunity results when the individual manufactures specific antibodies for a particular infectious disease by either (1) having an attack of the disease or (2) having an injection of an antigen stimulating the formation of antibodies for the specific disease. The antigen may be dead or weakened microorganisms or minute amounts of their toxins. *Passive* acquired immunity is used when the human body is not able to manufacture specific antibodies for a particular infectious disease. Then the specific antibodies are produced elsewhere and injected into the person. The specific antibodies may be found in the liquid part of a person's blood or in a constituent of the blood—gamma globulin. In some cases, the specific antibodies are produced by an animal that has received injections of the microorganisms or their toxins. The animal produces specific antibodies that are removed from its blood, concentrated, and standardized before injection into the person. Passive immunity lasts a relatively short time. It is given when a person is ill with a particular disease or needs immediate protection, such as when susceptible infants are exposed to a disease.

A booster dose works on the immunological principle that once bodily mechanisms producing antibodies have been stimulated by an immunizing agent, the

American Public Health Association: *Control of Communicable Diseases in Man.* 11th ed. New York: The Association, 1970, p. 68.
Charles L. Jackson: State laws on compulsory immunization in the United States. *Public Health Reports 84* (September, 1969):787; and United States Public Health Service, Center for Disease Control: Current trends in immunization requirements prior to school entry. *Morbidity and Mortality Weekly Report 19* (October 10, 1970):398-399.

## Table 1
### Immunization Requirements Prior to School Entry
### October 1970

| State | Is there a state law requiring immunization for a specific disease or diseases prior to school entry? | Diphtheria Immunization Required | Measles Immunization Required | Pertussis Immunization Required | Polio Immunization Required | Rubella Immunization Required | Smallpox Immunization Required | Tetanus Immunization Required | Dept. of Health | Dept. of Educ. | Have regulations been issued? | If yes, is compliance required? | Health | Education | If no state law at present, are there plans pending for proposing such a law? |
|---|---|---|---|---|---|---|---|---|---|---|---|---|---|---|---|
| Alabama | No | | | | | | | | | | | | | | No |
| Alaska | No | | | | | | | | | | | | | | No |
| Arizona | No | | | | | | | | | | | | | | Yes |
| Arkansas | Yes | Yes | Yes | Yes | Yes | | Yes | Yes | | X | Yes | Yes | | X | |
| California | Yes | | Yes | | Yes | | | | X | | Yes | Yes | | | |
| Colorado | No | | | | | | | | | | | | | | |
| Connecticut | Yes | | Yes | | Yes | | | Yes | | | | | | X | |
| Delaware | No | | | | | | | | | | | | | | No |
| District of Columbia | Yes | | | | | | Yes | | X | | Yes | | | | |
| Florida | No | | | | | | | | | | | | | X | No |
| Georgia | Yes | Yes | Yes | Yes | Yes | | Yes | Yes | X | | Yes | Yes | | | |
| Hawaii | Yes | Yes | Yes | Yes | Yes | Yes | Yes | Yes | X | | Yes | Yes | | | |
| Idaho | No | | | | | | | | | | | | | | No |
| Illinois | Yes | Yes | Yes | Yes | Yes | Yes | Yes | Yes | X | X | Yes | Yes | | | |
| Indiana | No | | | | | | | | | | | | | X | No |
| Iowa | No | | | | | | | | | | | | | | Yes |
| Kansas | Yes | Yes | Yes | Yes | Yes | Yes | Yes | Yes | X | | Yes | Yes | | X | |
| Kentucky | Yes | Yes | Yes | | Yes | Yes | Yes | Yes | X | | Yes | Yes | | | |
| Louisiana | Yes | Yes | Yes | Yes | Yes | | Yes | Yes | | | | | | | |
| Maine | No | | | | | | | | | | | | | | No |
| Maryland | Yes | | | | | | Yes | Yes | X | | Yes | Yes | X | X | |
| Massachusetts | Yes | Yes | Yes | Yes | Yes | | Yes | Yes | X | | Yes | Yes | | | |
| Michigan | Yes | Yes | Yes | Yes | Yes | Yes | Yes | Yes | X | | Yes | Yes | | | |
| Minnesota | Yes | | Yes | | | | | | X | X | Yes | Yes | | X | |
| Mississippi | Yes | Yes | Yes | Yes | Yes | | Yes | Yes | X | X | Yes | Yes | | X | |
| Missouri | Yes | Yes | | | Yes | | | Yes | X | | Yes | Yes | | | |
| Montana | No | | | | | | | | X | | No | | | X | Yes |
| Nebraska | No | | | | | | | | | | | | | X | No |
| Nevada | No | | | | | | | | | | | | | | No |
| New Hampshire | Yes | | | | | | Yes | | X | | No | | | | |
| New Jersey | Yes | Yes | Yes | | Yes | | Yes | | | | | | | X | |
| New Mexico | Yes | Yes | | Yes | Yes | | Yes | Yes | X | X | Yes | Yes | | | |
| New York | Yes | | Yes | | Yes | Yes | Yes | | X | | Yes | Yes | | | |
| North Carolina | Yes | Yes | | Yes | Yes | | Yes | Yes | X | | No | | X | | |
| North Dakota | No | | | | | | | | | | | | | | No |
| Ohio | Yes | Yes | Yes | Yes | Yes | Yes | Yes | Yes | X | X | Yes | Yes | | | |
| Oklahoma | Yes | Yes | Yes | Yes | Yes | Yes | | Yes | X | | Yes | | | | |
| Oregon | No | | | | | | | | | | | | | X | Yes |
| Pennsylvania | Yes | | | | | | Yes | | X | | Yes | Yes | | | |
| Rhode Island | Yes | Yes | Yes | Yes | Yes | Yes | Yes | Yes | | X | | | X | X | |
| South Carolina | Yes | | | | | | Yes | | X | | Yes | Yes | X | | |
| South Dakota | No | | | | | | | | | | | | | | No |
| Tennessee | Yes | Yes | Yes | Yes | Yes | Yes | Yes | Yes | X | | Yes | Yes | | | |
| Texas | No | | | | | | | | | | | | | X | No |
| Utah | No | | | | | | | | | | | | | | No |
| Vermont | No | | | | | | | | | | | | | | No |
| Virginia | Yes | | | | | | Yes | | | X | Yes | Yes | | X | |
| Washington | No | | | | | | | | | | | | | | No |
| West Virginia | Yes | Yes | Yes | Yes | Yes | Yes | Yes | Yes | X | | Yes | Yes | | | |
| Wisconsin | No | | | | | | | | | | | | | | No |
| Wyoming | No | | | | | | | | | | | | | | No |
| Puerto Rico | Yes | | | | | | Yes | | X | | Yes | Yes | | | |
| Virgin Islands | Yes | | Yes | | | | | | | X | Yes | | | | Yes |
| Total | 31 Yes / 22 No | 19 | 21 | 16 | 22 | 11 | 27 | 17 | Health: 20 / Education: 4 / Combined: 5 | | 25 Yes / 3 No | 22 Yes | Health: 2 / Education: 13 / Combined: 2 | | 5 Yes |

Source of Information: Immunization Projects, Immunization Branch, State and Community Services Division, Center for Disease Control, Atlanta, Georgia.

Note: Effective September, 1971, Texas required polio, diphtheria or tetanus, measles, rubella, and smallpox immunizations.

mechanisms become sensitized and react to a second or third injection of the immunizing agent. Each time these mechanisms manufacture a vigorous output of antibodies depending on the peculiarities of the disease. The booster dose may stimulate enough antibodies so that the disease cannot do any damage in the human body. The booster dose may work well, fairly well, or not at all.

Detection procedures indicate the person's susceptibility to a particular disease. The Schick, Dick, and tuberculin tests are examples of detection procedures. The Schick test is used to indicate whether a person is susceptible to diphtheria. The Dick test is used to discover whether the individual is susceptible to scarlet fever. The results of tuberculin tests reveal whether the tubercle bacilli have entered the human body.

## SOME COMMON DISEASES

For sixteen common diseases, the causes, occurrence, methods of transmission, incubation period, signs, susceptibility, and methods of control will be discussed. First, however, certain terms need to be defined:

*Carrier*—A person who harbors the causative agent of a specific disease, usually without the outward signs of the disease, and is a source of infection. A healthy carrier may be in the incubation period, convalescence, or postconvalescence.

*Chemotherapy*—Use of chemical agents to cure or limit the progress of a disease.

*Chemoprophylaxis*—Use of chemical agents, including antibiotics, to prevent the development of a disease.

*Disinfection*—Chemical or physical means to kill infective agents outside of the human body.

*Concurrent disinfection*—Measures taken during the course of a disease to dispose of or destroy all infectious secretions from the body of the ill person, particularly articles soiled with the secretions.

*Terminal disinfection*—Measures taken after the infected person has died, is taken to a hospital, is no longer a source of infection, or has had isolation discontinued.

*Incubation period*—The interval of time between exposure to the causative agent of the disease and the appearance of the first sign of the disease.

*Isolation*—During the period of communicability, the separation of the infected person from others so that the causative agent of the disease will not be spread to other persons.

*Quarantine*—Four types of quarantine may be enforced. *Complete quarantine* limits the freedom of movement of well persons who have been exposed to a communicable disease for a period not longer than the longest incubation period of the disease. *Modified quarantine* is a partial limitation of freedom of movement, such as exclusion of children from school. *Personal surveillance* is the close supervision of persons who have been exposed to a disease in order to facilitate immediate recognition of the signs of the disease. *Segregation* is the separation of a group of persons from other persons to assist in the control of a communicable disease. An example would be the removal of susceptible children from their homes to the homes of persons having immunity to the disease.[3]

*Vaccine*—Dead or weakened bacteria or viruses introduced into the body to stimulate the production of antibodies.

### Chicken Pox

Chicken pox is a universal disease reported among 75% of persons under 15 years of age and living in metropolitan communities. The virus is spread by droplets from the nose and throat and by articles freshly soiled by discharges from the skin and mucous membranes of infected persons. The average incubation period is from 13 to 17 days. Some of the signs are slight fever, mild constitutional symptoms, succession of skin eruptions leaving a granular scab, skin eruptions more abundant on covered parts of the body, and shedding of scabs. Chicken pox is more severe in adults than in children. There is no quarantine or specific treatment. Isolation includes exclusion from school for one week after first skin eruptions. Concurrent disinfection by proper disposal and thorough cleaning of articles soiled by nose and throat discharges and fluids of skin eruptions should be practiced.

### Common Cold

Many of our communicable diseases begin with the signs of a common cold.

[3]American Public Health Association: *op. cit.*, p. 288.

Having a worldwide distribution, colds are caused by 55 or more known viruses and some unknown viruses.

Discharges from the nose and throat of a person with a cold are the sources of infection. When an infected person coughs or sneezes, he sprays into the air thousands of tiny droplets. The droplets may be carried a distance of at least three feet. This is *droplet infection* or droplet spread. Not only are the viruses of colds spread by droplet infection but also indirectly by articles contaminated by discharges from the nose and throat of the infected person.

The incubation period is between 12 and 72 hours, usually about 24 hours. Everyone is apparently susceptible to the viruses of common colds. Many persons have two to six colds yearly.

Signs of the cold are easily observed, such as "stuffiness" in the nose, soreness and "scratchiness" in the nose and throat, coughing, sneezing and sniffling, "runny nose" and discharges from the nose, watery eyes, tickling in the throat, and sometimes a slight fever or a mild headache. Complications from colds are rare, but they can trigger acute sinusitis, middle ear infections, and other respiratory infections.

Several methods of control can be employed to protect the individual from becoming infected with the cold viruses. Infected people who are coughing, sneezing, and blowing their noses should be avoided as much as possible. Following simple hygienic measures such as (1) washing hands with soap and water before eating or handling food; (2) not using towels, eating and drinking utensils, and toilet articles used by other persons; and (3) having sufficient sleep, rest, and proper diet can assist in reducing the possibility of a common cold.

For the person infected with a cold, simple health practices should be followed. These practices include:

Going to bed at the first signs of the cold

Keeping warm and dry, avoiding undue exposure

Eating light meals of nourishing foods

Drinking larger quantities of fluids than usual

Covering the nose when sneezing and the mouth when coughing and properly disposing of paper handkerchiefs

Blowing the nose carefully

Washing eating and drinking utensils thoroughly

Consulting the family physician if the cold persists for more than a week

There is no effective prevention for common colds. Research in vaccine development is underway, but no vaccine is available.

## Infectious Hepatitis

Viral hepatitis includes both infectious hepatitis and serum hepatitis. Infectious hepatitis is caused by a virus which is spread by a person infected with the disease, person-to-person contact in a localized epidemic such as that in a school, or exposure to contaminated water, food, or raw shellfish. Serum hepatitis is spread by inoculation of blood or blood products exposed to contaminated syringes or needles.

The virus of infectious hepatitis may be found in feces and urine and is usually spread by the fecal-oral route in person-to-person contact. Contaminated waters and food such as sliced meats, salads, bakery products, raw or uncooked clams and oysters, and milk have been means of spreading the virus. The incubation period ranges from 10 to 50 days, commonly 30 to 35 days.

The onset of infectious hepatitis is usually abrupt with fever, discomfort, lack of appetite, nausea, and abdominal discomfort. Within a few days, jaundice (yellow appearance of the skin and the whites of the eyes caused by an excess of bile pigment in the blood) occurs. Everyone is susceptible, although a low incidence occurs among exposed infants and preschool children.

Infectious hepatitis may be a mild illness lasting one or two weeks or can be severely disabling lasting several months. There are no specific treatment and no vaccine for active immunization.

Every person should be considered a potential carrier of the hepatitis virus. Adequate water purification and continuous inspection of food, meat, and milk supplies assist in preventing the spread of the virus. Examination and regular checking of food handlers, sterilization of food receptacles, and good sanitary measures reduce the possibility of the spread of the virus. Serum hepatitis may be prevented by the use of disposable needles and syringes.

## Infectious Mononucleosis

This disease, commonly called "glandular fever" or "mono," occurs among children, college students, and hospital personnel, with it being widespread among children. The cause of infectious mononucleosis is unknown. It is believed that the disease is spread by direct contact, such as kissing, with an infected person. There is no means of prevention, and little is known concerning protection after the person has had the disease. Incubation period varies from two to six weeks.

Signs of infectious mononucleosis include a vague feeling of bodily discomfort, fever, sore throat, and a tired feeling. Fever is a constant sign except in the mildest cases. Half of the infected persons have sore throats. The lymph glands in the infected person's throat may or may not become enlarged. A pinkish red rash may appear on the trunk. In some persons, these signs are so mild that the disease is not recognized.

Infectious mononucleosis may continue for a long period of time. The infected person shows exhaustion, aching of legs, weakness, low blood pressure, low blood sugar, low-grade fever, and an increase in lymphocytes, as found in laboratory tests. The bases for the medical diagnosis are the persistent fever, sore throat, enlarged lymph glands, and increase in lymphocytes.

Most cases of infectious mononucleosis are mild. Future attacks are short-lived and not infrequent. There is no specific treatment. Plenty of fluids and bed rest help the infected person.[4]

## Influenza

Influenza occurs in periodic epidemics with the highest incidence among school children although all ages are susceptible. A self-limiting disease, the recovery period is two to seven days.

Viruses of similar biological properties cause influenza. However, the viruses are distinct and separate. They are spread by droplet infection or by articles soiled with discharges from the nose and throat of a person with influenza. The incubation period is usually 24 to 72 hours. Signs are chills, fever, headache, backache, malaise (vague feeling of bodily discomfort), loss of appetite, and muscular aching. Sore throat, nasal discharges, and cough are common. Laboratory tests confirm the presence of the influenza viruses.

Complications from influenza are reported when influenza becomes an epidemic in a community. Bacterial pneumonia is often reported. Isolation of the infected person will prevent the development of bacterial infections. Concurrent disinfection should be practiced. There is no quarantine and no specific treatment.

The most satisfactory means of preventing influenza is vaccination. The vaccination should be taken before influenza is reported within a community.[5]

## Mumps

Mumps is caused by a virus and occurs most often in children between the ages of five and fifteen years. Males acquire mumps more often than females. The virus is spread by droplet infection and by direct contact with the saliva of an infected person or indirectly through articles contaminated with the saliva of infected persons. The incubation period is from 12 to 26 days, commonly 18 days. Everyone is susceptible.

The salivary glands of the infected person are commonly involved in mumps. Signs of mumps include headache, loss of appetite, chills, and pain in the salivary glands. Swelling occurs in the parotid glands, the largest salivary glands, located just below the ears. Frequently, one parotid gland is affected first followed by involvement of the gland on the opposite side. When the swelling is great, the pain increases. The temperature varies between 100° and 104° F.

Complications from mumps are found among teenagers and adults. Orchitis (inflammation and swelling of the testicles) occurs in boys and men. The mammary gland, ovaries, and pancreas may be involved in females past puberty. Deafness has been known to follow mumps.[6]

From the onset of swelling, the patient should remain in isolation for nine days. Concurrent disinfection of articles soiled

Franklin H. Top: *Communicable and Infectious Diseases*. 6th ed. St. Louis: The C. V. Mosby Company, 1968, pp. 391-396.

[5]American Public Health Association, *op. cit.*, pp. 112-119.
[6]Top, *op. cit.*, pp. 397-405.

with secretions of the infected person's nose and throat should be undertaken. Quarantine is not necessary, and there is no specific treatment.

The live attenuated virus mumps vaccine is useful for children approaching puberty, for adolescents and adults who have not had mumps, and selected groups in the labor force who may be exposed to the virus. Males, particularly, should receive the vaccine.[7] In a study of nearly 3000 school children, the live attenuated virus mumps vaccine was proven to be 95.6% effective in protecting against mumps.[8]

## Pneumonia

Pneumococcal pneumonia is an acute bacterial infection of the lungs. It occurs most frequently among persons living in crowded conditions and during the winter and spring months. More cases of pneumococcal pneumonia are reported among men than women.

The cause of pneumococcal pneumonia is *Diplococcus pneumoniae*; these bacteria are spread by droplet infection, by direct oral contact with infected persons or carriers, or indirectly through articles contaminated with discharges from the nose and throat of infected persons. The incubation period is believed to be one to three days but is not well determined.

The signs of pneumonia are severe shaking chill, headache, aching, agonizing pain in the side, and dry cough. Breathing is more rapid than usual. Temperature may be 102° to 105°F. Pulse rate is elevated. Saliva is thick, scanty, and streaked with blood. There may be a loss of appetite, nausea, and vomiting. The skin is hot and dry. Fever may be 102°F for seven to ten days in untreated cases.

Complications from pneumococcal pneumonia can be expected in 15 to 20% of the infected persons. Recurrence of the disease is common. Pleurisy (inflammation of the membrane covering the lungs) is common with difficult or labored breathing and accumulation of fluid in the pleural space.

Susceptibility is widespread. Isolation is of dubious value, and there is no quarantine. Injection of penicillin is the usual treatment.

## Rheumatic Fever

Rheumatic fever can affect any region of the human body. The exact cause of rheumatic fever is not known, but it always follows a streptococcal infection, such as "strep throat," scarlet fever, or tonsillitis. Whether the cause of rheumatic fever lies within the streptococcus itself or in some unknown agent that the streptococcus carries with it is not known. A person who has had a streptococcal infection may develop rheumatic fever while another person will not.

The original signs of the streptococcal infection include a fever between 101° and 104°F, severe pain in swallowing, swollen glands below the jaw, pain when the throat is pressed under the angle of the jaw, headache, and possibly vomiting. Streptococci can infect anyone. A member of a family may be a carrier of the streptococci if sore throats repeatedly occur within a family. The family physician should obtain throat cultures and have the streptococci identified, by laboratory tests, so that the physician can follow the recommended treatment for streptococcal infections.

Rheumatic fever is not contagious and mimics other diseases. There is no test to determine susceptibility. A person is vulnerable to further attacks since no one becomes immune to rheumatic fever after one attack. Rheumatic fever results in inflammation of the heart, weakens the heart muscle, affects the valves of the heart, impairs the heart's pumping action, and enlarges the heart. Usually, the damage to the heart valves occurs on the left side of the heart. Often the heart valves are so affected that the valves cannot open and close as they should. Scar tissue forms in healing and may interfere with the opening or closing of the heart valves.

Swelling and tenderness of the joints are the sign from which rheumatic fever acquires its name. The knees, wrists, and elbows become hot, painful, and swollen. A high fever accompanies a pink rash on the skin. Painful hard lumps appear under the skin. Abdominal pains and nosebleeds may be present. *St. Vitus' dance* (or *chorea*) is a definite sign of rheumatic fever. St Vitus' dance consists of jerky, involuntary

[7]American Public Health Association, *op. cit.*, pp. 158-160.

[8]Live virus mumps vaccine tests 95 percent effective. *Public Health Reports 83* (March, 1968):208.

movements often seen in muscle twitching of the face and limbs.

Children and teenagers with active rheumatic fever are put to bed either at a hospital or at home. The bed rest may be a few weeks or a few months. The medical care is aimed at keeping the patient reasonably quiet in bed. There is no specific chemotherapy to cure rheumatic fever. Medications are prescribed to reduce the inflammation of the heart. When there is no heart inflammation, medications are given to reduce the signs of rheumatic fever.[9]

There is no isolation, concurrent disinfection, and quarantine. Persons who have had rheumatic fever should be placed on continuous chemoprophylaxis for long periods, possibly throughout life. Children receive the chemoprophylaxis until they are 18 years old and then five years beyond the last attack.[10]

*Rheumatic heart disease* is the result of scarring of the heart valves caused by rheumatic fever. During an attack of rheumatic fever, there may be mild or severe inflammation of the valves of the heart. The inflammation can lead to scar tissue, which leaves the valves roughened and sometimes deformed. When the valves do not open and close properly, the blood is kept from flowing into the chambers of the heart as it should. Scar tissue in the heart muscle may reduce the heart's strength. When a heart murmur develops during an attack of rheumatic fever, rheumatic heart disease may be present. A heart murmur can be described as a stream of blood rushing through a valve which has been scarred during the inflammation of the heart and valves.

Persons with rheumatic heart disease need additional chemoprophylactic measures before and following certain kinds of surgical and dental procedures, including tooth extractions.

## Rubella

Commonly known as "German measles," rubella is caused by the virus of rubella.

This disease occurs worldwide with extensive epidemics among children but also occurring among adolescents and adults. The virus is spread by droplet infection or direct contact with infected persons or indirectly with articles soiled with discharges from the nose and throat of the infected person and possibly from the blood, urine, or feces of the infected person. The incubation period is from 14 to 21 days.[11]

The signs of rubella include a rash that appears on the day when the person first becomes ill. The rash is first found on the face and neck and then on the arms and trunk. The rash is light pink to red in color and is characterized by spots which change size. In addition to the rash, there is a slight rise in body temperature.

Complications are not usually found in rubella, although women affected with rubella in the early months of pregnancy may have a miscarriage or give birth to a child with crippling defects. Arthritis is another common complication.[12]

The hemagglutination inhibition, or HI, test can confirm rubella infection even when there are no signs of rubella. Also, the HI test can detect immunity years after infection. The results of the HI test should be accepted only from laboratories which perform the HI tests regularly and have recognized competence.[13]

Isolation is practiced in the usual mild cases among children and adolescents. Concurrent disinfection and quarantine are not necessary, and there is no specific treatment.

A single dose of the live attenuated rubella virus vaccine can protect 90 to 95% of the persons susceptible against natural exposure. Children not having reached puberty and over one year of age are receiving the vaccine to ensure reduction of epidemics in the future.[14] A double-duty vaccine to give immunity to both rubella and mumps with a single injection has been approved for distribution by the federal government.

---

Ralph Bugg: Fighting the masked crippler: rheumatic fever. *Today's Health* 46 (March, 1968):36-40.
[9]American Public Health Association: *op. cit.*, pp. 203-205.

[11]*Ibid.*, pp. 210-213.
[12]Top, F.: *op. cit.*, pp. 506-511.
[13]United States Public Health Service: *Rubella* (#2041), 1970, p. 5.
[14]American Public Health Association, *op. cit.*, pp. 210-213.

## Rubeola

Many adults are not aware that rubeola is one of the most serious diseases occurring to children. Commonly known as the "red measles," the incidence of disease could be drastically reduced because of the availability of vaccines.

Rubeola is caused by the virus of measles which is spread by droplet infection and by articles freshly soiled by discharges from the nose and throat of the infected person. From exposure to the first sign of fever, the incubation period varies from eight to 13 days, and is usually about 10 days.[15]

Signs of rubeola include nasal discharges, sneezing, cough, fever, eye sensitivity to light, and a rash appearing on the second and third day. The rash begins on the face and neck, behind the ears, on the forehead, and later on the chest; it spreads rapidly over the body surface. The rash is a light pink color with small spots about the size of a pinhead. The spots increase in size and change color, followed by shedding and fading. A day or two before the rash, Koplik's spots (small, bluish-white spots surrounded by a bright red circle) appear on the mucous membranes inside the cheek and on the tongue.

One of commonest complications of rubeola is an inflammation of the middle ear. Other complications are inflammation of the brain, permanent deafness, blindness, and brain damage among children who are not vaccinated.[16]

To reduce the infected person's risk against other infections and to reduce the spread of the virus, isolation takes place from diagnosis until seven days after appearance of the rash. Concurrent disinfection should be practiced. Quarantine in large communities is impractical. There is no specific treatment.

Both a live attentuated (less virulent) virus vaccine and an inactivated vaccine can prevent rubeola. The physician decides which vaccine is appropriate for use. Children and teenagers under 15 years of age are the persons who should be vaccinated.[17]

[15]*Ibid.*, pp. 145-149.
[16]Top, F.: *op. cit.*, pp. 361-373.
[17]American Public Health Association: *op. cit.*, pp. 145-149.

## Scarlet Fever

The cause of scarlet fever is *Streptococcus pyogenes*, which has many distinct types. The highest incidence of scarlet fever occurs during late winter and spring, usually among 3- to 12-year-old children. The streptococci are spread by direct contact with the person ill with scarlet fever or by a carrier and occasionally, as a food-borne epidemic. Rarely are the streptococci spread by indirect contact with objects contaminated by the nasal or throat discharges of the infected person. The incubation period is one to three days.

The signs of scarlet fever are high fever, sore throat, tonsillitis, swollen lymph glands in the neck, skin rash (consisting of small, bright red spots), heavily coated or so-called "strawberry" tongue, nausea, and vomiting. The rash appears on the neck, chest, armpits, elbows, groin, and on the inner surfaces of the thighs. During convalescence, peeling is seen at the tips of toes and fingers and at the soles and palms. Persons of all ages are susceptible to scarlet fever.

The patient should be isolated in a single room, a small ward of a hospital, or a cubicle in uncomplicated cases until recovery or no less than seven days from the beginning of the disease. Concurrent disinfection of articles soiled with pus discharges from infected person should be practiced. There is no quarantine required, and no immunization is available. Early treatment, usually with penicillin helps prevent complications such as rheumatic fever.[18]

## Tetanus

Tetanus, or lockjaw, affects more males than females. Fatality varies from 35 to 70% according to the treatment, age of infected person, geographic area, and length of incubation of the tetanus bacillus growing at the site of an injury.

The cause of tetanus is the toxin of the *Clostridium tetani*. The toxin has an affinity for tissue of the central nervous system and for motor nerve cells from the spinal cord. The disease is not communicable from human to human. It is transmitted by contact with contaminated soil or street dust or by spores introduced into wounds.

[18]*Ibid.*, pp. 237-242.

caused by splinters, nails, or gunshot. Spores are formed by the tetanus bacillus and are found in earth, garden mold, and manure. The tetanus bacillus multiplies in closed wounds and lives without oxygen.

The signs of tetanus include pain or tingling at the point of the infection or the healed sore. Other signs include restlessness, stiffness of the neck, irritability, stiffness of the arms and legs, and tightness of the jaw. Profuse perspiration takes place. Painful stiffness of the jaw and spasm of facial muscles occur. Later, there is difficulty in swallowing and breathing. Fever may vary between 101° and 104° F.[19] The incubation period ranges from four days to three weeks depending on the location, type, and extent of the wound. The average length of the incubation period is ten days.

Active immunization with tetanus toxoid is preferably given in infancy or early childhood in combination with the diphtheria toxoid and pertussis vaccine. Booster doses are administered in intervals of ten years. A person who has been actively immunized against tetanus before an injury with possible exposure to the tetanus bacillus is given a booster dose of the tetanus toxoid. A person who has had no previous immunization against tetanus and is exposed to the tetanus bacillus is given tetanus immune globulin or tetanus antitoxin on the day of the injury providing there are no gunshot wounds, compound fractures, or wounds not readily cleansed of foreign matter. Isolation, concurrent disinfection, and quarantine are not required. There is specific treatment.[20]

## Tuberculosis

Although the incidence of tuberculosis has declined steadily in the United States, epidemics have been reported among children in crowded classrooms. More cases of tuberculosis are found in cities than in rural areas. However, the death rate from tuberculosis has been declining in recent years.

There are several types of *Mycobacterium tuberculosis*, but only the bovine and human types cause tuberculosis in man.

Bovine tuberculosis is spread through raw milk from tuberculous cows. Because all milk sold must be pasteurized and federal and state governments have effectively eliminated bovine tuberculosis in dairy cows, this source of the disease is not a factor in the United States. Human pulmonary tuberculosis, however, still concerns school personnel since this type of tuberculosis destroys lung tissue which is necessary in the exchange of oxygen and carbon dioxide in respiration.

Infection with tubercle bacilli takes place by swallowing the bacilli or by inhalation. Usually, the bacilli are spread through droplet infection. The incubation period from infection to the first lesion is about four to six weeks. For progressive pulmonary tuberculosis, the incubation period may be years.

The tubercle bacilli are spread by droplet infection. They may work their way to the lungs of a susceptible person where they attack the alveoli (the tiny air sacs of the lungs) and form microscopic lesions (alterations in tissue structure). Unless the body defenses slow down or stop the multiplication of bacilli, the bacilli will continue to multiply. In most cases, the body defenses do their work, and the multiplication slows down or stops within three to ten weeks. The infection becomes dormant. White blood cells surround the bacilli, and they, in turn, are surrounded by layers of other cells to form the *tubercle.* As healing occurs, the lesions become calcified. Calcification is a sign of healing.

Some persons with tuberculosis do not have the body defenses to stop the multiplication of bacilli. The bacilli spread through the lungs to the circulatory system. The bacilli are carried to the bones and joints, lymphatic system, kidneys, skin, and membranes which envelop the brain and spinal cord. This is *miliary tuberculosis.*

The healing of the lesion may be imperfect. Or, the bacilli may kill the cells surrounding them. Or, the bacilli may multiply more rapidly than body defenses can stop them. Defending cells die. Tissues are destroyed. A cavity is left in the lung. The disease-producing tubercle bacilli are released.

*Reinfection tuberculosis* is a new infection in a person in whom the first infection has healed. There is always a risk that the

⁹Top, F.: *op. cit.*, pp. 620-629.
⁰American Public Health Association, *op. cit.*, pp. 250-253.

dormant infection will become active. The most common form of tuberculosis is re-infection tuberculosis. It usually starts in the upper parts of the lungs, where the bacilli form lesions and spill into the small endings of the bronchi leaving a cavity in the lung.

The signs of pulmonary tuberculosis may include fever, chronic cough, blood spitting, loss of body weight, pain in the chest, and persistent fatigue. However, the disease must be confirmed by medical diagnosis, chest x-rays, and laboratory tests. At first, the cough is very slight, but later it becomes painful, exhausting, and lasts over a long period of time. The amount of blood found in the saliva is likely to be small. However, in far advanced cases of tuberculosis, hemorrhages may occur. Pain *in* the chest also may be due to other infections attacking the lung tissue.

## *Tuberculin Tests*

In tuberculin testing, the test material can usually indicate those persons who are infected by tubercle bacilli. A *positive reaction* reveals that infection has taken place, but it does not indicate the activity or inactivity of the infection or the location of the infection. In most cases, when a person with a positive reaction is given a chest x-ray, there is no tuberculosis in the lungs; therefore, the positive reaction only indicates that the person has been exposed to the bacilli sometime during his life. A *negative reaction* discloses that the person does not have and has not been exposed to the tubercle bacilli. The test material used in tuberculin testing contains *no* living tubercle bacilli.

**Mantoux Test.** The most commonly used tuberculin test is the Mantoux test. This is an interdermal test. The physician injects the test material between the layers of the skin, and after two or three days he reexamines the spot where the injection was made. If there is redness and swelling at the spot of the injection, the test is judged to be a positive reaction. Medical authorities consider the test to be reliable.

**Multiple-puncture Tests.** Two types of multiple-puncture tests are the Heaf test and Tine test. To administer the Heaf test, the test material is placed on the skin of the forearm; then a metal device with six tiny needles painlessly pushes the test material into the skin to a uniform depth of 1 mm. The Tine test consists of a plastic cartridge with four tips. The test material has been placed and dried on the four tips which are pressed against the skin.

**Jet Injection.** This method uses a jet gun to deliver the test material intradermally under high pressure. Jet injection is also used for survey and screening purposes.

## *Chest X-rays*

Chest x-rays and stained smears of sputum are used by the physician in the diagnosis of tuberculosis. The examination of sputum can indicate if the tubercle bacilli are in the nose and throat discharges of a suspected tuberculous patient.

## *Prevention*

Several methods of prevention are used to control tuberculosis. First, chemoprophylaxis by the administration of isoniazid for a period of one year has demonstrated to be effective for household associates of persons with active tuberculosis and for other persons whose risk of acquiring tuberculosis is great. Second, hygienic practices by the patient, such as covering the nose and mouth when coughing, spitting, sneezing, and laughing, are means of prevention and effective in breaking the chain of transmission of the tubercle bacilli. Third, the BCG (Bacillus Calmette-Guérin) vaccine, given to persons who are negative reactors to tuberculin tests, provides good protection in over 90% of the persons vaccinated. This protection may last up to 12 years according to evidence gathered in controlled trials. Fourth, those who live or work among groups of persons having a high tuberculosis rate should have routine x-ray examinations. School personnel, if infected, would be a special hazard to pupils; therefore, all should be screened by tuberculin tests with x-ray examinations for positive reactors. Fifth, persons who are known to have been exposed to the disease should have periodic x-ray screening. Sixth, tuberculin testing of pupils at school entrance and at the age of 14 years discovers infected cases. In addition, there should be periodic retesting of negative reactors to tuberculin tests and preventive treatment to those persons who become positive reactors.

A statewide school-centered tuberculin-testing program has been successfully implemented in Utah. Children entering school, eighth-graders, and school personnel who are negative reactors to tuberculin tests received tuberculin tests annually. Positive tuberculin reactors comprised .5% of the children entering school, 1% of the eighth-graders, and 11% of the school personnel.[21]

In a study reported by Hanzel, it is estimated that 85% of first-graders and ninth-graders will participate in tuberculin testing. About 1.5% of the first-graders will have positive reactions to the tuberculin tests. When the family members of these first-graders receive tuberculin tests, about 40% will have positive reactions. The ninth-graders will have 3 to 6% positive reactions, and 20 to 30% of the school personnel will have positive reactions.[22]

*Treatment*

The infected person should receive prompt chemotherapy. Concurrent disinfection of articles soiled by nose and throat discharges must be enforced. There is no quarantine.

Modern treatment of tuberculosis consists of chemotherapy, outpatient care, inpatient care, laboratory services, completion of chemotherapy regimens, supportive social services, case detection and prevention, and reporting tuberculosis cases. All infectious persons are placed under a well-planned *chemotherapy* regimen. Two drugs are used in the initial regimen. In severe cases, three or more drugs are prescribed. Every effort is made so that each patient completes his chemotherapy regimen.

For the tuberculous patient, most or all of his treatment is as an *outpatient*, either in a health center, clinic, or physician's office. Infectious persons with primary tuberculosis seldom need to be hospitalized. Infectious persons needing *inpatient care* or hospitalization are placed in selected general hospitals, not tuberculosis hospitals or sanatoriums. Many patients with tuberculosis have other diseases which need hospital care. The hospital stay for a tuberculous patient is usually short.

*Laboratory services* are of major importance as they are used to determine the susceptibility of the tubercle bacilli to specific antituberculosis drugs. *Completion of chemotherapy regimens* is the primary goal of every patient's tuberculosis treatment program. The patient's understanding of the program and his reliability in carrying it out must be evaluated. Supportive social services should be provided so that the patient can complete the chemotherapy regimen. If the patient follows the chemotherapy regimen faithfully, prolonged disability is not often experienced. Very few patients require vocational rehabilitation as in the past, and most patients return to their usual activities early in the course of the chemotherapy regimens. *Case detection and prevention* are important aspects of the tuberculosis-control program. Special emphasis is placed on those persons who are heavily exposed or who are thought especially susceptible. Also, the large number of persons who are infected with tubercle bacilli *and* have never received chemoprophylaxis are of great concern in case detection and prevention. *Reporting tuberculosis cases* is essential in the tuberculosis-control program. Every case must be reported to the local health department, which will make available the health department's nursing, laboratory, and roentgenographic services to the physician and will screen the patient's close contacts in order to avoid the spread of the disease.[23,24]

**Venereal Diseases**

Syphilis and gonorrhea are continuously reported among teenagers. Sometimes the teenager has both venereal diseases at the same time. Health departments and family physicians should be empowered to examine and treat persons of any age having a venereal disease or any person who has had contact with another person having a venereal disease. This authority exists in 37 states.[25]

[21]E. Newman: Tuberculin-testing among pupils and personnel in schools. *Amer. J. Public Health* 59 (May, 1969):778.

[22]George D. Hanzel: A program for tuberculosis control in the schools. *J. School Health* 40 (March, 1970):111.

[23]National Tuberculosis and Respiratory Disease Association: *Introduction to Respiratory Diseases*. 4th ed. New York: The Association, 1969, pp. 31-45.

[24]American Public Health Association, *op. cit.*, pp. 265-269.

[25]Donald A. Dukelow: An editorial-consent for care. *J. School Health* 40 (May, 1970):223.

*Syphilis*

Syphilis is caused by *Treponema pallidum*, a delicate spirochete. The chief means of spreading the treponemas is by sexual intercourse. The incubation period is ten days to ten weeks, usually three weeks.

There are several classifications of syphilis; among the most common are *primary*, *secondary*, *latent*, *late*, and *congenital*. Once the treponemas are beneath the surface of the skin or mucous membrane, they enter the lymph channels and migrate to the nearest lymph gland, where they multiply and grow. Later, they pass into the circulatory system, which carries them to every part of the body. The treponemas burrow deep into bone marrow. This stage is called "primary syphilis."

During primary syphilis, the treponemas start their destruction of tissues, bones, and organs after being firmly entrenched within the human body. From ten to 90 days after the treponemas enter the body, a chancre appears at the place of entry, nearly always on or near the genital organs. The chancre appears as a round, ulcerous lump with sharp, raised edges. It is not painful and disappears from one to five weeks later whether the syphilis is treated or not. To many people, the disappearance of the chancre means the syphilis is cured, but this is a false belief since the destructive organisms are rapidly multiplying within the infected person's body.

*Secondary syphilis* is the stage which begins about six weeks after the disappearance of the chancre. There may be fever, swollen lymph glands, small pink or white sores in the mouth and about the genital organs, and sore throat. Huge patches of hair come out with combing. The skin may become dry or scaly. Often these signs may be mild and overlooked. During secondary syphilis, the disease is in its most infectious state. After a short while, the signs vanish.

A latent period between secondary and late syphilis may last from one to 40 years while the treponemas are digging into deep tissues of the human body.

Late syphilis occurs with little or no warning. The central nervous system and the cardiovascular system are the main targets of late syphilis. The treponemas attack the central nervous system and destroy the optic nerve and brain tissue. They may also invade and cause inflammation of the walls of the heart and arteries. Firm, nodule-like tissues called "gummas" form in the skin, bones, muscles, and liver.

Treponemas can be passed by a syphilitic pregnant woman to her unborn baby. If the mother of the unborn baby is not treated, the baby receives the disease before birth. This is *congenital syphilis*. The baby may be blind, deformed, or dead at birth. If the baby is alive at birth, it may be cured of syphilis; however, the treponemas have already had ample opportunity to destroy the baby's tissues, organs, and nerves. Congenital syphilis can be prevented if the mother of the baby receives treatment early in pregnancy.

Over 200 blood tests for detection of syphilis have been developed, but only a few of these are used. The physician may select one test or several tests before a final diagnosis is made. After treatment, all patients are urged to continue having periodic blood tests. A person who has had syphilis does not build up any immunity. He can acquire the disease a second, third, or fourth time.

There is no isolation. Persons undergoing treatment should refrain from sexual intercourse with partners not under treatment. Concurrent disinfection should be practiced for the disposal of articles soiled with discharges from open lesions. There is no quarantine.

The objective of medical treatment is to maintain a desired level of antibiotics in the blood for a long enough period of time to kill the treponemas. If syphilis is treated early, the chances of killing the treponemas are greater than in latent and late syphilis, and the serious destruction of the later stages can be prevented.[26,27]

*Gonorrhea*

Gonorrhea is caused by *Neisseria gonorrhoeae*, the gonococcus. The gonococci are usually spread by sexual intercourse. Discharges of infected reproductive organs contain the gonococci. If gonorrhea is untreated, the gonococci work their way along the passages of the reproductive

[26] American Public Health Association, *op. cit.*, pp. 244-247.
[27] Top, F., *op. cit.*, pp. 604-619.

organs and may cause sterility in both men and women. The incubation period lasts usually three or four days, sometimes as long as nine days.

Three or four days after exposure to gonorrhea, a man has a burning pain during urination and a discharge of pus. There are often no early signs of infection in women. Months after exposure when the gonococci have progressed into the uterus, a woman will have pain in the lower abdomen and a vaginal discharge. Analysis of secretions from the cervix, vagina, and urethra can determine if the gonococci are present.

There is no immunity to gonorrhea, and a person can acquire gonorrhea many times. Gonorrheal arthritis may result when the gonococci attack the joints of the human body, and blindness may result in untreated cases.

If a pregnant woman has gonorrhea, the gonococci can infect the baby's eyes at birth. To prevent this infection, a chemoprophylactic agent is placed in the newborn baby's eyes.[28]

There is no isolation. Persons undergoing treatment should refrain from sexual intercourse with partners not under treatment. Concurrent disinfection is practiced in the disposal of articles soiled with discharges from lesions. There is no quarantine.[29]

Antibiotics are effective in the treatment of gonorrhea. After the treatment is completed, gonorrhea patients remain under a physician's care as other venereal diseases may also develop.

## Whooping Cough

This common disease, also called "pertussis," of children is found throughout the world. The incidence is highest in the late winter and early spring in large communities. The cause of whooping cough is the *Bordetella pertussis*, the pertussis bacillus. The bacillus is spread by droplet infection or indirectly by contact with articles contaminated with the throat discharges of infected persons. The incubation period is usually seven days or within ten days.

This bacterial disease involves the trachea, bronchi, and bronchioles (the major structures of respiration). The onset is an irritating cough which recurs or intensifies within one or two weeks and lasts for one to two months. The recurring cough becomes violent with a series of coughs without inhalation between the coughs and followed by the characteristic high-pitched whoop and expulsion of mucus. Everyone is susceptible.

Pupils infected with whooping cough are separated from susceptible school children and are excluded from school and public places. Isolation of children over two years of age is not practical. Concurrent disinfection takes place with all articles soiled with discharges from the nose and throat of the infected person. If school children are observed throughout each school day so that the first sign of whooping cough can be detected, quarantine is not necessary. There is specific treatment.

The proven effective procedure to control whooping cough is the active immunization of all susceptible preschool children. The pertussis (whooping cough) vaccine is combined with diphtheria and tetanus toxoids. Routine immunization can be started when an infant is two or three months old. A single booster dose is recommended one year after the initial immunization and again before entering school.[30]

## IMPLICATIONS FOR HEALTH EDUCATION

One of the areas of health education is "The Prevention of Diseases to All Parts of the Human Body." Units from this area and supplementary content in addition to this chapter might be as follows:

Unit: Causative agents of diseases
Unit: Immunization
Unit: Common cold, chicken pox, mumps, measles (rubella and rubeola)
Unit: Infectious hepatitis and infectious mononucleosis
Unit: Rheumatic fever and rheumatic heart disease
Unit: Influenza, pneumonia, scarlet fever
Unit: Whooping cough and tetanus
Unit: Tuberculosis
Unit: Syphilis and gonorrhea

The units on the causative agents of diseases; immunization; common cold, chicken

[28]*Ibid.*, pp. 260-266.
[29]American Public Health Association, *op. cit.*, pp. 97-98.
[30]*Ibid.*, pp. 280-282.

pox, mumps, and measles (rubella and rubeola); rheumatic fever and rheumatic
heart disease; and whooping cough and
tetanus could be taught in the intermediate
grades of the elementary school. In the
primary grades, units might have been
"ways in which diseases are spread," "simple ways to prevent diseases," "vaccinations of children in the primary grades,"
and "septic sore throat." In the junior or
middle and senior high school, the units
might be "infectious hepatitis and infectious mononucleosis;" "influenza, pneumonia, and scarlet fever;" "tuberculosis;"
and "syphilis and gonorrhea." Additional
units might include instruction about the
uses of chemotherapy in the treatment of
diseases, tuberculin tests, bacterial endo-
carditis, meningitis, cancers of the human
body, diphtheria, smallpox, malaria, and
amebic dysentery.

## References for Further Study

Adams, J. M.: *Viruses and Colds*. New York: American
Elsevier Publishing Company, Inc., 1967.
Anderson, G., Arnstein, M. G., and Lester, M. R.:
*Communicable Disease Control*. 4th ed. New York:
The Macmillan Company, 1964.
Boyd, W.: *An Introduction to the Study of Disease*.
6th ed. Philadelphia: Lea & Febiger, 1971.
Bureau of Disease Prevention and Environmental Con-
trol, National Communicable Disease Center: *Syph-
ilis: A Synopis*. Public Health Service Publication
1660, 1968.
Clark, D. W., and MacMahon, B.: *Preventive Medicine*.
Boston: Little, Brown and Company, 1967.
Cockburn, A.: *Infectious Diseases: Their Evaluation
and Eradication*. Springfield, Ill.: Charles C Thomas
Company, 1967.
Dauer, C. C., Korns, R. F., and Schuman, L. M.: *In-
fectious Diseases*. New York: American Public Health
Association, 1968.
Hanlon, J.: *Principles of Public Health Administration*.
5th ed. St. Louis: The C. V. Mosby Company, 1969.
Hilleboe, H., and Larimore, G. W.: *Preventive Medi-
cine*. 2nd ed. Philadelphia: W. B. Saunders Com-
pany, 1965.
Hoagland, R.: *Infectious Mononucleosis*. New York:
Grune & Stratton, Inc., 1967.
Kindig, E. L., ed. *Disorders of the Respiratory Tract
in Children*. Philadelphia: W. B. Saunders Com-
pany, 1967.
Krugman, S., and Ward, R.: *Infectious Diseases in
Children*. 4th ed. St. Louis: The C. V. Mosby Com-
pany, 1968.
Landon, J. F., and Sider, H. T.: *Communicable Dis-
eases*. 8th ed. Philadelphia: F. A. Davis Company,
1964.
Sartwell, P. E., ed.: *Preventive Medicine and Public
Health*. 9th ed. New York: Appleton-Century-Crofts,
Inc., 1965.
Schwartz, W. F.: *An Introduction to Syphilis and
Gonorrhea*. Atlanta, Ga.: Communicable Disease
Center, 1965.
Smillie, W. G., and Kilbourne, E. D.: *Preventive Medi-
cine and Public Health*. New York: The Macmillan
Company, 1969.
Smith, I. M.: *Infectious Diseases*. Baltimore: The
Williams & Wilkins Company, 1967.

# Chapter 5

# *DENTAL HEALTH*

## AN INCIDENT

Elementary school classroom teachers have discovered that 25% of children have never been to a dentist. Also, when these teachers have encouraged tooth brushing after lunch, the children have indicated that the only time that they brush their teeth is before breakfast. Junior high or middle school teachers have discussed among themselves the number of students with speech problems due to missing permanent front teeth. Also, these teachers have seen a high intake of candy and sweetened soft drinks at lunch. Teachers of health education in high schools have taken notice of the number of students who suck breath sweeteners, of the decreased intake of foods high in calcium and vitamin C, and of the loss of permanent teeth among students.

Dental caries (tooth decay) is one of the most serious health problems of the school-age child. It is estimated that by the time children reach the age of 7, they have at least three decayed deciduous teeth. The average high school student has seven missing, filled, or decayed permanent teeth involving 14 tooth surfaces.[1] Ninety-eight percent of all Americans have dental caries at some time during their lives. At any one time, there may be a billion unfilled cavities in the mouths of Americans. One-sixth of an American family's budget for professional health services goes toward dental care.[2]

[1]American Dental Association: *Dental Health Facts for Teachers.* Chicago: The Association, 1966, p. 11.
[2]National Institute of Dental Research: *Research Explores Dental Decay.* 1967, p. 1.

## DECIDUOUS TEETH

By the time the child is 3 years old, he has 20 teeth called the "deciduous" (sometimes called "baby," "first," "foundation," "milk," "primary," or "temporary") teeth. These teeth consist of central incisors, lateral incisors, cuspids, first molars, and second molars.

As soon as the deciduous teeth have appeared, a child should be taught how to brush his teeth and should develop the habit of cleaning his teeth immediately after eating. His first visit to the family dentist should occur when he is between the ages of 2 and 3 years. Dental examinations and x-rays assist the dentist to detect dental caries. It is important that there be no premature loss of deciduous teeth or their retention beyond the normal time of shedding. Permanent teeth can erupt out of position when there is early loss or late retention of deciduous teeth. Neglect of deciduous teeth is very common because often parents do not understand their importance, and no attention is paid to early loss or late retention, and to decay and infection.

The deciduous teeth perform the following functions. First, they assist in the chewing of food. Second, they contribute to facial development. Third, they preserve the space for the incoming permanent teeth. Fourth, they are a part of the child's speech equipment.

## SIX-YEAR MOLARS

The first of the permanent teeth to appear are the six-year molars. These teeth do *not* replace deciduous teeth but erupt in back of the second deciduous molars. They are the largest teeth in the mouth and

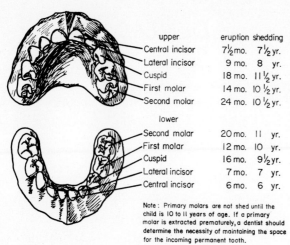

| upper | eruption | shedding |
|---|---|---|
| Central incisor | 7½ mo. | 7½ yr. |
| Lateral incisor | 9 mo. | 8 yr. |
| Cuspid | 18 mo. | 11½ yr. |
| First molar | 14 mo. | 10½ yr. |
| Second molar | 24 mo. | 10½ yr. |

| lower | | |
|---|---|---|
| Second molar | 20 mo. | 11 yr. |
| First molar | 12 mo. | 10 yr. |
| Cuspid | 16 mo. | 9½ yr. |
| Lateral incisor | 7 mo. | 7 yr. |
| Central incisor | 6 mo. | 6 yr. |

Note: Primary molars are not shed until the child is 10 to 11 years of age. If a primary molar is extracted prematurely, a dentist should determine the necessity of maintaining the space for the incoming permanent tooth.

Figure 3. Eruption and shedding of primary teeth

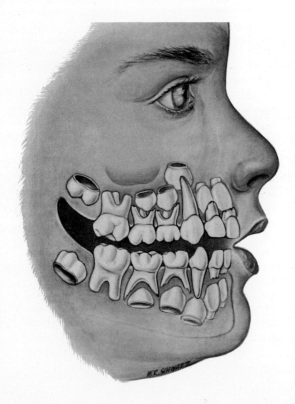

Figure 4. Dentition of six-year-old child. The child has all twenty of his primary teeth, plus four permanent teeth—the six-year molars. The other permanent teeth are developing under the primary teeth. (Copyright by the American Dental Association. Reprinted by permission.)

decay easily. There are four of them. The six-year molars are often mistaken for deciduous teeth because they slip into the mouth before any of the back teeth appear. To locate the six-year molar, find the exact middle front space between the two center teeth and count backward either right or left, on the upper or lower jaw. The sixth tooth from the center is the six-year molar, provided that no teeth are missing. When a six-year molar is lost, the contour of the face is affected, other teeth tend to "drift," and dental caries, malocclusion, and pyorrhea may result.

## MIXED DENTITION

When the child is between the ages of 6 and 12, the roots of the deciduous teeth are gradually dissolving, while the permanent teeth are undergoing the final stages of development. When the permanent tooth is fully formed and ready to erupt, the deciduous tooth become loose. Permanent teeth appear in the lower jaw before corresponding teeth in the upper jaw. In some instances, there may be variations in the time of eruption of the permanent teeth in upper and lower jaws.

If a second deciduous molar is lost too soon, the dentist may insert a space maintainer so that there is room for the incoming second bicuspid. Dental care during the period of mixed dentition is essential. Parents may not realize that the four first deciduous molars are needed until the tenth year, and that the four second deciduous molars are needed until the twelfth year.

## PERMANENT TEETH

By the time a person reaches 21 years of age, he should have 32 permanent teeth, 16 in each jaw. The incisors, located in the center front of the mouth, cut food. The cuspids, located at the corners of the mouth, tear food. The bicuspids, with two cusps in back of the cuspids, tear and crush food. The molars, located in the back of the mouth, are used to grind food. The incisors and cuspids have one root; the bicuspids may have one or two roots. Molars have two or three roots. When the jaws are closed, the upper front teeth should slightly overlap the lower front teeth. The upper and lower molars should fit snugly together. These permanent teeth should be retained throughout life.

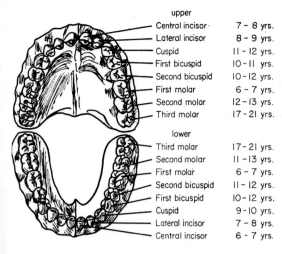

| upper | |
|---|---|
| Central incisor | 7 - 8 yrs. |
| Lateral incisor | 8 - 9 yrs. |
| Cuspid | 11 - 12 yrs. |
| First bicuspid | 10 - 11 yrs. |
| Second bicuspid | 10 - 12 yrs. |
| First molar | 6 - 7 yrs. |
| Second molar | 12 - 13 yrs. |
| Third molar | 17 - 21 yrs. |
| lower | |
| Third molar | 17 - 21 yrs. |
| Second molar | 11 - 13 yrs. |
| First molar | 6 - 7 yrs. |
| Second bicuspid | 11 - 12 yrs. |
| First bicuspid | 10 - 12 yrs. |
| Cuspid | 9 - 10 yrs. |
| Lateral incisor | 7 - 8 yrs. |
| Central incisor | 6 - 7 yrs. |

Figure 5. Eruption of the permanent teeth

## STRUCTURE OF THE TOOTH

Into the bony sockets of the upper and lower jaws are the hard, calcified structures—the teeth. A tooth is divided into two parts: crown and root. The *crown* appears above the gum and is separated from the root by the neck of the tooth. The root anchors the tooth in a bony socket of the jawbone. The crown consists of enamel, dentin, and pulp cavity. The hard, glistening substance that covers the crown is the *enamel.* Below the enamel and cementum is an ivory-like substance which forms the body of the tooth. This is the *dentin.* The hollow space in the center of the tooth is the *pulp cavity,* which contains nerves, blood vessels, and lymphatics.

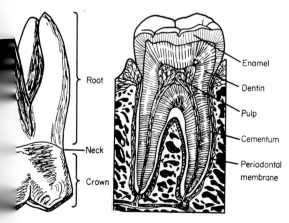

Figure 6. The structure of the tooth

The *root* consists of the periodontal membrane, cementum, dentin, and pulp cavity. The *periodontal membrane* acts as a shock absorber as the teeth come together in the chewing process. Also, many diseases of the teeth have their origin in the periodontal membrane. The *cementum* is a thin layer of bony tissue covering the root of the tooth, between the periodontal membrane and the dentin.

## SOME SIGNS OF POSSIBLE DENTAL HEALTH PROBLEMS

The following signs are easily observable by the teacher or by the nurse in the elementary school student and the secondary school youth:

Swollen jaws
Poor oral habits, such as thumb sucking, nail biting
Toothache
Tartar
Bleeding gums
Malocclusion
Ulcerated gums
Brown or black spots at edge of tooth
Missing teeth
Unusual placement of teeth
Use of only one side of the mouth for chewing
Refusal to eat hard food
Abnormal sucking
Loose teeth

*Tartar,* or dental calculus, is the crust-like material formed by deposits of calcium and phosphate from saliva on the teeth. Tartar cannot be removed by tooth brushing; however, the dentist can remove tartar at regular intervals.[3]

## DENTAL EXAMINATIONS

One of the most important phases of the health appraisal of a pupil is the diagnostic dental examination. It can be performed by the family dentist in his private office or by a cooperating dentist in the school.

Because of the incidence of dental caries among children and youth, regular visits to the family dentist are necessary in order to detect and correct tooth defects and dental diseases in their early stages. Irregularities in the growth of teeth can thus be observed and corrected, and pain can be prevented by early detection and correction of defects and diseases. The overall

[3]National Institute of Dental Research: *Research Explores Pyorrhea and Other Gum Diseases.* 1967, p. 4.

cost of dental care is considerably reduced when there is early correction of diseases and defects.

A form, such as that below, can be sent to all parents. If there is no family dentist, the school health services' staff may suggest cooperating dentists from a list provided by the local dental society.

---

**DENTAL EXAMINATION CARD**

*To the Parent:* Our school health program is designed to promote and protect the health of the student. We urge parents to have their children visit their dentist at least once a year for a dental examination and treatment advised by the dentist. When your son or daughter visits the dentist of your choice, please see that the dentist receives this card. When the dentist has completed the examination and treatment, this card should be returned to the school.

_____

Date                           Principal

(front)

---

**REPORT OF DENTAL EXAMINATION**

This report certifies that I have examined the teeth of _____ and:
                              Pupil

☐ 1. Dental treatment is in progress.

☐ 2. All necessary dental treatment has been completed.

☐ 3. No dental treatment is required at this time.

Further recommendations _____
_____
_____
                                        D.D.S.
Date              Signature of Dentist
PLEASE RETURN THIS CARD TO THE TEACHER

(back)

Figure 7

## X-Rays

Thorough diagnosis of the condition of the teeth by the family dentist often involves the use of x-ray equipment. Tiny cavities, not visible through ordinary examinations, can be detected by x-ray. New decay beneath old fillings, and abscessed teeth can be found. In addition, x-ray pictures can reveal an impacted tooth, a tooth with crooked roots, or a hidden permanent tooth that cannot erupt. Early periodontal disease can be also disclosed in x-rays. The full-mouth x-ray can be used to detect early defects and diseases so that correction can be made promptly. The American Dental Association has advised dentists that x-rays "should be kept at a minimum and should come after careful consideration of both the dental and general health needs of the patient." Also, the Association has recommended that x-rays should not be a part of every dental examination.[4]

## Topical Fluoride Applications

Fluoride solutions may be applied by the dentist to the teeth of children in early childhood and who have not had access to fluoridated drinking water supplies since birth. Topical fluoride applications will not halt decay already started but will help to prevent new decay. First, the dentist cleans the teeth. He removes stains and tartar, which might irritate the gums, and then, he applies a fluoride solution to the teeth. The applications should be repeated at intervals. Topical fluoride application may result in a 30 to 40% reduction of caries.[5] Many research studies have shown that topical fluoride applications among large groups of children have given considerable protection against dental caries. In those communities with fluoridated water supplies, the dentist may recommend topical fluoride applications for some children as an additional preventive measure.

## COMMON DENTAL HEALTH PROBLEMS

Dental health problems are dental caries, periodontal disease, malocclusion, and accidents that injure the teeth or supporting tooth structures. Less than 5% of the school-age population is spared the ravages of dental caries.

## Dental Caries

*Dental caries,* commonly called "tooth decay," is a destructive and progressive

---

[4]Dental x-rays. *Science 195* (February 2, 1968):515.
[5]National Institute of Dental Research: *Research Explores Dental Decay, op. cit.,* p. 6.

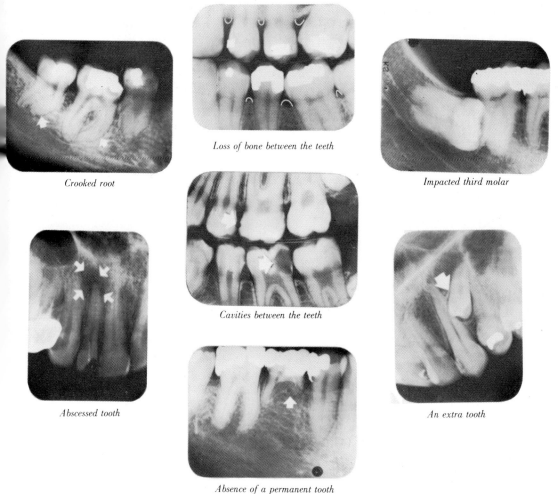

Crooked root

Loss of bone between the teeth

Impacted third molar

Cavities between the teeth

Abscessed tooth

An extra tooth

Absence of a permanent tooth

Figure 8A. Dental X-rays. (Copyright by the American Dental Association. Reprinted by permission.)

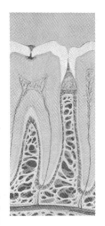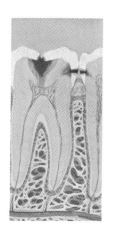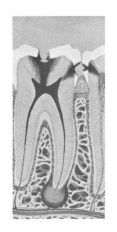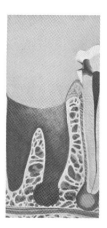

Figure 8B. Progress of decay. Left to right: Early stage of dental decay. The enamel has been penetrated. The softer dentin has been attacked. The pulp has been killed and an abscess formed. The molar is extracted. The bicuspid is abscessed. Redrawn from Dental Health Facts for Teachers. (Copyright by the American Dental Association. Reprinted by permission.)

process that destroys tooth structure and produces cavities in teeth. Children and youth have sugar on their morning cereal, sugar-sweetened crackers with their mid-morning snack, cookies for lunch, peanut butter and jelly sandwiches after school, cake for dinner, and a handful of dried raisins before going to bed. In addition, they may drink two to three bottles of sweetened soft drinks. Average per capita consumption of sugar in a year in the United States is about 100 pounds.

There are four factors necessary to produce dental caries: the presence of decay-producing bacteria, a caries-producing diet with large amounts of sugar, dental plaque, and a susceptible tooth surface. Certain types of decay-producing bacteria are found in the mouths of most persons. They form deposits on the tooth surfaces when the surfaces are not free of food residues. The bacteria grow and multiply into bacterial colonies called plaque. Colorless and transparent, the plaque is constantly developing and sticking to the teeth. When the bacteria come in contact with foods high in sugar, they produce gummy substances called dextrans which help the plaque to stick to the teeth. More bacteria lodge in the sticky plaque and multiply. Many of the bacteria act on the sugar to produce acids. These acids begin to dissolve the enamel of the tooth and start decay. Acid production begins within five minutes after foods high in sugar are eaten and continues for long periods of time even when the sweet foods are not in the mouth. Caries can also develop without the plaque, since food residues collect in pits and fissures of the teeth and begin to ferment. Frequent between-meal eating of foods or liquids high in sugar increases the chances of dental caries.[6]

Caries may begin underneath the plaque, in the sheltered areas between the teeth, near the gum line, and in many pits and fissures which are structural flaws of the teeth, as these areas are all hard to clean Left undetected, the decay will penetrate the enamel and reach the dentin. The decay progresses rapidly into the dentin and reaches the pulp cavity. When the pulp cavity becomes infected, an abscess may form either within the tooth or at the tip of the root. Soreness, swelling, and pulsating pain accompany the abscess; usually the tooth must be removed. Often adjoining teeth are affected with caries, and abscesses become evident.

Failure to remove the plaque may lead to the formation of *tartar* or *calculus* on the crown surfaces of the teeth or the root surfaces beneath the gum margins. Tartar is covered by a layer of living bacterial plaque. The tartar must be removed by the dentist because it may be the forerunner of gingivitis and pyorrhea.

There is definite need for teaching about dental caries and about the relation of daily sugar intake to dental caries in our schools. School personnel should be aware that the availability of candies and sweetened soft drinks in lunchrooms and in dispensing machines has an adverse effect on student dental health. For this and other reasons, the Council on Food and Nutrition of the American Medical Association, the American Dental Association, and the National Congress of Parents and Teachers have all issued statements urging school personnel not to sell candies and sweetened soft drinks on school premises.

## Periodontal Diseases

Studies have revealed that periodontal disease is one of the most widespread diseases of mankind. More than 20 million adult Americans have lost teeth from this cause, and at least 67 million have periodontal disease. Periodontal disease affects the tissues and membranes surrounding the teeth rather than the teeth themselves.

In *gingivitis,* the gums become tender, inflamed, and swollen. They bleed easily and stand away from the teeth. Gingivitis is frequently the result of deposits of tartar and plaque; however, a host of mouth and other diseases and conditions can cause gingivitis. It is estimated that 90% of 11-year-olds and 85% of children between 11 and 18 have gingivitis.[7] Neglected gingivitis can result in periodontitis.

*Periodontitis* (pyorrhea) is due to debris and neglected tartar. Debris consists of soft particles of food remaining on the teeth and gradually turning into plaque.

[6]National Institute of Dental Research: *Research Explores Plaque.* 1969, pp. 1-3.

[7]Theodore Berland and Alfred E. Seyler: Teeth care for teenagers. *Today's Health* 46 (March, 1968):66.

Heavy tartar is deposited on the inside surfaces of the lower incisors and outside surfaces of the upper molars. Tartar has rough, rock-like edges which make it easier for plaque to accumulate on the teeth. Gum and bone can be seriously harmed by tartar, especially when the tartar works into spaces where it cannot be removed by tooth brushing. The tartar irritates the gums so that the gums separate from the teeth leaving pockets into which food debris can accumulate. Particles of food decay in the pockets, and pus begins to form.[8] As periodontitis worsens, the inflammation spreads. Pockets deepen, and more pus forms. Infected gums bleed and

disease. The disease is not readily communicable, and many persons harbor the causative agents without ever having the disease.[10]

## Malocculsion

Irregularities of tooth position and poor occlusion (fitting together of the teeth when the jaws are closed) are malocclusion. Facial deformities and increased susceptibility to infection and dental caries can result from malocclusion.

Malocclusion most commonly occurs during the time the deciduous teeth are being shed and the permanent teeth are erupting. An investigation of more than 1000

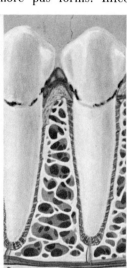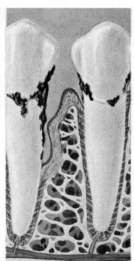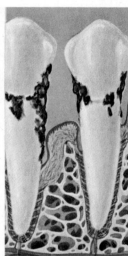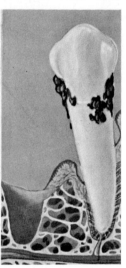

Figure 9. Progress of periodontal disease. Food debris and tartar deposits have irritated the gums, causing them to withdraw from the teeth. Bacteria grow and multiply in the gum pockets. Infection progresses. The support for the teeth is destroyed, and the teeth are eventually lost. (Copyright by the American Dental Association. Reprinted by permission.)

ulcerate, and tissue damage increases. In the final stages of periodontitis, the bone is attacked and destroyed causing the teeth to loosen and to come out.[9]

*Vincent's infection* (trench mouth) is a disease characterized by extreme inflammation and soreness of the gums. It is accompanied by ulceration of the gums, pain, bleeding, and a foul odor. Unhygienic mouth conditions tend to increase the spirochete *Borrelia vincentii* and the bacillus *Bacillus fusiformis* associated with the

Michigan school children indicated that about 30% of the children in all age groups had some degree of malocclusion.

There are two general types, inherited and acquired. Four factors are involved in heredity: (1) deciduous teeth may be shed too early; (2) deciduous teeth may be retained too long; (3) permanent teeth may erupt before the jaws have reached the growth sufficient to support the permanent teeth; and (4) the dental arches of the mouth may be too narrow.

Acquired malocclusion is mainly the result of bad habits. Abnormal thumb or

Theodore Berland: Periodontal disease: hidden threat to grown-ups' teeth. *Today's Health* 47 (August, 1969):28.
National Institute of Dental Research: *Research Explores Pyorrhea and Other Gum Diseases, op. cit.,* pp. 1-2.

[10]Franklin H. Top: *Communicable and Infectious Diseases.* 6th ed. St. Louis: The C. V. Mosby Company, 1968, pp. 694-695.

finger sucking, tongue thrusting, lip sucking, and certain sleeping positions can bring abnormal pressure on the teeth and bones of the face. Poor dental care may result in early loss of deciduous or permanent teeth. As a result, teeth adjacent to or opposite the space left by the lost teeth may drift out of position. If a deciduous tooth is lost too early, the adjoining teeth drift and reduce the space for the oncoming permanent tooth.

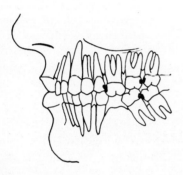

Figure 10. Effects of loss of a permanent molar

Malocclusion can have several harmful effects. Facial deformities and speech defects can result. The child may select foods not suitable for his nutritional needs because his malocclusion interferes with the chewing of food. Later in life, periodontal diseases may develop. Irregular or protruding teeth detract from appearance and can cause social and emotional disturbances. The child or adult with malocclusion cannot accept the statement, "an attractive smile is a person's greatest asset."

Acquired malocclusion can be prevented with the aid of the dentist. He can inform the patient of poor dental habits, prevent premature loss of teeth, provide space for teeth that will erupt later, and extract teeth that have been retained too long. Some of these preventive measures, however, should not be taken until conditions warrant.[11] Often the family dentist may refer his patient to an orthodontist—the dental specialist who detects, prevents, and corrects irregularities in the teeth and jaws.

The best preventive measure is regular dental care started at an early age and

[11]American Dental Association, *op. cit.*, pp. 19-20.

continued throughout a lifetime. Regular dental care can prevent the need for more complicated treatment at a later date.

## CAN YOU REMOVE THE DENTAL PLAQUE?

In order to demonstrate how effective tooth brushing is, the following experiment can be done.

1. Obtain disclosing wafers from one of the following:
   a. Amural Products Company
      1200 East Chicago Avenue
      Naperville, Illinois 60540
   b. Colgate-Palmolive Company
      Professional Services Departments
      P.O. Box 7994
      Chicago, Illinois 60677
   c. Proctor and Gamble Distributing Company
      Professional Relations Division
      Winton Hill Technical Center
      Cincinnati, Ohio 45224
2. Ask students to bring small mirrors so that they can see the results of this experiment.
3. Have each student chew a disclosing wafer. The wafer is swished around the mouth and teeth for about a minute. The wafer may be swallowed.
4. The dye of the wafer dissolves in the mouth fluids and colors the clumps of bacteria red.
5. The red clumps sticking to the teeth can be seen by looking in the mouth with a mirror.
6. Students should be able to remove the red clumps with a toothbrush. The dye can be swallowed.

The dye indicates the areas where plaque is most likely to persist. The dye does not stain clean tooth surfaces or fillings, but it will stain tongue and lips for two hours. If the students repeat the experiment daily they will witness the plaque and accumulation of food particles—all indicating the necessity of thorough tooth brushing after eating.

### Tooth Brushing

Correct tooth brushing can be demonstrated by the dental hygienist or teacher in school, as well as by the family dentist. The method pictured in Figure 11 is recommended by the American Dental Association.

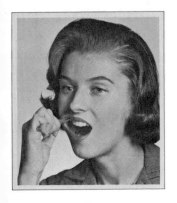

1

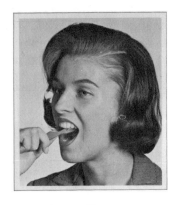

2

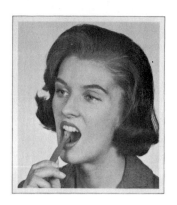

3

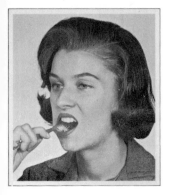

4

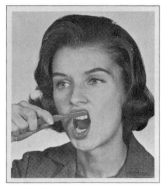

5

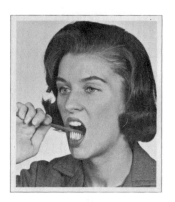

6

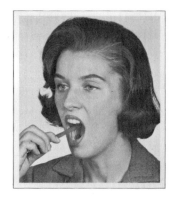

7

Figure 11

1. Clean the outside surfaces of the upper back teeth.
2. Clean the inside surfaces of the upper (and lower) back teeth.
3. Clean the inside surfaces of the upper front teeth.
4. Clean the outside surfaces of the lower back teeth.
5. Clean the outside surfaces of the upper (and lower) front teeth.
6. Clean the inside surfaces of the lower front teeth.
7. Clean the grinding surfaces of the upper and lower teeth.[12]

For correct tooth brushing, a toothbrush with a "flat brushing surface, firm bristles and a head sufficiently small to permit access to all surfaces of the teeth"[13] should be used. Care of the toothbrush as well as its use should be taught. To demonstrate correct tooth brushing, the teacher can use models of teeth. Children and youth can be encouraged to bring their toothbrushes for tooth brushing after lunch and after the snack period. Watching himself in a mirror can help the student while he practices the correct method.

After the teeth are brushed, the mouth should be rinsed thoroughly with lukewarm water forced back and forth between the teeth several times. Toothbrushes should have time to dry between use and must be kept clean.

The family dentist is the best person to advise the student about the use of electric toothbrushes, some of which have been proven to be safe and effective.

The *when* and *how* of tooth brushing are more important than the choice of a particular brand of dentifrice and dental floss. If the student desires to use a dentifrice (tooth paste or powder), the family dentist can recommend a dentifrice. The use of dental floss after tooth brushing should be taught to the student by the family dentist or by a dental hygienist.

Hayden[14] has suggested that proper tooth brushing would be greatly encouraged if school buildings had oral hygiene stations in classrooms or other specific areas. Supervised tooth brushing with a therapeutic dentifrice and with periodic use of disclosing wafers could reduce dental caries and periodontal disease significantly.

## WHAT CAN THE TEACHER DO?

When the signs of dental health problems have been observed among students, what can be done? Following the school system's procedures, teacher or nurse should inform parents of children of elementary school age of possible dental health problems in parent-teacher or parent-nurse conferences. With secondary school students, dental health problems should be discussed in teacher-pupil conferences. Parents should be encouraged to take the younger child to the family dentist, but secondary school pupils should be encouraged to seek their own care from their family dentists. The teacher should inform the nurse, who can check the dental care given by the dentist. School personnel should be alert for further possible dental health problems among pupils. Teachers should evaluate their own dental health practices and should regularly visit their own dentists (Chapter 8). School personnel can remove soft drink and candy-vending machines from the school premises. They should also be familiar with school nutrition and its importance to dental health (Chapter 10). All teachers can assist in promoting dental health by:

1. Encouraging tooth brushing after the noonday school meal and snacks
2. Encouraging proper nutritional habits
3. Discouraging concentrated sugars in the diet
4. Discouraging thumb sucking and nail biting
5. Discouraging the placement of pencils, pens, and other objects between the teeth
6. Warning against cracking nuts and biting hard candy with the teeth

Elementary teachers and teachers of health education can include dental health units in the area "Care of All Parts of the Human Body." In addition, certain concepts in dental health might be stressed in the elementary school:

1. Daily health practices and regular visits to the dentist are important to good dental health.
2. Understanding the structure and function of the teeth and gums can contribute to a clean and healthy mouth.
3. Daily food selection and eating patterns are vitally important to the promotion of dental health.
4. Protecting the mouth from disease and deformity involves the use of a variety of health products and services.
5. Promoting dental health and preventing dental diseases are worthwhile, valuable goals throughout life.

[13]American Dental Association: *Dental Health Facts for Teachers, op. cit.*, p. 14.
[14]Charles H. Hayden: Preventive dental procedures adaptable to school health programs. *Amer. J. Public Health* 59 (March, 1969):522.

6. Prevention of dental diseases and deformity is important to the quality of total health.[15]

## Implications for Health Education

Units in the intermediate grades, junior high or middle school, and high school can be taught about the following: dental caries; malocclusion; periodontal disease; teenagers' dental health problems; and fluoridation of drinking water supplies. An outline of content of a dental health unit is found in Chapter 14, and the content within a lesson plan on dental health is found in Chapter 15. The unit on fluoridation could include not only the scientific evidence for fluoridation but also the arguments against fluoridation.

## FLUORIDATION OF WATER SUPPLIES

More than 4000 American communities with a total population of more than 82 million have fluoridation of drinking water. Natural fluorides are found in the drinking water of more than 10 million additional people in the United States. Seven states have legislation requiring fluoridation.

There have been more than 3000 clinical and experimental reports on the biological effects of fluorides. These reports substantiate the value of adding one part of fluorine to one million parts of water as a means of reducing dental caries. Also, these reports indicate that there is no health hazard. Fluoridation of drinking water does not affect the color, odor, or taste of water, and costs about ten cents per person a year. A review of legal questions raised by opponents of fluoridation reveals that the constitutionality of fluoridation has been well established by many court decisions.[16]

Grand Rapids, Michigan, and Newburgh, New York, are two of the many communities studied to validate statistics about the reduction of dental caries among children having access to fluoridated water. One part of fluorine was added to one million parts of fluoride-free lake water used by the people of Grand Rapids. Two groups of children of the same age level were compared: those born in Grand Rapids prior to fluoridation and those born in Grand Rapids having access to fluoridated water since birth. The children who had access to fluoridated water had 65% less dental caries than the other children had. In Newburgh, children drinking fluoridated water since birth had 60% less dental caries, over a period of 10 years, than children in Kingston, New York, who did not use fluoridated water.[17] In a study by Ast and others, the cost of dental care of 735 children in a fluoridated and non-fluoridated area was compared during a three-year period. The study revealed that fluoridation of community water supplies reduces the cost of dental care for children and the hazard of tooth loss.[18]

Extensive studies by the United States Public Health Service have shown that one part of fluorine added to one million parts of water can bring about 60% less dental caries among children having access to the fluoridated water than among children living where the water did not have the desirable fluoride content.[19] The American Dental Association, American Medical Association, National Research Council, American Public Health Association, and other qualified professional health groups have urged that all communities provide fluoridated drinking water.

## EVALUATION OF DENTAL HEALTH CONSUMER PRODUCTS

For more than 35 years, the Council on Dental Therapeutics of the American Dental Association has been evaluating every type of dental health product, including toothpastes, tooth powders, and mouthwashes making therapeutic claims in advertising. Dentists as well as nonprofessional health personnel have profited from this information. These evaluations are given in *Accepted Dental Remedies*, published by the American Dental Association.

[5]Division of Dental Health, Texas State Department of Health: *Texas Teachers' Handbook on Dental Health Education, Grades 1-6.* Austin, Texas: The Department, 1971, p. 118.
[6]George A. Strong: Liberty, religion, and fluoridation. *J. Amer. Dental Assoc.* 76 (June, 1968):1398-1409.

[17]Fluoridation. *J. Amer. Dental Assoc.* 65 (November, 1962):578-718.
[18]David B. Ast, Naham C. Cons, James P. Carlos, and Adele Polan: Time and cost factors to provide regular periodic dental care for children in a fluoridated and non-fluoridated area. *Amer. J. Public Health* 57 (September, 1967):1635.
[19]National Institute of Dental Research: *Research Explores Dental Decay, op. cit.,* p. 5.

Breath sweeteners and mouthwashes have gained tremendous popularity by advertising. Most breath sweeteners have flavoring or sugar in them. The sugar promotes the formation of dental plaque and acid. Cervical caries or cavities near the gum line have been noted to increase in persons who use breath sweeteners continuously. Mouthwashes serve no greater purpose than to aid in removal of loose food and debris, and rinsing with plain water does a more effective job.

## References for Further Study

American Dental Association: *Scientific Reasoning and the Fluoridation Controversy*. Chicago: The Association, 1962.

————— : *Answers to Criticism of Fluoridation*. Chicago: The Association, 1964.

Arnim, S. S.: An effective program of oral hygiene for the arrestment of dental caries and the control of periodontal disease. *J. So. Calif. Dental Assoc.* 35 (July, 1967):264.

Berland, T., and Seyler, A. E.: *Your Children's Teeth*. New York: Meredith Press, 1968.

Ciba Foundation: *Caries-resistant Teeth*. Boston: Little, Brown and Company, 1965.

Lauterstein, A. M., and Barber, T. K.: *Teeth, Their Forms and Functions*. Boston: D. C. Heath & Company, 1965.

Morrey, L. W., and Nelsen, R. J., eds.: *Dental Science Handbook*. Washington, D.C.: National Institute of Dental Research, 1969.

Muhler, J. C.: *Fifty-two Pearls and Their Environment*. Bloomington: Indiana University Press, 1965.

Stoll, F., and Catherman, J.: *Dental Health Education*. 4th ed. Philadelphia: Lea & Febiger, 1972.

Young, W. O., and Striffler, D. F.: *The Dentist, His Practice, and His Community*. 2nd ed. Philadelphia: W. B. Saunders Company, 1969.

# Chapter 6

## *CHRONIC HEALTH CONDITIONS*

**AN INCIDENT**

Teachers in elementary schools have noticed that several children hesitate when speaking and reading. The children may stare vacantly or have a nodding spasm. Then, the children continue doing whatever they were doing. Teachers naturally have been disturbed about this behavior.

Junior high or middle school teachers have become alarmed at students who show signs of sweating, dizziness, trembling, blurred vision, mental confusion, and shallow breathing. Students ask for candy bars. These signs appear when the students have not eaten lunch or after the students have had strenuous exercise in physical education classes.

Teachers in high school have become frightened by the behavior of certain students in classrooms. These students suddenly cry or groan and appear to faint. Their bodies twitch violently for a few minutes, and saliva may appear on their lips. When the behavior subsides, the students lie quietly and relax.

Throughout recorded history, there has been evidence of health conditions with unknown origins and with no known treatments. Julius Caesar and Alfred the Great were epileptics. A century ago, many children and adults had diabetes, cerebral palsy, glaucoma, structural scoliosis, and muscular dystrophy, but little was known about these conditions. Today, some of these conditions are controlled by medical care; others have neither a definite known cause nor a treatment. They have *no* relation to the causative agents of diseases, such as bacteria, but rather, they are caused by a malfunctioning of some part of the body. Medical science continuously probes why these chronic health conditions exist, how best to provide care for victims of the conditions, and what is involved with each.

Of utmost importance in assisting any child with a chronic health condition is the acceptance of the pupil by the teacher and his classmates. A student having diabetes, for example, should have a sense of belonging within his group. To foster this acceptance, the teacher has three tasks. First, the other pupils, regardless of age level, should realize that these health conditions can occur to anyone. Second, these pupils should be informed about the different types of chronic health conditions so that misinformation cannot overrule specific health facts. Third, all persons should accept the fact that they, too, may develop a chronic health condition. When there is an epileptic pupil in the class, his classmates should be aware of the epileptic's behavior during a seizure and should be able to assist him so that he does not injure himself. Persons who are aware of their own health conditions can be better adjusted to society than can those who are unaware of their health problems.

**DIABETES MELLITUS**

As the seventh leading cause of death, diabetes is reported among 4.5 million Americans, and it is estimated that there are more than 1.6 million undetected cases in the United States. A diabetic cannot change carbohydrates into energy or store sugar for future use. These inabilities are caused by a lack of insulin, which is produced by the islands of Langerhans (clusters of cells in the pancreas). The islands of Langerhans may not produce sufficient insulin, or they may not be able to release the insulin that is produced.

Diabetes mellitus can be divided into two types: juvenile diabetes and maturity-onset diabetes. About 200,000 children and teen-agers in the United States have juvenile diabetes which must be controlled by regular insulin injections. At least 75% of all diabetics have maturity-onset diabetes, which has its clinical start after the age of 40 and is less severe than juvenile diabetes.

Recent research has revealed that hypoglycemia (an abnormally low blood sugar level) may be the first stage of some cases of diabetes. Authorities estimate that the number of persons with hypoglycemia are several times more numerous than known diabetics. In hypoglycemia, there is an excessive production of insulin. The person with chronic low blood sugar may be continuously hungry, jittery, fatigued, restless, and confused. Some diabetics have normal and even abnormally high levels of insulin since researchers believe that diabetes is not entirely due to the failure of the pancreas to produce insulin. Most cases of hypoglycemia are due to one form or another of hyperinsulinism—excessive production of insulin. Hyperinsulinism may be due to a benign or malignant tumor in the islands of Langerhans.

## Signs

Everyone should be aware of some of the possible signs of diabetes. These signs, when called to the attention of the family physician, may assist him in the diagnosis of the condition. The physician, however, is the only person who can determine whether the person has diabetes. Some signs of *possible* diabetes mellitus:

Abnormal thirst
Frequent urination
Constant hunger
Loss of weight and strength
Dry skin
Pains in the legs
Slow-healing infections
Boils on the skin at times
Sugar in the urine when a urinalysis is performed
Sugar in the blood when a blood test is given

In some cases there may be no easily recognized signs of diabetes. The person may not feel quite well, may tire easily, and have infections that are slow to heal.

An eye examination by an ophthalmologist may reveal unusual eye conditions related to diabetes.

## Medical Detection Procedures

Physicians have many procedures for determining the presence of diabetes mellitus. The procedures include a thorough medical examination, analysis of the urine, analysis of the blood, the glucose-oxidase skin test, and the glucose tolerance test. The last test measures the ability of the normal liver to absorb and store large quantities of glucose.

## Control of Diabetes

Once the physician has determined the presence of diabetes mellitus, he institutes five basic measures to *control* diabetes mellitus. These essentials are continuous medical supervision, diet, exercise, medication, and urine testing. Throughout the life of the diabetic he must maintain close and intelligent cooperation with his physician. Contrary to popular misconceptions, the diabetic usually eats the same foods as those eaten by the rest of the family. Daily diet may include lean meats and fish, cheese, eggs, vegetables, fruits, breads, cereals, milk, and butter. Some diabetics need a more restricted diet, which will be determined by the physician. It is important that the diabetic have food at regular times, such as a three-meal-a-day schedule. The daily diet should not contain extra nourishment; it should remain the same from day to day.

Exercise plays an important role in the control of diabetes mellitus, because muscular activity assists in the conversion of carbohydrates into energy. In elementary and secondary schools, the diabetic student should learn the skills of individual and dual sports, not only so that he can enjoy these sports during his schooling but also so he can continue to engage in them as an adult. Some recommended sports are tennis, golf, badminton, swimming, bowling, and archery. The diabetic should have about the same amount of exercise each day.

Insulin administered to diabetics is a preparation made from the pancreas of animals. It is given by *injection* to enable the diabetic to utilize carbohydrates. In addition to regular insulin, there are long-lasting types of insulin mixtures that enable the frequency of injections to be reduced. Sometimes these long-lasting mixtures are used alone, sometimes in combination with regular insulin. Since 1957, oral compounds have been used for mild cases of diabetes mellitus; they reduce the blood sugar to safe levels without the injection of insulin and encourage the self-active insulin-producing parts of the pancreas to secrete the necessary quantities of insulin.

Diabetic educational programs are engaged in teaching diabetics and their families the importance of continuous medical supervision, proper diet, and daily exercise; the technique for self-injection of insulin; and how to perform simple 30-second urine tests each day. Physicians instruct the diabetic in the type of urine test to do. One mother enrolling in a diabetic educational program indicated one of her teenage daughters had died of diabetes because neither the daughter or mother knew about the importance of urine testing each day.

In addition, a well-regulated life and good body hygiene are important. The diabetic's schedule should be about the same every day, although an unusual situation, such as sickness, may create changes in his diet and medication. To maintain good body hygiene, he should take every precaution to prevent infection from cuts, bruises, or other injuries. Children should receive immediate American Red Cross First Aid for wounds that might develop infection.

## Complications

The five basic essentials—medical supervision, diet, exercise, medication, and urine testing—must be followed without fail; otherwise complications result. Diabetic acidosis (diabetic coma) occurs when sugar is not burned because of an insufficient amount of insulin in the body. Signs of diabetic acidosis are nausea, vomiting, fruity breath, flushed and dry skin, deep and labored breathing, and drowsiness. The physician should be contacted, and the diabetic should go to bed. The diabetic should be kept warm and drink a cupful of hot liquid. The easiest way for the diabetic to avoid diabetic acidosis is to follow rigorously his physician's prescriptions for insulin injections or oral compounds.

An insulin reaction occurs when the diabetic takes too much insulin or too many of the oral compounds, or does not eat enough food, or waits too long to eat after taking insulin, or takes too much exercise. In other words, there is not enough sugar in the diabetic's blood. Signs of insulin reaction are mild hunger, sweating, dizziness, trembling, blurred vision, mental confusion, and shallow breathing. Most diabetics recognize the early signs of the reaction and take measures to prevent its developing into anything more serious. Eating a little sugar and drinking fruit juice are common ways to prevent insulin reaction. Physicians urge diabetics to carry lump sugar with them, as well as an identification card stating that they are diabetics. To avoid an insulin reaction, the diabetic should eat at regular hours and take his medication at the same time each day.

## Facts not Fallacies

Teachers should be aware that many misconceptions exist concerning diabetes mellitus. The teacher should be acquainted with these facts:

1. Diabetes is *not* a contagious disease.
2. Diabetes is *not* caused by eating too many sweet foods.
3. Diabetics can marry, can be employed for most occupations, and can buy life insurance.
4. Diabetics can be useful citizens living a full life.
5. There are more instances of diabetes among married women than among single women. There are more instances of diabetes among women than among men.
6. Adults who are overweight should realize that their chances of becoming diabetics are greater than those of adults who are underweight or who maintain a normal weight.
7. Heredity plays an important role in diabetes. If both parents are diabetic, all children may be diabetics. If one parent is diabetic and the other parent has a family history of diabetes, there is a 50% chance that the children will become diabetics. If neither parent has diabetes but there are histories of diabetes in the family, the children have a 25% chance of becoming diabetics.
8. Medical detection procedures, new sources of insulin, methods of con-

trolling diabetes, and facilities to assist diabetics are continuously being improved.

### What Can the Teacher Do?

A teacher has observed certain possible signs of diabetes among her pupils. What can be done to assist such pupils? According to the school system's procedures for referral medical examinations, the parents of elementary school children should be informed of signs of possible diabetes and encouraged to take the child to the family physician. The older student, in secondary school, can become acquainted with the possible signs of diabetes during a teacher-student conference. This adolescent should be encouraged to seek medical care from his family physician. Usually the nurse is sought out, and the follow-through begins. The teacher of the diabetic should be informed that her student is receiving medical care so that he can be alert for diabetic acidosis or coma and insulin reaction.

The teacher can assist the diabetic pupil by:
1. Encouraging him to participate in physical education activities
2. Being aware that the diabetic pupil can take care of himself
3. Understanding the reasons for accessibility of fruit, candy, and sugar to the diabetic pupil
4. Encouraging meticulous health habits
5. Preventing unusual physical exercise
6. Teaching facts concerning diabetes in direct health instruction
7. Giving American Red Cross First Aid to the diabetic pupil after injury

It is of utmost importance that the teacher become familiar with the basic facts concerning diabetes; he will then be able to dispel fallacies through direct health instruction.

The teacher should be aware of the five major objectives of the American Diabetes Association: professional education, patient education, diabetes detection, education, and research. The annual Diabetes Week is for the purpose of finding the "unknown" diabetics during the association's Diabetes Detection Drive.

### EPILEPSY

Most children and youth with epilepsy belong in school. Epilepsy is the only health condition where the student is more handicapped by the attitude of society than by epilepsy itself! At least 2,000,000 Americans have epilepsy. About 75% of the known cases of epilepsy are persons under 20 years of age.

"Epilepsy" is the general name given to a number of disorders of the nervous system occurring when brain cells discharge too much nervous energy into the brain. Normally, brain cells release energy in small amounts which stays limited in proper nerve channels. In epilepsy, the cells release energy in a great flood, and the energy overflows the nerve channels. The repeated releases of abnormal amounts of energy result in the *seizure*.

Epilepsy is generally divided into two forms: if there is no evidence of specific brain damage, the case is *idiopathic epilepsy*; if there is specific brain damage, the case is *symptomatic epilepsy*.

More than nine possible causes of epilepsy are given. An adverse prenatal condition which resulted in faulty development of the brain before birth may be a cause. Complications and injuries occurring during birth may be causes. Complications resulting from diseases of early childhood may injure the brain and cause a high fever. Severe or prolonged head injuries may be causes. Tumors of the brain, blood and vascular disturbances, chemical poisonings, and certain endocrine and metabolic disorders may be causes. In addition, other causes of unknown origin are listed by medical science.

Seizures occur in both sexes, at any age, and in any race. Seizures may range in severity from momentary impairment to major convulsions. Seizures are classified as *petit mal*, *grand mal*, and *psychomotor*.

Children and youth with *petit mal* epilepsy have seizures more frequently than persons with grand mal epilepsy. Seizures for petit mal last only a few seconds during which the epileptic may have a fixed staring look, and his eyebrows or eyelids may twitch. Often the petit mal seizure takes place in the midst of a conversation. The epileptic suddenly stops speaking; then, a few seconds later, he picks up where he left off. He does not seem to be the least confused by the interruption.

Pronounced behavior occurs during a

*grand mal* seizure. The epileptic appears to faint. He may cry out or groan, or he may fall down. His face turns pale, and his body twitches violently for about a minute. He may breathe deeply. Saliva may appear on his lips. He feels no pain. The epileptic relaxes and lies quietly for a few minutes. Some epileptics sleep deeply for hours after the seizure. Others may be confused after the seizure.

The epileptic undergoing a *psychomotor* seizure seems withdrawn and intent with something going on within himself. He may tug at his clothing. He is neither bothersome or angry. Often, the epileptic wanders around the room. The seizure lasts only a few minutes, and the epileptic has no recollection of what he did during the seizure.

About half of the persons with epilepsy have a definite warning, called an "aura," that a seizure is on its way. These epileptics may become nauseated or feel nauseated, or see strange lights, or hear strange sounds.

## What Can the Teacher Do?

Teachers can assist the pupil having a petit mal seizure by:

1. Being patient with the pupil during periods when he has the seizure
2. Preventing injuries to the pupil that might occur during the seizure
3. Limiting the class size in physical education
4. Supervising the epileptic closely in science and home economics laboratories, in physical education and industrial arts classes, and in group activities of the elementary school.

Teachers should be aware of the epileptic's behavior during a grand mal seizure; they can help the epileptic by:

1. Remaining calm
2. Providing a place where he can lie down, perhaps a cot behind a screened corner of the classroom
3. Staying with him during the seizure
4. Lowering him gently to the floor so that he does not hurt himself in a fall
5. Placing a pillow under his head or holding his head so that he does not injure his head
6. Moving objects out of his way as his body twitches violently

7. Guiding but *not* restraining his movements
8. Allowing him to sleep
9. Notifying the parents of a young child so that they may take the child home where he can have additional rest
10. Supervising him carefully during physical education activities
11. Informing his classmates through direct health instruction of the basic facts concerning epilepsy.

The epileptic pupil should have a sense of belonging within his group. To foster this acceptance, the teacher must let the epileptic's classmates know how he may behave during a seizure and what procedures they can follow to assist him when he undergoes the seizure. Pupils in the intermediate elementary school grades are old enough, if well instructed, to assist an epileptic who has a seizure on the school bus or on the playground.

## Additional Facts

The severity and frequency of seizures can be lessened with anticonvulsant drugs. A control diet may also be prescribed by the physician. Important to the care of the epileptic is acceptance by his family, friends, and associates.

An epileptic under continuous medical supervision can be employed for most occupations. He has a chronic health condition which he can learn about and accept, and he can adjust to the situation. Seizures may gradually become less frequent and severe with proper medical care. Most epileptic pupils can attend school and college, and they can marry and have children.

Nearly all states permit the licensing of epileptics whose seizures are controlled for driving, but the length of the seizure-free period required for qualification varies. Accidents resulting from drivers undergoing seizures are extremely rare.

Idiopathic epilepsy has been termed "genetic" as a tendency to seizures seems to be transmitted through inheritance. Even though no absolute proof of inheritance exists, it is well known that a high percentage of persons who have had the onset of their seizures in the early years of life have a family history of seizures.[1] The

[1] Inheritance of epilepsy? *Today's Health* 48 (March, 1970):20.

Epilepsy Foundation of America is one of many agencies working to eliminate social, legal, emotional, and educational barriers.

## CEREBRAL PALSY

A child with cerebral palsy is not able to control voluntary muscles effectively because of damage to the motor area of the central nervous system. There may be as many as 750,000 persons with cerebral palsy in the United States. At least 25,000 babies are born with cerebral palsy each year.

Damage to the motor area of the central nervous system is likely to occur before, during, and just after the birth of the baby. There is mounting evidence that the lack of oxygen in the unborn child's brain is often among the primary reasons for cerebral palsy. The brain of the unborn child is sensitive to the lack of oxygen and to any interference with circulation of blood in the brain tissues. Other probable causes of damage are birth injuries, Rh incompatibility between the mother and unborn child, infection of the mother with German measles during the first three months of pregnancy, and faulty development of brain cells before birth.

Damage to the motor area of the brain may interfere with normal walking, running, writing, or talking. Damage may impair the body's balancing mechanism so that one set of muscles does not counter another set. About 33% of persons with cerebral palsy have speech problems; at least 16% have hearing defects; and about 62% suffer from emotional stress.

There are different types of cerebral palsy, and mixed types are common. The most common types are *spastic, athetoid, ataxic, tremorous,* and *rigid*. Spastics, the largest group of patients, have tense, contracted muscles. The athetoid individual lacks control and makes many unorganized and involuntary movements. The athetoid and spastic cases account for more than 75% of those afflicted. The ataxic person has a disturbed sense of equilibrium which causes many falls. The tremorous individual has a rhythmic pattern of uncontrolled movements or shaking which makes the use of his hands and feet difficult. In rigid cerebral palsy, stiffness due to muscle contraction makes the victim

slow-moving. A CP child may be spastic and ataxic, or of mixed type.

One or more of the limbs may be affected. Monoplegia involves one limb and is rare. Paraplegia involves the legs only and usually is the spastic or rigid type. Hemiplegia affects the arm and the leg on one side and usually is the athetoid type. Triplegia (involving both legs and one arm) and quadraplegia (affecting all four extremities) usually are the spastic type.

Much can be done to help the child with cerebral palsy. Certain types of surgery, new medications, eyeglasses, hearing aids, braces and other specially designed aids, and physical and speech therapy help the cerebral palsy patient. Many people work with the child having cerebral palsy: physician, teacher, physical therapist, special education personnel, speech therapist, and psychologist to name a few.

Bakwin and Bakwin[2] list conditions favorable to the development of a socially acceptable personality in the child. He should experience friendship, affection, and acceptance. He should not be expected to assume too much responsibility, yet not be too dependent. He should have a permanent home so that he is not changing schools throughout his school years, thus, finding his niche among friends. The child should have the opportunity for new experiences and receive help as he adjusts to new situations. He should be able to succeed within the limits of his type of cerebral palsy. He should have ample chance to use his energy. Last, the child with cerebral palsy should have a sense of responsibility, be independent, have courage, and develop a social sense.

The United Cerebral Palsy Associations, Inc., have as their goal a long-range attack on the entire problem of cerebral palsy. They help to provide treatment, care, and education, and they provide training for employment and find jobs for the cerebral palsied.

## VISION DEFECTS

By the end of the fifth grade 80% of children have some type of visual difficulty

[2]Harry Bakwin and Ruth M. Bakwin: *Clinical Management of Behavior Disorders in Children.* 3rd ed. Philadelphia: W. B. Saunders Company, 1966, p. 153.

Most eye defects occur between the ages of one to seven years. About four million Americans have some degree of amblyopia. Each year, the eyes of about 100,000 children are damaged beyond help of treatment. Unfortunately, very little information concerning vision defects is found in public school textbooks.

## Amblyopia ex anopsia

Amblyopia ex anopsia or "lazy eye blindness" is a dimness of vision from the disuse or nonuse of an eye. Children may have a tendency to amblyopia at birth or may acquire it soon afterwards. Amblyopia may be due to muscular imbalance, refractive error, or other visual defect when the infant is still learning to focus his eyes. If the child sees a double image, he tends to use the stronger eye and suppress the weaker one. The vision in the weaker eye fails to develop properly or is lost.

Before the child reaches the age of six, the central part of the eye which discriminates small details should develop. Thus, the child with improper development due to amblyopia cannot read because he cannot discriminate one word or letter from another word or letter. The child can see with the weak eye, but details of vision that should appear in sharp focus are lost. Amblyopia tends to get slowly worse until the child's eyes reach a certain point in their development. Amblyopia does not improve without medical treatment.

If amblyopia is discovered before the age of three, treatment is successful. After the age of six, treatment provides improvement for only a small percentages of cases. Thus, all children should have an eye examination at the age of three or earlier. Correction of amblyopia in a young child consists of placing the good eye at an optical disadvantage and forcing the child to use the weak eye. Continual use of the weak eye helps to improve it only if the treatment is started in time. Normal vision may be recovered. However, after vision has been recovered, the basic cause, such as muscular imbalance or other visual defect, must be corrected. If not corrected, double vision will return.[3]

## Strabismus

Strabismus, squint, or "crossed eyes" does not correct itself as the child grows older. Vision in the crossed eye will fail to develop, and the child will be partially blind without knowing it. In strabismus, external eye muscles do not function correctly in focusing both eyes on an object at the same time. There are three types of strabismus: (1) crossed eyes in which the eye turns inward; (2) wall eyes in which the eye turns outward; and (3) vertical in which the eye turns upward. The student with strabismus has double vision because he receives two images, and he has no depth perception. Usually he gives up trying to see with both eyes and subconsciously eliminates the image in one eye. If detected and treated early, strabismus can be corrected by an ophthalmologist.

## Retinitis pigmentosa

In childhood, retinitis pigmentosa produces its first sign, night blindness, which gradually decreases the ability to see at night. Later side vision is lost, and the adult has "tunnel vision." Changes in the retina include an overgrowth of supporting connective tissue and atrophy of blood vessels and the part of the optic nerve which passes through the retina. An ophthalmologist can detect retinitis pigmentosa by using an ophthalmoscope to look into the interior of the eye. If black pigment deposits are scattered around the edges of the retina and throughout the retina, retinitis pigmentosa is present. No known treatment can halt the progress of retinitis pigmentosa. Adults, with medical supervision, can usually keep their reading vision throughout their lives, even though the reading vision is restricted to a small central part of the visual field. Some cases of retinitis pigmentosa result in total blindness.[4]

## Glaucoma

Ophthalmologists, until recently, conducted screening surveys to detect glaucoma only in persons over 40 years of age. Today, they hope to detect susceptibility to glaucoma at an early age before permanent changes have taken place in the eye. Ten-

---

National Institute of Neurological Disease and Blindness: *Eye Research.* 1967, pp. 37-38.

[4] *Ibid.,* pp. 17-18.

dency towards glaucoma can be detected in childhood.

Glaucoma is an intense intraocular pressure of the eyeball and cupping of the optic disc. Within the aqueous chamber of the eyeball is a watery fluid, the aqueous humor. Most of the fluid drains through the canal of Schlemm, which is located at the junction of the sclera and cornea. The absorption and escape of this fluid must be at the same rate so that the pressure within the eyeball remains constant. If the pressure does not remain constant, the optic

cruciating headache and vomiting since the pressure inside the eye rises to a dangerous level in a matter of hours. The pressure must be reduced immediately, or blindness may result. The standard medical treatment for acute glaucoma is surgery. *Chronic* glaucoma occurs with its victim usually unaware of its development. There is no pain, and the loss of side vision is gradual. *Secondary* glaucoma is related to infection, injury, tumor, or cataract (lens become opaque or foggy). Infection may occur in the iris, ciliary body, or choroid. Injury to

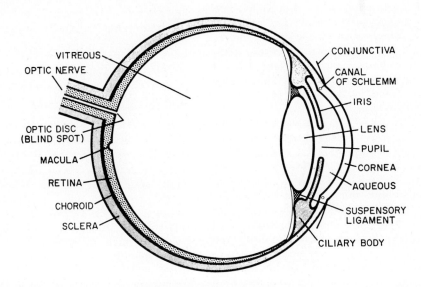

Figure 12. Cross section of the eye

disc will show a "cupping" caused by pressure from the front of the eyeball. As the optic disc is the site of entrance of optic nerves into the retina, any damage to the optic disc affects the retina. There are several reasons why the pressure does not remain constant: (1) the iris may be pushed too close to the cornea; (2) the canal of Schlemm may be obstructed; (3) an infection, tumor, or cataract may hinder the escape of the aqueous humor, and (4) the structure of the eyeball may not permit the escape of the aqueous humor.

There are four types of glaucoma. *Infantile* glaucoma occurs at birth or during the first years of life and is recessively inherited. Blindness can occur if medical treatment does not halt the progression of glaucoma. *Acute* glaucoma causes an ex-

the eyeball may cause malfunctioning of the canal of Schlemm. A tumor within the anterior portion of the eyeball may obstruct the passage of aqueous humor. A cataract may change the structure of the lens to such a degree that the flow of aqueous humor may be blocked.

A family history of glaucoma should alert everyone to the signs of glaucoma. No one sign would mean glaucoma. Any loss of side vision, seeing rainbow halos around lights, eye aches after seeing movies or television in the dark, unexplained pain in and around the eyes, fuzzy or blurred vision which comes and goes, watering of the eye, and any change in eye color are some of the signs of glaucoma.

Instruments which measure the intraocular pressure are used by the ophthamologist in diagnosing glaucoma. The most commonly used instrument is Schiotz' tonometer. The ophthalmologist drops a local anesthetic in each eye. The patient sits in a chair with his head tipped back or the patient lies down. The ophthalmologist carefully places the tonometer on each eyeball because the pressure differs in the right and left eye. Usually, the ophthalmologist will ask the patient to return for other pressure readings. Other instruments used to measure intraocular pressure are the applanation tonometer and tonograph, a four-minute continuous recording of the pressure.

In some communities, public health personnel and physicians have established clinics to assist in the detection of glaucoma. Early detection of glaucoma can prevent blindness. A person with glaucoma will need continuous medical supervision by an ophthalmologist to prevent further damage to the optic disc and retina by some form of medication or by surgery.

It is imperative that through direct health instruction the student be made to realize that blindness from glaucoma can be prevented. However, the glaucoma must be detected early, because sight destroyed by glaucoma cannot be restored. Glaucoma has no relation to cancer or to high blood pressure. Glaucoma is not contagious, and it is not caused by too much reading. Excessive intake of fluids or smoking can cause additional harm to those who have glaucoma.[5,6]

## Dyslexia

Two types of dyslexia are common: congenital, or developmental, and secondary. Congenital, or developmental, dyslexia is a reading disability which probably is a dysfunction, possibly genetic in origin, in males of average or above-average intelligence, due to a neurological deficit in that area of the brain which receives the visual image. Secondary dyslexias are due to such factors as (1) brain damage as in cerebral palsy; (2) hyperactivity with accompanying short attention span; (3) anx-

iety, depression, emotional disturbances; and (4) environmental conditions such as cultural and economic deprivations with poor exposure to reading, language, and knowledge.[7]

The dyslexic child may suffer from a muscle imbalance or a refractive error such as myopia, which can be corrected. Rarely does a visual defect produce dyslexia, but a visual defect often accompanies dyslexia.

The National Society for the Prevention of Blindness is the oldest voluntary health agency nationally engaged in the prevention of blindness. The Society's comprehensive program includes community service, public and professional education, and research. The Society emphasizes community glaucoma detection, preschool and school vision screening, and school and industrial eye safety.

## HEARING DEFECTS

At least 15 million adults and three million children have a hearing loss of some degree. Very few children are totally deaf. A hearing loss should be discovered before the child reaches school age.

There are three common types of deafness: conductive, perceptive, and mixed. *Conductive* deafness is caused by an obstruction of sound vibrations. The obstruction may be brought about by dirt and wax in the outer ear canal, adhesions, scar tissue, perforations of the eardrum, an abscess in the middle ear, or congestion of the eustachian tube. Infected tonsils, complications following measles or pneumonia, chronic sinusitis, or repeated sore throats may bring about the conditions leading to the obstruction of sound vibrations. Many cases of conductive deafness are attributed to the victim's early disregard of noises in the head, dull pain in the ear, and diminished hearing, as well as neglect of ear infections.

*Perceptive* deafness is due to abnormality or disease of the inner ear. It may be either congenital or acquired. There is no cure for perceptive deafness since segments of the auditory nerve are destroyed. If a woman has German measles during the

*id.*, pp. 11-13.
National Society for the Prevention of Blindness: *Glaucoma*. New York: The Society, 1969; and Everett Kiers: *So You Have Glaucoma*. New York: Grune & Stratton, Inc., 1958.

[7]Arthur H. Keeney and Virginia T. Keeney, eds.: *Dyslexia Diagnosis and Treatment of Reading Disorders.* St. Louis: The C. V. Mosby Company, 1968, pp. 49, 175.

first three months of pregnancy, her child may be born with a congenital hearing loss. Toxins produced by focal infections, such as pyorrhea, or resulting from diseases, such as influenza, can damage the nerve endings of the inner ear. Other diseases which may damage the nerve endings are meningitis, scarlet fever, whooping cough, and typhoid fever. Accidents, such as birth injuries and skull fractures, may injure the nerve endings of the inner ear. Certain drugs and high body temperature also can produce perceptive deafness.

Many persons with poor hearing have *mixed* loss—a combination of conductive and perceptive deafness.

Any sign of a hearing difficulty in children and teenagers should be called to the attention of the parents and the family physician. If preventive measures are taken as soon as the hearing difficulty is detected, the degree of hearing loss may be reduced. The National Association of Hearing and Speech Agencies promotes high standards of professional service and of community organization in identification, diagnosis and assessment, treatment, rehabilitation, education, and research in the various areas of communication disorders.

## SEVERE POSTURE CONDITIONS

Structural scoliosis is a severe lateral spinal deviation. It may be a result of vitamin deficiency (rickets or osteomalacia), polio, or other causes. The resulting effects may be a C-shaped left-total curve, an S-shaped combined curve, or right lumbar curvature. In the C-shaped left-total curve, the left shoulder is high; *or* the left shoulder is high and the left hip is prominent. With the S-shaped combined curve, the left shoulder is high with the right hip prominent *or* the right shoulder is high with the left hip prominent. In right lumbar curvature, the right hip is prominent. Functional scoliosis is caused by poor walking, standing, and sitting posture.

Occasionally, anterior-posterior curvatures of the spine can be severe. In kyphosis, there may be an extreme curvature in the thoracic region of the spine. In lordosis, there may be an extreme curvature in the lumbar region of the spine. These anterior-posterior curvatures may be the result of a slumped walking posture, shoulder blades pushed forward, a protruding abdomen, or sinking at the hips.

In all severe posture conditions, treatment by the family physician and an orthopedic physician is indispensable. Because posture conditions can affect the physiological functions as well as the mental health of the patient, they need expert medical care.

## MUSCULAR DYSTROPHY

At least 200,000 persons in the United States have some degree of muscular dystrophy. Males are affected five to six times as often as females. Muscular dystrophy can begin at any age. Children afflicted early in childhood rarely live to adulthood.

Muscular dystrophy is a progressive wasting of muscles, particularly skeletal muscles. The teacher may notice that a small boy may waddle as he walks with his abdomen sticking out. Later, the boy finds he has trouble getting to his feet after playing on the floor. He must "climb up his legs" to stand up. He teaches himself to roll over on his abdomen, get up on his hands and knees, and "climb up his legs" with his hands. Then, he can stand up. Other signs of muscular dystrophy are enlarged calf muscles which are abnormally weak. The arms are limp because the muscles of the shoulder girdle are weak.

The family physician can determine muscular dystrophy from clear-cut signs and from the health history of the patient and family. The patient's muscle reactions and movements are observed as a part of an extensive medical examination, and laboratory tests of the blood and urine are completed. Often the family physician will refer his patient to a neurologist. Biopsy of tissue from a big muscle, x-ray of a muscle, and an electromyograph (which records electrical activity in the muscles) may be used in diagnosis. At times, muscular dystrophy is difficult to diagnose.

Muscular dystrophy may be classified as (1) childhood; (2) juvenile; or (3) facioscapulohumeral. Childhood muscular dystrophy affects more boys than girls. It usually attacks when the boy is about three years old. The boy has enormous calf muscles. Juvenile muscular dystrophy may begin in childhood, but it more often begins in adolescence. Both sexes are equally affected. The muscle-wasting starts in the shoulder girdle affecting the use of the arms and in the pelvic girdle affecting the use of the legs. Facioscapulohumeral mucular dystrophy may appear in either sex during childhood or adolescence. Muscles of the face, shoulders, and upper arm are affected. Weak facial muscles may be the only sign of muscular dystrophy. The child may not be able to drink through a straw or to whistle. The child has a "flat" smile because of the weak face muscles which cannot raise the corners of his mouth.

Rare types and mixed types of muscular dystrophy also occur. The usual patient can continue to use his fingers even though he will probably be confined to a wheel chair eventually.

Treatment, especially by a physical therapist, is intended to keep the patient active as long as it is possible. Parents can learn simple physical therapy methods to help the dystrophic child.[8]

The Muscular Dystrophy Associations of America, Inc., provide assistance to patients needing braces, wheelchairs, and invalid-lifts. Also, local chapters organize transportation for the dystrophic child to and from clinics, schools, and recreational facilities. They also provide funds for research to determine the cause of muscular dystrophy and to find effective methods in the care of the dystrophic patients.

## IMPLICATIONS FOR HEALTH EDUCATION

One of the areas of health education is "Chronic Health Conditions." Units in this area might be:

    Unit: Diabetes mellitus
    Unit: Epilepsy
    Unit: Cerebral palsy
    Unit: Amblyopia ex anopsia, strabismus, and retinitis pigmentosa
    Unit: Glaucoma

National Institutes of Health: *Muscular Dystrophy, Hope Through Research.* 1968, pp. 1-22.

Unit: Conductive and perceptive deafness
Unit: Muscular dystrophy

Other chronic conditions to be discussed might be cystic fibrosis, myasthenia gravis, Parkinson's disease, multiple sclerosis, asthma, inflammatory neuromyopathies, PKU (phenylketonuria), mental retardation, and speech defects. Unfortunately, units from this area of health education too often have been omitted or casually discussed so that the public school student does not accept the person with the chronic health condition, does not realize that these health conditions can occur to anyone, and has misinformation based on fear and prejudice about these chronic health conditions.

## References for Further Study

American Public Health Association: *Services for Children with Cerebral Palsy.* New York: The Association, 1968.

Cruickshank, W.: *Cerebral Palsy—Its Individual and Community Problem.* Syracuse, N.Y.: Syracuse University Press, 1966.

Duncan, G.: *Modern Pilgrim's Progress with Further Revelations for Diabetics.* 2nd ed. Philadelphia: W. B. Saunders Company, 1967.

Epilepsy Foundation of America: *You, Your Child and Epilepsy.* Washington, D.C.: The Foundation, 1968.

Ford, F.: *Diseases of the Nervous System in Infancy, Childhood, and Adolescence.* 5th ed. Springfield, Ill.: Charles C Thomas, 1966.

Keats, S.: *Cerebral Palsy.* Springfield, Ill.: Charles C Thomas, 1965.

Mecham, M., et al.: *Communication Training in Childhood Brain Damage.* Springfield, Ill.: Charles C Thomas, 1966.

Rosenthal, H., and Rosenthal, J.: *Diabetic Care in Pictures.* 4th ed. Philadelphia: J. B. Lippincott Company, 1968.

Schmitt, G.: *Diabetes for Diabetics: A Practical Guide.* Miami, Fla.: Diabetes Press of America, n.d.

Scott, D.: *About Epilepsy.* New York: International Universities Press, 1969.

Schulman, J., et al.: *Brain Damage and Behavior.* Springfield, Ill.: Charles C Thomas, 1965.

United States Public Health Service: *Diabetes Source Book,* 1969.

Waife, S., ed.: *Diabetes Mellitus.* Indianapolis: Eli Lilly and Company, 1967.

# Chapter 7

# *EMERGENCY CARE*

## AN INCIDENT

At a meeting of teachers and principals, some questions have been asked about procedures to be followed when a pupil is injured or ill. Teachers and principals are aware that they are *in loco parentis* during school hours and that they share the responsibility of the pupil's care with the parent. Is the teacher considered negligent if the teacher did not give American Red Cross First Aid to the injured or ill pupil? Is the teacher considered negligent if the teacher did not anticipate risks which caused the pupil's injury? Is the teacher considered negligent if no reasonable steps were taken to prevent the pupil from being exposed to those risks? Is the teacher considered negligent if the care given to the injured pupil aggravated the severity of the injury?

A pupil's illness or injury raises many questions concerning the care of the pupil, notifying the parents, medical attention, transportation of the pupil to his home or family physician, recording of first aid procedures followed by the teacher, and the role of the school nurse. School personnel must be able to provide emergency care in order to avoid legal liability for negligence.

## TORT LIABILITY

Negligence is defined as "the failure to act as a reasonably prudent and careful person would under the circumstances involved."[1] This definition is used to measure teacher conduct whether the teacher

failed to do something to avoid the pupil's injury or whether the teacher was acting carelessly, ignorantly, or ineptly. There is no legal negligence unless an injury has occurred.

*Torts* are injuries or civil wrongs between common citizens for which the injured person has a claim for compensation. Tort liability is of far greater concern among teachers than other forms of liability. The National Commission on Safety Education clearly states the differences between negligence of commission and omission. In *negligence of commission*, there is unreasonable risk of harm even though the act is done with reasonable care, preparation, skill, and warning. In *negligence of omission*, there is lack of care, preparation, skill, or warning resulting in injury.[2] Liability for acts of negligence of either type is not disregarded by the courts simply because the teacher is employed by a governmental agency (the board of education). Tort liability for injuries occurring to pupils can involve any school employee. Bird[3] has placed the liability status of states into four general categories: (1) immunity from liability; (2) general immunity from liability for governmental functions (3) permission to purchase liability insurance with immunity waived up to amount of insurance; and (4) abrogated immunity.

The courts have indicated that a teacher has the duty to exercise reasonable care and prudence. If the teacher is negligent

[1]Harry N. Rosenfield: *Liability for School Accidents.* New York: Harper and Brothers, 1940, p. 3.

[2]National Commission on Safety Education: *Who is Liable for Pupil Injuries?* Washington, D.C.: National Education Association, 1963, p. 11.
[3]Patrick J. Bird: Tort liability. *J. Health, Physical Education and Recreation 41* (January, 1970):38.

and a pupil is injured, the teacher may be found liable, as any private person would be under similar circumstances. Because the teacher is employed by a board of education, it is often argued that any liability need not rest solely on the teacher but may also be placed upon the board of education. Many states have so-called "save harmless" statutes in the event a teacher is held liable for injury to a pupil from acts in the teacher's "line of service." The legislation has been created so that the teacher does not bear the full brunt of financial loss from damages awarded the plaintiff.

With few exceptions, a school district, as an agency of the state, has been immune from liability in damages for pupil injuries resulting from negligence of school employees. However, recently there has been a trend to apply this immunity doctrine *only* when boards of education, as the governing bodies of school districts, prepare, publish, and impose standards of care by reasonable and prudent teachers.

## WRITTEN EMERGENCY CARE PROCEDURES

Boards of education must prepare, publish, and enforce written emergency care procedures. When a pupil becomes ill or is injured, the teacher is expected to give proper American Red Cross First Aid, notify the parents, seek medical care if needed, arrange transportation to the physician or to the pupil's home, and provide information regarding the emergency care procedures on a permanent record. If the teacher follows all these regulations, the teacher is not negligent. If the teacher provides no emergency care or inadequate emergency care, there is the possibility of the teacher's liability for negligence.

The following information for all students should be accessible to the teacher: the student's home address and telephone number, the hours when at least one parent is usually at home, the parents' business addresses and telephone numbers, and the family physician's address and telephone number. There should also be a roster of teachers with their daily activities and the pupils' daily class schedules. Information concerning students, parents, and physicians should be in each teacher's classroom or laboratory.

At the beginning of each school year, the parents should sign a *waiver* permitting school personnel to transport the pupil to a physician if the pupil needs medical care and the parents cannot be reached. Waivers should be similar in content for grades 1 through 12, be filed in a central location, and dated for a period of one year.

## GENERAL DIRECTIONS

When providing emergency care, non-medically prepared school personnel must not attempt to diagnose an illness or injury. Emergency care for a pupil must be restricted to American Red Cross First Aid. Internal medication is avoided.

Most schools have forbidden school personnel to use antiseptics, internal medications relieving pain, and stimulants. In rare instances, however, a student's family physician may prescribe the use of antiseptics, medication, and stimulants, and the directions for their use. In these cases, written directions are forwarded to the school or public health nurse from the physician. School personnel must *not* give pupils headache tablets, laxatives, painkillers, or home remedies.

If a pupil refuses emergency care, parents should be notified and assume their responsibilities. In these instances, the teacher must decide if the illness or injury is serious enough to warrant immediate American Red Cross First Aid or immediate medical care regardless of the pupil's wishes.

Emergency care for the ill or injured pupil may be needed for a wide range of illnesses and injuries. Illnesses and injuries common to school-age children will be discussed in this chapter. Detailed instructions for possible illness and injury should be familiar to school personnel. Prevention of further illness or injury, relief from pain, proper transportation, and placing the responsibility for treatment with the physician are important. American Red Cross First Aid is intended only for immediate and temporary care until medical care is provided.

In Chapter 4, procedures for the isolation and exclusion of the pupil having communicable diseases and his readmission to school were discussed. These measures of

| Emergency | Description |
|---|---|
| ucts, petroleum products, rat poisons, etc. | and vomiting, visual disturbances, headache, convulsions, and deep sleep. Breath odor may reveal poison. |
| Rabid animal bite | Puncture wound; teeth marks on skin; saliva around wound. Bites on face, neck, and head especially dangerous; bites through clothing, such as a coat sleeve, not as dangerous as bites on exposed skin surface. |
| Shock | Failure of normal circulation of blood, creating depression of all body functions. |
| Skin irritations caused by poisonous plants, such as poison ivy, oak, and sumac | Small, swelling, red itchy spots; blisters. |
| Snake bite | |
| Nonpoisonous | Scratches rather than puncture wound; some pain; no swelling; marks of upper teeth; no large fang holes. |
| Poisonous Copperhead, coral snake, cotton-mouth (or water moccasin), rattlesnake | Puncture wound; swelling; discoloration. One or two large fang holes. There may or may not be marks of upper teeth. Victim shows general weakness, nausea and vomiting, shortness of breath, rapid and weak pulse, and possible dimness of vision. Possible unconsciousness. |
| Sprain | Violent stretching or twisting of a joint, causing partial or complete tears of some supporting ligaments of that joint. Swelling; pain on motion; tenderness; discoloration. |
| Strain | Overstretching or overexertion of a muscle or tendon. Soreness and stiffness of a muscle or muscles. |
| Unconsciousness—cause unknown | Person unconscious; may or may not be breathing. |
| Vomiting | Expulsion of matter from the stomach through the mouth. |
| Wounds | Break in the skin or mucous membrane. |
| Abrasion | Skin or mucous membrane rubbed or scraped off. |
| Incised | Straight, sharp cut; bleeds freely. |
| Lacerated | Jagged or torn, having extensive tissue damage. |
| Puncture | Deep, penetrating wound. |
| Gunshot | Small surface wound. Bullet may be deep or close to skin surface. Bullet may cause bone fracture. Extensive wound in some cases. |

## AMERICAN RED CROSS FIRST AID

School personnel should be encouraged to complete American Red Cross First Aid preparation. When a pupil is asphyxiated, the mouth-to-mouth method of artificial respiration cannot be successful if used by someone who has merely read the directions from a textbook. Previous practice is essential, because the pupil's life depends on correctly administered artificial respiration. School personnel should be able correctly to control bleeding by digital pressure at designated pressure points, by direct pressure, or by a tourniquet. A pupil with a broken leg should be given American Red Cross First Aid for the fracture until a physician arrives. Competence in performing the procedures for the first aid

care of fractures, as well as for all American Red Cross First Aid techniques, cannot be acquired from a textbook, but must be practiced over a period of time. American Red Cross First Aid courses provide opportunities to learn and to practice the proper procedures. For every six members of the school staff, three should have had recent American Red Cross First Aid courses.

## PARENTS NOTIFIED

Following administration of American Red Cross First Aid, the teacher must notify the pupil's parents of the illness or injury. The notification is usually by telephone and the conversation should be informative but not dramatic. The teacher should describe the signs of the illness or the nature of the injury, inform the parents that American Red Cross First Aid has been given, and stress the need for further medical care. During the conversation, the teacher will determine the method of transportation—whether school personnel will take the pupil to his home, to the family physician, or to a hospital, or whether the parent will come to the school for the pupil. The teacher should inform the parents that he will telephone them the next day to inquire about the pupil's condition.

## TRANSPORTATION OF THE PUPIL AND THE NURSE'S ROLE

Occasionally, school personnel must transport the pupil to his home. A member of the instructional or administrative staff who has a free period may do this. If a secondary school youth is injured or becomes ill, he should be provided with some form of transportation from school and should not be allowed to go home by himself.

Whenever a pupil is injured or becomes ill, the teacher should notify the school nurse. The nurse can then visit the pupil's home to check on parental care and to ascertain when the pupil will return to school. In secondary schools, the follow-through might be a telephone call rather than a home visit.

## EMERGENCY CARE RECORD

Immediately after the emergency is over, the pertinent data should be recorded on the emergency care record. When there is no school nurse, one copy is filed in the principal's office and another copy in the teacher's desk. If there is a school nurse on the staff, an additional copy should be filed in her office. A sample emergency care record is shown on page 92. Many state departments of health and school districts have developed emergency care records.

## FIRST AID SUPPLIES

For proper emergency care there must be adequate first aid supplies available. Lists of recommended supplies can be found in the *American Red Cross First Aid Textbook*. Similar lists have also been developed by state departments of health,

and some have been published by the Joint Committee on Health Problems in Education of the NEA and the AMA.

## SUMMARY OF PROCEDURES

For proper emergency care of an ill or injured pupil, these procedures are recommended:

1. Procedures of emergency care for the ill or injured pupil should be known to all school personnel

| For Illness | For Injury |
|---|---|
| a. Be aware of the possible types of illness occurring to the pupil | a. Be aware of the possible types of injuries occurring to the pupil |
| b. Recognize the signs of the particular illness | b. Recognize the signs of the particular injury |
| c. Give appropriate ARC First Aid for the particular illness | c. Give appropriate ARC First Aid for the particular injury |

   d. Notify the parent
   e. Secure medical or hospital care if needed
   f. Provide transportation so that the pupil can reach his home or family physician
   g. Follow-through
   h. Emergency care record

2. Continuous evaluation of the effectiveness of these procedures is made by school personnel.
3. Revision of these procedures follows evaluation.

In order to inform all school personnel about specific procedures for emergency care, an "Emergency Care Handbook" should be provided by the school administration. Procedures for a particular elementary school or high school should be considered in the light of specific factors, such as, the proximity of hospitals. Some of the procedures will involve details that need to be agreed on by all school personnel; for example, if school personnel-owned automobiles are to be used for transporting a pupil, they might be covered by special insurance paid by the local board of education. The particular days and hours that the drivers of these automobiles are available for emergency care purposes should also be known to school personnel.

PUBLIC SCHOOL
_____

STATE

EMERGENCY CARE RECORD

Name of Student _____ Age _____ Sex _____

Home Address _____ Phone _____

Student's Teacher _____ Grade _____

Location and Time of Accident or Illness _____
_____
_____

Possible Cause of Illness or Injury _____
_____
_____

Description of Illness _____
_____
_____

Description of Injury (Part of body injured, degree of injury) _____
_____
_____

American Red Cross First Aid Rendered for the Accident or Illness _____
_____
_____

Notification of Parents _____ at home _____ at business _____

Transportation of the Student to His Home? _____

To His Family Physician? _____ To a Cooperating

Physician _____ To the Hospital? _____

Have the Parents Been Encouraged to Seek Medical Care? _____

Has the Follow-through Taken Place? _____

Comments Upon the Accident or Illness _____

WITNESSES PRESENT:   Name and Address _____

Name and Address _____

Date_____ Your Signature_____

(Use other side of this record for additional comments)

Figure 13

## IMPLICATIONS FOR HEALTH EDUCATION

Emergency care is especially relevant to two areas of health education: "American Red Cross First Aid" and "Safety Education." Some suggested units are:

Other units from the area of safety education may be suggested from accidents occurring on the playground from bicycling, indicating a unit on bicycle safety; or high incidence of accidents among high school students riding motorcycles indi-

| Type of emergency | Area of health education | Unit from the area |
|---|---|---|
| Serious bleeding | American Red Cross First Aid | Wounds and control of bleeding |
| Fracture of the lower arm | American Red Cross First Aid | Fractures and ARC First Aid |
| Snake bite | American Red Cross First Aid | Poisonous and nonpoisonous snake bites and ARC First Aid |
| Sprained ankle | American Red Cross First Aid | Injuries to bones and muscles (other than fractures) and ARC First Aid |
| Poisoning by mouth | American Red Cross First Aid | Poisoning and ARC First Aid |
| Burns from the use of chemicals | Safety Education | Proper handling of chemicals |
| Gunshot wound | Safety Education | Gun safety |
| Lacerated wounds | Safety Education | Self-preservation in event of tornado |
| Falls | Safety Education | Accidents in the school |

cating a unit on motorcycle safety; or panic seen at an unscheduled fire drill and need for a unit on fire drills at school.

## References for Further Study

American Medical Association: *First Aid Manual.* Chicago: The Association, 1967.

Brennan, W., and Ludwig, D. J.: *Guide to Problems and Practices in First Aid and Civil Defense.* Dubuque, Iowa: Wm. C. Brown Company, 1971.

Byrd, O.: *School Health Administration.* Philadelphia: W. B. Saunders Company, 1964.

Florio, A. E., and Stafford, G.: *Safety Education.* 3rd ed. New York: McGraw-Hill Book Company, 1969.

Gauerke, W. E.: *School Law.* New York: Center for Applied Research in Education, Inc., 1965.

Henderson, J.: *Emergency Medical Guide.* 2nd ed. New York: McGraw-Hill Book Company, 1969.

Joint Committee on Health Problems in Education of the National Education Association and the American Medical Association: *School Health Services.* Washington, D.C.: National Education Association, 1964.

Leibee, H.: *Tort Liability for Injuries to Pupils.* Ann Arbor, Mich.: Campus Publishers, 1966.

Lewis, A. M., ed.: *Immediate Care of the Sick and Injured.* Sedgwick County, Kansas: Kansas Medical Society and Medical Society of Sedgwick County, 1966.

Mayshark, C., and Shaw, D. D.: *Administration of School Health Programs.* St. Louis: The C. V. Mosby Company, 1967.

National Safety Council: *Accident Facts.* Chicago: The Council, yearly.

Seaton, D., Stack, H., and Loft, B.: *Administration and Supervision of Safety Education.* New York: The Macmillan Company, 1968.

Stack, H., and Elkow, J. D.: *Education for Safe Living.* 4th ed. Englewood Cliffs, N.J.: Prentice-Hall, Inc., 1966.

Strasser, M., Aaron, J., Bohn, R., and Eales, J.: *Fundamentals of Safety Education.* New York: The Macmillan Company, 1964.

United States Public Health Service: *Emergency Health Services Selected Bibliography.* 1970.

# Chapter 8

# HEALTH OF
# SCHOOL PERSONNEL

## AN INCIDENT

A new teacher has been told that she must have a medical examination and chest x-ray by her family physician before receiving a teaching contract. She had never been required to have a medical examination or chest x-ray to enter college, before student teaching, or previous to other employment. She sees no reason to comply with the request for a medical examination and chest x-ray.

At a teachers' meeting, the new teacher has been asked to join the group health insurance plan for hospital services and medical-surgical services. She has indicated that she has no need for these plans since she never had these plans previously. What can the other teachers do?

All those employed by a local board of education should be considered school personnel, including teachers, principals, superintendents, counselors, supervisors or consultants, secretaries, clerks, nurses, physicians, dental hygienists, school lunch workers, custodians, matrons, bus drivers, and other school personnel. Special school personnel may be part-time employees, nurses employed by the local health department, medical and dental specialists, psychometrists and psychologists, and school social workers. None of these personnel should be excused from adhering to regulations promoting the physical and mental health of employees. Established by the board of education, these regulations are formulated to promote the welfare of the total school population, and no one, despite length of employment, salary, or legal status, should be considered exempt from their requirements.

In this chapter, the health of the teaching and administrative staffs will be stressed, even though health requirements for other school personnel will be included. Thus the college health program, preservice teacher education, health requirements of school employees, and welfare practices will be mentioned.

## COLLEGE HEALTH PROGRAM

The college health program consists of college health services, healthful college living, and health education. College health services are usually administered by student health centers. Healthful college living encompasses the total environment encountered by the student and its effects on the student's physical and mental health. Health education relates to the basic college health education course for all students *and* professional school health education courses for all prospective teachers.

Since 1920, the American College Health Association has participated in programs designed to improve the health of *all* college students. Today's college student has available well-staffed and well-organized student health centers with diversified services. Clinical medicine, as now practiced in our student health centers, includes services by those in many medical specialties, such as otorhinolaryngology, allergy, dermatology, urology, gastroenterology, proctology, psychiatry, and orthopedics. It is possible that, in the future, college medicine *per se* will become a medical specialty.

Not only the student's illnesses, injuries, and psychological problems but also the student's environment are of growing interest to the staffs of our student health centers. It is possible, for example, that environmental conditions are unsanitary or contribute to accidents. The staff must consider not only where the student lives but also where he dines, attends classes, studies, participates in physical education, and enjoys his leisure time on the campus. Thus, staffs of student health centers have joined forces with staffs of student life activities, administrative personnel and faculty, and counseling and guidance services to eradicate any campus environmental causes of student illness, injury, or emotional problems.

The American College Health Association has indicated that there are 19 services and activities of health programs. These services and activities include outpatient services, provisions for emergencies or disasters, inpatient services, record-keeping, laboratory services, radiological services, pharmacy (medication) services, mental health, athletic medicine, dental services, rehabilitation or physical medicine, health promotion or preventive medicine, environmental health and safety, occupational health, health education, research, communications, extramural resources, and special problems. Outpatient services should provide care for the student's physical and emotional health problems, be available at regularly scheduled hours, and be provided in a location convenient to all students. Inpatient services should provide hospitalization when students are too ill to take care of themselves, when bed care is necessary for physical or emotional illness, and if seasonal epidemics occur. Laboratory services should be readily available to make the standard laboratory evaluations, such as in the areas of hematology, microbiology, urinalysis, and clinical chemistry. Pharmacy (medication) services provide medications of a uniform high quality dispensed in a "manner consistent with the pharmacy code or other pertinent laws or administrative regulations of the state in which the college is located." Prompt recognition and effective treatment are important objectives of the mental health service. Emergency care in the mental health facility should be available on a 24-hour basis. Athletic medicine services include evaluation of the health of the college student before participation in physical education, intramural sports, and intercollegiate athletics. Dental services consist of these essential activities: (1) emergency treatment

of mouth infections and accidents involving the teeth and supporting structures; (2) diagnosis and consultation; (3) prophylaxis and preventive services by dental hygienists; (4) patient education; and (5) provision of protective devices for students participating in contact sports. Rehabilitation or physical medicine is intended for (1) students, staff, and faculty who have an impairment of function from injury or illness; and (2) students who enter the college with a physical or emotional handicap. Health promotion or preventive medicine includes evaluation of the student's health status at the time of admission to the college; immunizations and screening procedures; and prevention of complications to students with diabetes, epilepsy, or cardiovascular disease. Environmental health and safety should (1) provide continuous surveillance of environmental health and safety hazards; (2) report findings of health and safety hazards to the central administration of the college; (3) recommend means of controlling these hazards; and (4) furnish consultation concerning these hazards. Health education may include (1) formal health education through organized courses; (2) informal learning experiences through health services; and (3) programmed development and research affecting the student's health behavior.[1] Formal health education includes the basic college health education course and the professional school health education courses.

A basic college health education course dealing with the health problems of college students should be available to all freshmen on a college campus. Students should be made aware of the incidence of diseases, injuries, emotional health problems, and other factors that influence their personal and family health. Students can discuss mental illness, drug abuse, alcoholism, contraception, abortion, homosexuality, venereal diseases, nutrition, water and air pollution, and the purchase of health products and services. Decisions concerning sexual behavior face every student. Newly wedded husbands and wives are confronted with each other's health problems, unexpected illnesses of infants and young chil-

[1]American College Health Association: *Recommended Standards and Practices for a College Health Program.* rev. ed. Evanston, Ill.: The Association, 1969, pp. 6-11, 14-19, 21-22, 24-25, 26-29, 33-36.

dren, and emotional difficulties in marriage. To many college administrators, the most crucial problem is drug abuse. Experimentation with marijuana, LSD, or heroin may, however, be a result of health problems among students.

Professional school health education courses deal with the health problems of elementary school children and secondary school youth. Not only are there courses for the elementary school classroom teacher but also for the teacher of health education in the secondary schools and for the physical educator. The Joint Committee on Health Problems in Education of the NEA and the AMA recommends health education courses for *all* prospective teachers. These courses are offered at the undergraduate and graduate levels.

## PRESERVICE TEACHER EDUCATION

Many questions can be asked about the role of teacher education in the health of future teachers. What optimum physical and mental health should teachers have? What physical and mental health factors adversely affect teaching? Should the type of teaching or grade level be considered in evaluating the prospective teacher's physical and mental health? Is there a realistic attempt to discover emotional disturbances in prospective teachers? What physical and mental health deviations should disqualify a prospective teacher? What are the mental health variables and personality problems that can have a detrimental effect on teaching? Does the prospective teacher need professional school health education courses?

To find some of the answers to these and other questions, a screening selection committee should be available to investigate all students entering the teacher education program. For those not entering teacher education until their junior year, this selection would necessitate the cooperation of the faculty in the subject-matter fields in order to screen prospective teachers. The committee could include representatives of the teacher education faculty, and of subject-matter fields, members of counseling and guidance services, administrative personnel, and a representative of the student health center. The screening committee might demand more objective data for selecting teachers than are available to the faculty.

The prospective teacher should be required to have:

1. A thorough medical examination at admission, prior to student teaching, and at graduation
2. Tuberculin testing annually; positive reactors would have chest roentgenograms
3. Complete cumulative health records on mental and physical health, designed to include a summation of pertinent facts to be used by school employment officials
4. Continuous faculty advisement with the assistance of counseling and guidance services to "screen out" students with emotional health problems so that psychiatric aid can be had early in the undergraduate years
5. Screening of vision, hearing, and speech during the freshman year so that remediable defects can be corrected; all screening should be repeated before student teaching
6. Physical education, utilizing health grade classifications given by family or college physicians, physical education tests, and posture screening
7. A health grade classification for participation in college intramural sports
8. A college environment that promotes sanitary measures and accident prevention
9. A basic college health education course followed by the professional school health education courses
10. A college health council to assist in solving health problems
11. Professional school health education courses to provide the subject matter basic to the school health program; these are to be taught by professors prepared in school health education and with appropriate teaching experiences.

The Joint Committee on Health Problems in Education of the NEA and the AMA made this statement in 1924: "Every prospective teacher, even when not specializing in Health Education, should be required to take one course where the health program as a whole is considered, synthesis indicated, and methods of securing desired results are discussed."[2] Forty-two years later, the same committee indicated that institutions preparing teachers should provide opportunities for prospective teachers to develop competencies in school health services, healthful school living, and health education. All prospective teachers were to have preparation in the school health program so that these teachers had "an understanding of the different aspects of the school health program."[3] If the preparation of the prospective elementary school classroom teacher, physical educator, and secondary school teacher omits the school health program, how can we expect these teachers to fulfill their responsibilities in recognizing and helping to solve the health problems of their own students?

In addition to the school health program, prospective teachers should have courses in health education subject matter appropriate to the elementary and secondary schools. Courses should include instruction in these *areas* of health education:

> Prevention of diseases of the human body
> Chronic health conditions
> American Red Cross First Aid
> Safety education
> Mental health
> Nutrition
> Community health
> Consumer health
> Adult health problems
> Family life and sex education
> Drug abuse, narcotic addiction, smoking, and misuse of alcoholic beverages
> International health

Familiarity with the subject matter in these areas of health education and an understanding of the school health program are essential to the basic preparation of the teacher of health education. In a 1970 study[4] of the certification requirements of teachers of health education in the 50 states and District of Columbia,

courses about the school health program and personal hygiene were the most frequently required or suggested. Certification requirements are the minimum standards of preparation for the teacher, however, and both the elementary school classroom teacher and the physical educator could benefit from several areas of health education. Members of some state legislatures have become alarmed over the lack of instruction against drug abuse in the public school and have passed legislation that *all* teachers, grades 4 through 12, teach about drug abuse. Other state legislators have become aware of the need for health education about venereal diseases, nutritional deficiencies, emotional health problems, family life and sex education, fluoridation of drinking water supplies, quackery, alcoholism, accident prevention, and smoking, to name a few topics. Therefore, future requirements for certification may well demand more thorough preparation in health education.

## COMMON SIGNS OF POSSIBLE DEFECTS, DISEASES, ILLNESSES, OR INJURIES OCCURRING TO SCHOOL PERSONNEL

Absenteeism among school personnel is due to many health problems. Mental and emotional illness may be the most frequently reported health problem. Other health problems include heart disease, kidney infections, cancer, obesity, arthritis, venereal diseases, diabetes, anemia, orthopedic deviations, glaucoma, cataracts, periodonitis, vision and hearing difficulties, menstrual problems, difficulties during menopause, skin infections, prostatic problems, and tuberculosis. Repeated respiratory infections are often overlooked because they have the same signs as common colds.

Some signs of possible defects, diseases, illnesses, or injuries occurring to school personnel are

1. Recurring pain in the joints, muscles, chest, sinuses, and lower back
2. Unexplained nausea and vomiting
3. Recurring fatigue
4. Change in weight, sudden or extreme
5. Recurring headaches
6. Continuous fever
7. Bleeding from the skin, nose, or body opening
8. Recurring chills
9. Extreme weakness
10. Recurring indigestion
11. Sleeplessness

[2]Joint Committee on Health Problems in Education of the National Education Association and the American Medical Association: *Health Education.* New York: The Committee, 1924, p. 76.

_____: *Suggested School Health Policies.* 4th ed. Washington, D.C.: National Education Association, 1966, pp. 48-49.

Jessie Helen Haag: Certification requirements in health education. *School Health Review* 2 (February, 1971):11-15.

12. Changes in color or appearance of the skin or a growth on the skin
13. Abnormal restlessness, inattentiveness, aggressiveness, or shyness
14. Continuous stumbling or falling
15. Recurring bruises
16. Changes in vision such as squint, seeing double, losing side vision, and seeing "halos" or "rainbows" around lights
17. Continuous swelling in the abdomen, at the joints, or in other parts of the body
18. Unusual lumps or growths which increase in size
19. Breathlessness after very little exertion
20. Persistent coughing
21. Persistent sore throat
22. Loss of appetite and strength
23. Excessive thirst and hunger
24. Painful or excessive urination
25. Repeated dizziness
26. Changes in bowel habits, such as constipation and diarrhea
27. Changes in personality
28. Loss of hearing
29. Recurring skin infections or disorders such as psoriasis
30. Loose teeth, swollen jaws, or refusal to eat hard food
31. Difficulty in swallowing and talking
32. Proneness to accidents

These signs should be brought to the attention of the family physician or dentist. These signs may be the result of the teacher's failure to assume his responsibilities for promotion and protection of his physical and mental health.

## MEDICAL EXAMINATION

Boys and Infram[5] have found that complete medical examinations of school personnel are more common in large school systems and that there generally is a relationship between the size of the school system and the stringency of medical requirements for personnel. A complete medical examination not only includes a thorough examination itself but also laboratory tests and special examinations.

Before discussing when the examination should be given and what the examination should consist of, three concepts should be stressed. Responsibility for the medical examination of school personnel is shared by both the employee and the board of education. The information on the employee's health record is confidential. Medical examinations of school personnel should be given periodically.

The Joint Committee on Health Problems in Education of the NEA and the AMA urges periodic medical examinations or an examination at any time when there is "warrantable suspicion of poor health."[6] The examination gives the staff member an opportunity to learn about his health problems. Also, the examination provides the members of the board of education, superintendent of schools, and principals the assurance of knowing that school personnel are fit for their jobs.

The medical examination should include blood pressure and pulse; height and weight; skin; external eye structures, distant visual acuity and muscle coordination of the eyeballs; nasal passages; ear canals, membranes of the ears, and hearing acuity; tooth structure, occlusion, and gums; mouth and pharynx, thyroid gland; bones of the thoracic area; breasts; lungs; heart; abdomen; function and structure of bones and muscles; lymph nodes; reflex actions; body temperature; nutritional status; and tests for detection of organic heart disease. The male school employee should be given rectal and prostate examinations by the physician in addition to examination of the penis and testicles. The female school employee should be given the rectal and pelvic examinations by the physician in addition to the examination of the breasts. The medical examination can be made either by the family physician or by a physician designated by the school.

## LABORATORY AND OTHER TESTS

Tuberculin tests and chest x-rays should be used to detect the presence of tubercle bacilli in school personnel. Laboratory tests may include urinalysis, serologic tests, and other tests such as the "Pap" test.

A report of the United States Public Health Service recommended that all school personnel should be given tuberculin tests. It was further suggested that nonreactors have annual tuberculin tests and positive

[5]Floyd E. Boys and Adnan F. Infram: Health standards for the employment of school personnel—a national study. *J. School Health* 35 (May, 1965):224.

[6]Joint Committee on Health Problems in Education of the National Education Association and the American Medical Association: *Health of School Personnel.* Washington, D.C.: National Education Association, 1964, pp. 8-9.

reactors have chest x-rays.[7] The American School Health Association's Study Committee on Tuberculosis made this statement in November 1969: "If all school personnel having any contact with school children were to submit to annual study for signs of tuberculosis," tuberculosis could be controlled in schools.[8] An annual chest x-ray may be required of each school employee. Routine 14" x 17" chest films are considered the most satisfactory method of detecting pulmonary tuberculosis.

A serologic test for syphilis should be included with each medical examination. If the results of the test are positive, treatment for syphilis should be started immediately by the family physician.

Other serologic tests can reveal the presence or the effects of the causative agents of bacillary dysentery, typhoid fever, infectious mononucleosis, and certain rickettsial and viral diseases. These tests are especially necessary for food workers, custodians, and home economics teachers.

Laboratory tests should include the "Pap" test for women employees to detect the presence of early signs of uterine cancer. A vaginal specimen containing cells shed from the uterus is studied through a microscope to determine if any cancer cells are present. The test, which is highly reliable, is a quick and painless procedure.

One of the most informative of laboratory tests is the urinalysis. It indicates the status of the kidneys and, to some degree, the health of other organs. Common tests check the urine for acidity, specific gravity, presence of epithelial cells and leukocytes, albumin, and presence of sugar or glucose. The presence of blood and pus is also determined.

Skin tests may be used for diagnosing allergies, for determining natural or acquired immunity, and for investigating a person's susceptibility to certain diseases. The physician may include an examination of fecal material or request that the patient have an electrocardiogram.

[7]United States Public Health Service: *A Child Centered Program to Prevent Tuberculosis*, No. 1280. 1965.
[8]The Study Committee on Tuberculosis, American School Health Association, November 7, 1969. *J. School Health 50* (March, 1970):158.

## OTHER EXAMINATIONS

School personnel should be aware that other examinations can reveal their physical and mental health status. An annual eye examination by an ophthalmologist or optometrist can indicate unobserved changes in vision, early signs of visual defects and diseases, and signs of health conditions in other parts of the body, such as diabetes and syphilis. Glaucoma in its early stages can also be detected during the ophthalmological examination.

Psychiatric examinations are not uncommon among school personnel. Such examinations may be desirable if certain behavior has been observed by the family physician, family, friends, school associates, or pupils. Some of the behavior patterns that may be signs of mental and emotional health problems are as follows:

1. Sulking or being too aggressive
2. Being sorry for oneself and self-centered
3. Having no regard for others
4. Displaying meanness, cruelty, and hostility
5. Taking advantage of associates and family
6. Revealing overdependence on other persons
7. Being lazy
8. Failing to fulfill one's obligations
9. Having few interests and hobbies
10. Failing to make decisions
11. Being easily defeated and accepting failure
12. Violating social and moral codes
13. Being irritable and moody
14. Failing to help others
15. Seeking only one's own desires
16. Being inflexible and unable to adapt to new situations

To avoid some of these behavior patterns, the adult's basic psychological needs must be satisfied; he must be able to meet adult problems with mature techniques and attitudes, and he must be able to cope with adverse conditions. Some of the psychological needs are affection, security, recognition, self-esteem, and creative opportunities.

An annual dental examination and roentgenographic survey can reveal dental diseases and defects unseen in a regular inspection by the family dentist. Oral cancer may be detected by x-ray surveys. If dental diseases and defects are detected and treated early, the adult may improve his appearance and avoid the necessity of dentures.

## HEALTH RECORD

The school employee's health record should be accessible only to certain administrative personnel as it is confidential. The record may consist of several parts, including the results of medical examinations, chest x-rays, laboratory tests, and other examinations. The *first* part of the health record might consist of the health history of the candidate or employee. The health history can be a record of immunization procedures; health habits inventory; record of previous illnesses; record of serious injuries and operations; irregularities in daily health, such as headaches, nosebleeds, and diarrhea; dates of the last visits to the family physician and dentist and reasons for the visit; and record of illnesses within the immediate family. The health history could be completed before the medical examination.

The *second* part of the health record might include the results of the medical examination by the family physician or designated physician and the results of any laboratory tests by that physician. The second part of the record should be detachable so that it can be kept in the physician's office. The *third* part of the health record might include the results of chest x-ray procedures and tuberculin tests. This third part should also be detachable. The second and third parts of the record should provide for successive annual results and thus become a cumulative record. The *fourth* part of the record should be removable for the employee's use and be separate from other parts. On the fourth part, the employee records data pertinent to illnesses, injuries, operations, and health disturbances occurring since employment. The *fifth* part of the health record contains information about the employee's physical and mental fitness and possible health conditions needing correction following employment. This last part of the health record can be used in conference with the employee if he has a physical or mental health difficulty needing correction. The purpose of the conference would be to encourage the employee to seek correction of the health difficulty.

A standard employee health record can be designed by a school system so that data can be recorded. Suggestions for an employee health record can be obtained from other school districts or local and state health departments. Physicians, counselors, school principals, and employee officials should keep confidential all data concerning the employee's physical and mental health.

The second part of the employee's health record, sent to the family physician, should remain in the physician's office. The physician should determine what data are needed by the employment official. These data should be forwarded to the employment official and filed with the confidential records of the employee. If the physician indicates that an employee's physical or mental conditions affect the health of other school personnel and pupils, the employment officer should inform the employee in order to seek correction of the conditions.

## WELFARE PRACTICES

Many school systems have retained outstanding teachers because of beneficial welfare practices. Superintendents are aware that such practices promote a sense of security among school personnel. Some of the benefits provided are sick leave, group health insurance plans, teacher retirement plans, salary schedule and standards for promotions, continuing contract policy, and tenure.

### Sick Leave

*Sick leave* is the specified number of days that the school employee may be absent from his job because of personal illness or injury, with partial or no loss in salary. The length of time may be stated on the employee's annual contract. Superintendents must establish definite procedures for notifying school officials of absences and dates of return, and school personnel should be informed of these procedures. In some instances, a principal may be notified by the school employee. The principal then either contacts a designated school official who obtains a substitute employee or the principal himself obtains a substitute. In some school systems, officials of the central administrative offices are notified, and they secure a substitute. All school personnel should be informed of these varying procedures regarding the date of return. At the time of return, the procedures may require the employee to submit a certificate issued by a family physician or by a physician employed by the board of education; it indicates whether the employee has recovered from illness. Some school systems require that the employee absent from his job for three or more days submit a physician's certificate stating the nature of the illness or injury and whether the employee has fully recovered.

The number of days granted for sick leave varies. Sick leave policy may be decided by boards of education or by state-wide mandatory regulations. The number of days usually ranges from 5 to 10. Sick leave may be cumulative; that is, days of sick leave not used by the employee in one year are added to the number available in the following year as cumulative sick leave.

Sick leave policies may need interpretation to school personnel. Policies about sick leave for an illness or injury requiring hospital care will probably differ from those dealing with sick leave for a slight illness or injury not requiring medical attention. Time for quarantine, dental surgery and treatment, and convalescence from illness may be included in sick leave. Maternity absence may be treated as sick leave, usually without pay. A beginning teacher may need assistance in understanding the conditions under which sick leave is granted and the procedures for notifying school officials about absence and date of return.

## Leave of Absence Other Than Sick Leave

Death or illness in the family, a wedding in the family, personal business, attendance at professional education meetings, obligations of an officer to a professional organization, jury duty, emergencies arising within families other than illness or death, and other unusual situations may require that the school employee be absent from his job. A leave of absence for reasons of this sort is not, of course, the same as a sabbatical leave, when the teacher is absent from his job for an entire semester or year. Personal business requiring absence might include the taking of examinations given by a university or college to an employee registered for graduate courses or military obligations.

Boards of education should develop definite policies. School personnel should be informed of the conditions under which leave of absence is granted, of procedures to be followed for notification of absence, and of procedures reporting the date of return.

## Group Health Insurance Plans

Krantz reports that 59% of teachers in urban school districts pay all the premiums for hospitalization insurance. In all school districts in the United States, 79% of teachers pay all of the premiums for medical-surgical insurance. It was estimated by Krantz that over 50% of non-school employees in the U.S. have their premiums for health insurance, "paid for, at least in part, by their employers." Krantz urges teachers to become aware of their need for medical, dental, and hospital care and to have premiums paid by local boards of education.[9]

Insurance plans offered should be voluntary, because school personnel should be able to choose to join or refuse to join the different types of group insurance plans available to them. The type of insurance plan the school employee wishes to join is left entirely to his own choice and is not a requirement for the retention of his job. This voluntary decision on the part of the school employee has both advantages and disadvantages.

Annual premiums for members of a group plan are less expensive than annual premiums for individuals who are not members of a group. In small communities, the number of school personnel in one school district or in a single building may be inadequate for membership in a group insurance plan. In such instances, personnel within several school districts may join one group. Group insurance may provide broader coverage because of fewer exclusions. A shorter waiting period before benefits become effective is usually another advantage of group plans. There are disadvantages to group insurance. First, benefits are limited to the basic needs of the majority of the group. Second, benefits apply only so long as the individual remains an employee. Third, employees retiring after being members of a group may

[9]Goldie Krantz: The selection of health coverage for school employees. *J. School Health* 36 (June, 1966):291.

not be able to continue their coverage as members of a group. Individual insurance, though more costly, may offer coverage to meet individual needs not included in group plans.

The following types of health insurance plans are commonly used by school personnel: prepaid hospital benefits, prepaid medical-surgical benefits, accident insurance, and disability income insurance.

Plans for prepaid hospital benefits usually cover hospital care for a stated length of time; meals and special diets; general nursing services; x-ray examinations, all drugs and medicines; laboratory examination; operating room; surgical dressings and plaster casts; use of cystoscopic room; oxygen and oxygen therapy; anesthetic materials and services; electrocardiograms; physiotherapy and hydrotherapy; radiation therapy; and blood transfusion service. The purpose of a plan for prepaid hospital benefits is to assist a person in paying for hospital care. Before subscribing to any hospital benefits plan, the subscriber should be familiar with the services offered by the plan.

Prepaid medical-surgical benefits are designed to assist the individual in paying for unexpected surgical or medical care. In these plans, there are schedules which state the amount of money alloted toward defraying surgical costs. Surgical procedures include surgery of the abdomen; amputations; surgical repair of dislocations and fractures; surgery of the eyes, ears, nose, and throat; general surgery, such as treatment for varicose veins and thyroidectomy; gynecological procedures such as hysterectomy; neurosurgery; and surgery involving many other specialized branches of medicine.

Group accident plans cover death or dismemberment of an insured individual due to an accident. Payments for loss of life, a hand, a foot, an eye, speech, hearing, and so forth are typical benefits. Benefits for total disability as a result of an accident are paid. These plans have no coverage for suicide or self-inflicted injury; bodily or mental infirmity or disease; or medical or surgical treatment not connected with accident. Subscribers should read their policies carefully and be aware of stipulations for temporary layoff, leave of absence, the termination of insurance,

and the monthly contribution of the employee.

Long-term disability insurance is income insurance. It guarantees the subscriber a monthly income if he is so disabled by illness or injury that he cannot work for a living. Long-term disability insurance supplements ordinary disability insurance and protects the subscriber for those total disabilities which last for years. Long-term disability insurance usually guarantees 60 to 70% of the subscriber's monthly income at the time of the disability. As with all other insurance subscribers need to be familiar with the provisions of the plan: monthly contribution, amount of monthly income received, length of time monthly income will continue, exclusions, and so forth.

## Retirement Plans

Teacher retirement plans vary regarding the benefits received, age when teachers must retire, and annual amount paid by the teacher into the retirement plan. Every state has some form of teacher retirement plan, and most states have provisions for teachers who become permanently disabled. There is need for constant re-evaluation of these retirement plans by state education associations to determine inadequacies in retirement benefits.

The teacher close to retirement faces many problems. The amount of retirement income and the age when the teacher must retire differ from state to state. The retirement income may lower the former teacher's standard of living if the retirement plan is not geared to a cost-of-living index. Age limit is another problem facing the teacher. During a shortage of teachers, teacher retirement plans might extend age limits so that teachers capable of performing their jobs and having satisfactory physical and mental health could be retained.

Boards of education with gradual retirement plans have added years to the active life of the teacher. Whereas retirement means a complete separation of the teacher from his job, gradual retirement plans adjust the teacher gradually both emotionally and financially to retirement. Some school systems start the gradual retirement plan when the teacher reaches the age of 61, when the plan may go into effect voluntarily. When he reaches the age of 65, the gradual retirement plan becomes compulsory. A teacher may decide to accept voluntarily the gradual retirement plan at 61 years of age. For a two-year period, he teaches four-sixths of the regular school day and is paid four-sixths of his regular salary; for the next two-year period, he teaches one-half of the school day and is paid one-half of his former salary.

## Salary and Promotions

The school employee's salary influences not only his job performance but also his sense of security. Inadequate salaries force school employees to seek part-time employment outside their school jobs. Nine-month salary plans, lack of policies governing increases in salaries, and an absence of cost-of-living adjustments are some of the factors which have made the teaching profession unattractive to many.

Local boards of education and state education departments should establish salary schedules so that elementary teachers are paid salaries equivalent to those of secondary teachers. Instructional supervisors and administrators should receive salaries that recognize years of successful teaching experience, competencies on the job, and advanced study. Counselors, special education teachers, and health educators or coordinators should be compensated for the advanced specialized study needed for their jobs. The school nurse should be compensated according to her professional preparation, her aptitudes in school nursing, and the fulfillment of her role in the total school health program.

A salary schedule permits the school employee to estimate his future salary and be aware of his obligations regarding competencies on the job, advanced study, and meritorious service. Salary increments should be carefully considered by boards of education before decisions are made for "across-the-board" increases or for advances in salary as rewards for outstanding performances. A school superintendent, before increasing a school employee's salary, should have pertinent information to help him evaluate the employee's services properly.

Promotions need the careful attention of school superintendents and boards of education. Promotional policies designed by school employee committees can do a great deal in promoting *esprit de corps*. Recognition of problems facing the employee, proficiency in handling the job, and efforts to improve the job should be accepted as some of the bases for promotion policies. Meritorious work can be used as a basis for promotion, if instructional positions receive equal recognition. Promotion policies need continuous evaluation by employee committees.

## Continuing Contract Policy

The policy of a continuing contract assures the school employee of a position for at least a period of two years and allows him to know a year in advance if his services are to be terminated. Some school boards and superintendents feel that school employees should be employed each year for a two-year period. Knowing that his services terminate at the end of two years, the teacher has a full year to seek employment elsewhere.

## Tenure

Tenure provides security for the school employee. For teachers, tenure removes the possibility of abrupt termination of a job. The teacher is employed for a two- or three-year probation period and, if competent, is assured of permanent employment. As long as the teacher remains competent, continuing employment is assured through continuing contract policies, annual contracts, or state tenure laws. If annual contracts are used, the competent teacher is more concerned about next year's salary than whether a contract will or will not be received. States having tenure laws assure permanency of employment unless tenure is ended by court action or by action of the school board after an open hearing. Tenure can have both advantages and disadvantages. Disadvantages are evident when poorly qualified and incompetent teachers retain their positions because of tenure.

Other beneficial welfare practices include provision for legal counseling, credit unions, aid for disabled and retired teachers, placement services, and library services for teachers. Welfare practices need constant evaluation, and sound practices provide a sense of security among school personnel.

## References for Further Study

American College Health Association: Evaluative criteria for health education in colleges and universities: a guide for self-appraisal of the college health education program. (1965); *Journal of the American College Health Association*; Recommended standards and practices for a college health program. (1969); Statement on health rights and responsibilities of students. (1968). Evanston, Ill.: The Association.

Association of State and Territorial Health Officers, Association of State and Territorial Mental Health Authorities, and Council of Chief State School Officers: *Mental Health in the Schools*. Washington, D.C.: Council of Chief State School Officers, 1966.

Byrd, O. E.: *School Health Administration*. Philadelphia: W. B. Saunders Company, 1964.

Farnsworth, D.: *College Health Administration*. New York: Appleton-Century-Crofts, 1964.

Joint Committee on Health Problems in Education of the National Education Association and the American Medical Association: *Healthful School Environment*. (1969); *Health of School Personnel*. (1964). Washington, D.C.: National Education Association.

Maltz, S.: *Critical Issues for College Health*. Dubuque, Iowa: Wm. C. Brown, 1970.

Mayshark, C., and Shaw, D. D.: *Administration of School Health Programs*. St. Louis: The C. V. Mosby Company, 1967.

Metropolitan Life Insurance Company: *Statistical Bulletin*. (monthly) New York, New York.

National Commission on Community Health Services: *Report of the Task Force on Environmental Health. Changing Environmental Hazards*, 1967.

Turner, C.: *Study Guide on Teacher Preparation for Health Education for WHO and UNESCO*. New York: Columbia University Press, 1967.

# Part II
## *HEALTHFUL SCHOOL LIVING*

# Chapter 9

## *ENVIRONMENTAL FACTORS*

### AN INCIDENT

Community action groups have become concerned with the health problems of their community. These problems include water pollution, sewage and solid waste disposal, and emergency procedures in the event of a natural disaster. However, teachers and students in the elementary and secondary schools have not considered that the schools have these problems also. Nor has instruction about water pollution and purification, sewage treatment, proper disposal of solid waste, and self-preservation in the event of a tornado and hurricane been included in health education courses.

> *Healthful school living* simply means living within a school where all environmental conditions, every social relationship, and every curriculum experience is carried on with due attention to health. None of these conditions or experiences should be allowed to endanger health or safety; they all should contribute to well-being.[1]

In this chapter, the following environmental factors will be considered: water supply; sewage and solid waste; heating, ventilation, and air conditioning; noise and acoustical design; light and color; school furniture; and safety.

### WATER SUPPLY

Water is utilized in a school building in many ways: to quench thirst, to prepare school noonday meals, to sanitize dishes and silverware, to clean corridors and toilet rooms, to launder towels, to prepare class materials, to bathe, and in countless other ways. In every instance, water must be pure and not polluted. Polluted water can be the source of such water-borne diseases as typhoid fever, bacillary dysentery, diarrhea, and amebic dysentery.

*Typhoid fever* is characterized by continuous fever, slow pulse, rose-colored eruptions or rash, and enlargement of the spleen. The disease is spread by fecal material and urine of persons infected with *Salmonella typhosa*. Protection, purification, and chlorination of public water supplies are vital for prevention of the disease. *Bacillary dysentery* is caused by the Shigella bacilli of which there are at least 30 serotypes. It is an intestinal disease characterized by diarrhea, fever, vomiting, and straining at stool or in urination. The stool may be bloody and contain mucus and pus. Bacillary dysentery is spread by the fecal-oral route from an infected person. Purification of water supplies reduces the possibility of this disease. *Diarrhea* may be caused by an enteric virus infection spread from the fecal material of an infected person. Liquidity and abnormal frequency of fecal discharges are the common characteristics. *Amebic dysentery* is caused by the *Entamoeba histolytica*, which is spread by intestinal discharges of infected persons into contaminated water. Signs of the disease vary. There may be slight abdominal discomfort and diarrhea, or the diarrhea may be severe with blood and mucus discharged in the fecal material. Public water supplies should be protected against fecal contamination.

To provide a water supply free from pol-

[1]Joint Committee on Health Problems in Education of the National Education Association and the American Medical Association: *Healthful School Environment.* rev. ed. Washington, D.C.: National Education Association, 1969, p. 7.

lution for a school building, the supply should be obtained from a public water system. The basic minimum supply of water needed in buildings fully equipped with cafeteria, gymnasiums, and showers is 25 gallons per pupil a day.[2]

The most common use of water in a school is for satisfying thirst. It is desirable to have at least one drinking fountain for each 100 pupils and one fountain on each floor. The most satisfactory type of fountain does not allow the mouth of the student to come in contact with the nozzle nor does the waste water fall on the nozzle. Drinking fountains placed in the corridor should be recessed into the corridor wall. In most instances, angle-jet fountains are preferable to vertical bubbler-type fountains.

As part of health education, teachers of the primary grades can show children how to use drinking fountains. The operation of the pressure control valve and the use of the angle-jet fountain can be part of a health education lesson.

Hand washing facilities should be provided outside the lunchroom. The habit of hand washing before and after the noonday meal should be established early in the life of the elementary school child. For effective hand washing, the school should provide warm water, soap, and single-use paper towels.

The lunchroom must have water for the preparation of food and for dishwashing. Toilet rooms for food workers also utilize water. Hot and cold water with mixing faucets should be provided at all sinks and washbasins. To provide 180°F. water for dishwashing, special water heaters and storage tanks are usually required. Cooled drinking water, from either a drinking fountain or cooled-water unit, should be provided in the dining area.

In modern elementary schools, sinks and work counters are a part of the classroom facilities. Attached to some elementary school classrooms are toilet rooms having toilets and washbasins. With available toilet rooms, hand washing and tooth brushing can become routine procedures for elementary school children.

The physical education facilities need a water supply. This water supply furnishes the warm, tepid, and cool water for showering. Water must be available for swimming pools, outdoor playing surfaces, and cleaning purposes. In the shower rooms, the number of shower heads depends on the enrollment of the physical education classes during each of the class periods. The "gang" or group shower is preferred.

Water is also needed for use with disinfectants in cleaning. Disinfection is the process for destroying infectious agents by chemical or physical means. Chlorine, iodine, bromine, ozone, and other substances possessing germicidal properties are used as disinfectants. Toilet facilities, shower and locker rooms, lunchroom, and all similar surfaces need disinfection.[3,4]

## SEWAGE AND SOLID WASTE

Sewage includes the waste water from dish washing, washbasins, toilet facilities, showers, sinks, laundry, drinking fountains, and instructional equipment such as at work counters in classrooms and laboratories. It includes surface drainage water and human body wastes. When there is improper sewage disposal and inadequate sewage treatment, diseases such as typhoid fever, amebic dysentery, hookworm, and other intestinal infections occur. *Hookworm disease* is caused by the hookworm which attaches itself to the wall of the human's small intestine. The female hookworm lays a large number of eggs which are discharged into the fecal material. Within 24 hours, the eggs in the fecal material become larvae which exist in moist soil. The larvae pass through five stages. In the third stage, the larvae may pierce the skin of a human, usually between the toes. The larvae pass to the circulatory system and then to the respiratory system. In the lungs, the larvae penetrate the walls of the air sacs and get into the bronchi and trachea. If the larvae reach the mouth, they are swallowed. They then lodge in

[2]Edward S. Hopkins, W. McLean Bingley, and George W. Schucker: *The Practice of Sanitation.* 4th ed. Baltimore: The Williams & Wilkins Company, 1970, p. 145.

[3]American Public Health Association: *Control of Communicable Diseases in Man.* 11th ed. New York: The Association, 1970, p. 289.
[4]E. Hopkins *et al., op. cit.,* pp. 9-10.

the small intestine to repeat the cycle. Anemia, malnutrition, and weakness may result.[5] Sewage should be discharged from the school into a public sewer system.

Solid waste includes garbage, rubbish (paper, metal, or glass used for food or drink containers), ashes, sweepings (tree branches, leaves), construction wastes (lumber, masonry), and industrial wastes (metal scraps, chemical wastes). In schools, this solid waste is most often wastepaper from classrooms, single-use paper towels, used drinking cups, scraps of metal and wood from shops, tin cans, bottles, used containers, chemical waste, and garbage. Improper disposal of garbage allows a breeding place for flies and other insects and feeds rats and stray animals.

Many communities require that garbage be wrapped in paper before being placed in the container. The garbage must be drained before wrapping, and the garbage containers must be kept clean. Metal containers with tight-fitting lids should be used. The containers should be water-tight, easy to wash, fly-tight, convenient to handle, and easy to clean.

The waste receptacles placed in the toilet rooms, home economic laboratories, shops, chemistry laboratories, art rooms, and lunchroom should be entirely covered with a swinging top that opens on pressure and swings shut when pressure is released. These receptacles should be large enough so that students cannot accidentally push them over and empty the contents. All receptacles should be emptied into galvanized iron cans with tight-fitting covers. In some communities, waste is collected by the municipality and chemically treated. School systems may have an outside incinerator where the waste is burned daily. Such an incinerator, brick-lined and screened over the opening, should not be accessible to stray animals and rodents.

Garbage should be placed in galvanized iron cans separate from waste. A multiple-can system permits satisfactory disposal. There may be local health regulations about the storage of cans. For example, these rules may require that garbage cans be kept on a well-drained platform within a screened area. Garbage from a school building should be collected daily. Garbage

cans should be cleaned, disinfected, and dried each time they are emptied.[6]

## HEATING, VENTILATION, AIR CONDITIONING

Proper classroom temperatures fall within a narrow range of dry bulb temperature. During the heating season and winter months, the classroom temperature should be 68° to 76°F. Lower temperature is desirable when students are moderately active. Students who are less active will be more comfortable in rooms with higher temperature. The recommended temperature for gymnasiums is 65°F. or slightly lower. In the primary school classroom in which there is considerable physical activity, the temperature may be 70°F. or lower. In the intermediate elementary school classroom, the temperature may be 76°F.[7]

Children at the elementary school level can participate in checking the room temperature, keeping hourly and daily charts, comparing room temperatures during the winter and spring seasons, and helping the teacher to maintain constant room temperature. A classroom thermometer should be at seat level on an inside wall.

Climate, locality, floor area, height of rooms, window area, number of occupants, type and use of the building, and operation of air-supply system determine the amount of air needed to circulate in a building. Warm-air heating, ventilating, and air conditioning also depend upon correct air distribution. Not less than 15 cubic feet of air per minute per person should be supplied in a room where students are doing light activity. The amount of air per person per minute should be raised to 20 cubic feet as the activity increases. A practical minimum under normal conditions is about 10 cubic feet of air per minute per pupil.[8]

In determining thermal comfort, the rate of movement of air in a room is important. The American Society of Heating, Refrigerating, and Air Conditioning Engineers

[5]American Public Health Association, *op. cit.*, pp. 4-6.

[6]Hopkins *et al.*, *op. cit.*, pp. 226-228.
[7]Joint Committee on Health Problems in Education of the National Education Association and the American Medical Association, *op. cit.*, p. 190.
[8]*Ibid.*, pp. 191-192.

recommends that room air velocities be kept below 20 to 50 feet per minute when heating a room.[9]

Various heating and ventilating techniques are used, such as window gravity and unit ventilators, hot-air arrangements, and panel heating. In the window gravity and unit ventilators, there is an intake of fresh air through open windows. On the opposite side of room from the windows, there is a gravity exhaust through windows or corridors. In the hot-air arrangements, hot air is circulated through ducts from a central hot-air furnace. In panel heating, heating is accomplished by warm-water piping or low-temperature electrical resistance components. The components are located behind or embedded in the back surfaces of walls, floors, or ceilings.[10]

*Air conditioning* is a "process of treating air so as to control simultaneously its temperature, humidity, cleanliness, and distribution to meet the requirements of the conditioned space."[11] Two types of air conditioning equipment are used in schools: (1) unit or room conditioners; and (2) central air conditioning system. Most of the room units are designed for air cooling only. When new buildings are constructed and a central forced hot-air system is used for heating, central air conditioning is preferred.[12]

## NOISE AND ACOUSTICAL DESIGN

*Noise* is unwanted sound. Sources of noise in schools can be activities in gymnasiums, motion picture projectors, mechanical ventilators, typewriters, activity in music rooms, equipment in the school kitchen, shop machines, custodial maintenance equipment, activities in home economics laboratories, and simply movement and conversation of pupils and teachers. Automobiles and trucks on adjoining

streets, airplanes, nearby construction work, and business activities create disturbing noise. The *decibel* is the unit of measurement of sound intensity or loudness of noise. The use of a number of typewriters in a closed room or office can produce nearly 80 decibels. Exposure to 95 to 100 decibels is hazardous.

Noise levels outside and within a building need to be considered. Acceptable noise level for classrooms is 40 decibels or less. School health services unit should be below 45 decibels. Thirty decibels may have to be absorbed by the various building materials used in wall and ceiling construction.

In classroom acoustics, the most important single factor is the control of reverberation of sounds. The absorptive and reflective surfaces in the room influence reverberation. Acoustical material can be applied to ceilings and walls to reduce reverberation while room surfaces, such as floors, may be covered with highly absorbent material.[13]

## LIGHT AND COLOR

A high quality of lighting and an adequate level of illumination are necessary for efficient performance of visual tasks. In the elementary and secondary school, visual tasks are numerous. Such tasks vary in direction, viewing distance from the eye, size, length of time for viewing the visual tasks, brightness difference, and the like.

Several variables must be considered when visibility of school tasks is to be determined: contrast, brightness level, size, time, and quality of the lighting. In *contrast*, the total task is the page of the book. The task detail includes the printing on the page viewed against the page of the book. Contrast of the task detail should be at a maximum, whereas contrast of the total task should be at a minimum. As to *brightness level*, the brightness of the task should be equal or slightly greater than the brightness of the entire visual environment. For visual comfort and efficiency, the brightness of surfaces immediately adjacent to the visual task is more important than that of remote surfaces in the visual background. As for *size* of the task detail, the larger the task detail, within a given

[9]American Society of Heating, Refrigerating, and Air-Conditioning Engineers: *ASHRAE Guide and Date Book: Fundamentals and Equipment for 1965 and 1966.* New York: The Society, 1965, p. 538.

[10]Joint Committee on Health Problems in Education of the National Education Association and the American Medical Association: *op. cit.,* pp. 196-197.

[11]American Society of Heating, Refrigerating, and Air-Conditioning Engineers, *op. cit.,* p. 951.

[12]Joint Committee on Health Problems in Education of the National Education Association and the American Medical Association, *op. cit.,* p. 193.

[13]*Ibid.,* pp. 171-179.

range, the easier and more accurate is the reading. Limitations are placed on the *time* for performing any seeing task. In the art of rapid and accurate reading, the seeing task is not to be overlooked. In seeing, the eye moves, pauses, picks up what is seen, transmits the information to the brain, and moves on again. If the object to be seen is available for 1/5 of a second, the eye works at the rate of five assimilations per second, if one object is gained per pause.

*Quality of illumination* depends on reflectances and glare. Desk tops and other furniture, floors, chalkboards, walls, and ceilings will be considered in the discussion of reflectance. Desk tops and other furniture should fall within the range of 35 to 50% reflectance. Distracting reflections on desk tops can be avoided if the desk tops are nonglossy. Natural-finished light wood floors and light-colored floor materials may produce reflectance up to 50%. Chalkboards should be light enough to blend well with the background and dark enough to afford adequate contrast to chalk writing. Colored chalkboards should not exceed 20% reflectance, but black chalkboards should have 5 to 10% reflectance. Walls should have a median of 50% reflectance. A 40 to 60% range allows a wide choice of pastel colors on the walls. Ceilings should have 70 to 90% reflectance, with a nonglossy or flat finish. High reflectance assures good utilization of light. Most white painted ceilings, with no acoustical materials, measure as high as 90% reflectance.

*Glare* is unwanted brightness causing discomfort, distraction, and reduction invisibility. Two classifications of glare are direct and reflected glare. *Direct* glare is related to conditions in the visual area directly associated with the source of light and its immediate environment. Windows and luminaires (complete lighting units with all appurtenances) are two common sources of direct glare. The degree of direct glare is governed by the angular displacement, visual size of source, brightness of source, and adaptation brightness. In angular displacement, a glare source close to the line of vision is more distracting than a glare source above the head. In visual size of source, large brightness areas are more distracting than small areas. As for the brightness of the source, there is more glare as the source becomes brighter. In adaptation brightness, on the other hand, the glare effect from light sources is decreased as the environmental level of brightness is increased. *Reflected* glare is related to conditions associated with the visual tasks and their immediate environment. Reflected light is used for most visual tasks. Glossy backgrounds can produce losses in contrast caused by reflected glare. These losses may be reduced by altering the light distribution. In this manner, more light comes to the task from outside the zone of reflected glare. Also, these losses may be reduced by spreading the downward light over a larger area or by increasing the illumination level.

Research reveals that the brightness of the task increases visual performance, but the quantity of illumination needed for efficient, accurate seeing varies far more than expected. Sixty-four percent of the student's total time is spent on such tasks as writing with pencil, reading, and working with duplicated materials.[14] Because many different tasks are being performed at the same time in a classroom, it would be impractical to provide a quantity of light on the basis of each given task. Also, the entire classroom must be provided with a satisfactory minimum level of illumination. Thus a general lighting level for a classroom is difficult to ascertain. In addition, certain classrooms, such as shops, sewing and art rooms, gymnasiums, and classrooms for children with physical disabilities, have special problems of illumination. The Illuminating Engineering Society recommends the following to improve seeing:[15]

1. The use of low-gloss ink rather than pencils and ball-point pens
2. The use of low-gloss ink, adequate spacing between lines of type, and minimum type size of 10-point Bodoni in textbooks
3. The use of matte paper for both working paper and printed materials
4. Requiring high opacity and high reflectance in paper

---

[14]*American Standard Guide for School Lighting.* New York: Illuminating Engineering Society, 1962, pp. 8-18.
[15]*Ibid.*, p. 17.

5. Proper combination of illumination, chalk, and chalkboards with supplementary lighting for chalkboards
6. The use of high-quality duplicated materials

There is a trend to avoid having direct sunlight in a classroom. The arrangement of windows, overhanging roofs, trees and bushes, and louvers or other shielding devices prevent direct sunlight from entering a classroom.

Electric lighting systems can be divided into five classifications: indirect, semi-indirect, general diffuse, semi-direct, and direct. *Indirect* lighting systems send from 90 to 100% of the light from luminaires to the ceiling and the upper part of the walls. Matte high-reflectance room surface finishes are essential. Indirect lighting systems produce fewest shadows. *Semi-indirect* lighting systems send from 60 to 90% of the light from the luminaire to the ceiling and the top of the walls. Light not sent to the ceilings and upper walls is directed downward. There are low brightness ratios between the ceiling and luminaire when luminous surfaces are used with semi-indirect units. Direct or reflected glare may result because the amount of light directed to the floor is greater. *General diffuse* lighting systems send about the same percentage of light upward as downward. These luminaires direct light equally in all directions. Shadows may be more noticeable. Direct and reflected glare may result. *Semi-direct* lighting systems send from 60 to 90% of light toward the work surface. There is a reduction of the brightness ratio between the luminaire and the ceiling. Shadows and reflected glare result. Light sources with large areas minimize shadows and reflected glare. High reflectance and matte finish on furniture and equipment reduce reflected glare. *Direct* lighting systems send from 90 to 100% of the light downward. Disturbing shadows and reflected glare may be produced. High-reflectance room and furniture surfaces redirect light to the ceiling.

No single lighting system can be recommended for all purposes because each system has characteristics that may be needed in different teaching environments. Combinations of two or more of these systems in the same classroom have been used.

## Promotion of Eye Health

In utilizing classroom light to promote the students' eye health, a teacher should:

1. Never seat a student with a bright window area in his direct field of vision
2. Keep the upper portion of windows unshaded except when the sun shines on the window surfaces
3. Make special seating arrangements for left-handed students
4. Keep window sills free of all objects
5. Not paste pictures on window panes
6. Use multiple seating arrangements
7. Check to be sure that no student works in his shadow
8. Check the conditions of all shades so that
   a. Daylight does not enter at the midpoint or at the sides of the shades
   b. No cracks or tears are found in translucent shades
9. Eliminate from the classroom all wall charts and maps that have become faded, dirty, or worn
10. Report and have replaced all defective incandescent bulbs and fluorescent tubes
11. Report and have cleaned dirty luminaires
12. Report and have cleaned dirty window glass
13. Keep chalkboards clean and free from accumulated chalk dust
14. Stand or sit in positions directing students' sight lines away from the windows
15. Check the illumination levels periodically in all parts of the room
16. Provide copyholders and easels for vertical-plane desks to maintain optimum lighting for close eye tasks
17. Make all board writing clear, large, and consistent
18. Plan the daily school program so that close visual tasks alternate with activities requiring a lesser degree of visual concentration
19. Use artificial light to supplement daylight when brightness levels fall below standard in any part of the room
20. Place students with visual difficulties in classroom positions that give them the best light in accordance with their individual visual difficulties

21. Allow students to change their seats when they desire more or less light
22. Provide library areas of classrooms with ample brightness levels
23. Check to be sure that pictures, cabinets, bookshelves, tables, and other room surfaces have been treated with nonglossy finishes
24. See that shrubbery and trees in the vicinity of classroom windows are trimmed to permit entrance of a maximum of natural light
25. Cover chalkboards not in use
26. Cover glass surfaces in cabinets, and remove glass covers on pictures
27. Select and use teaching aids having nonglossy surfaces
28. Select student textbooks and supplementary reading materials having appropriate type size, nonglossy surfaces, and desirable contrasts
29. Be aware of glare on black slateboard surfaces
30. Have blackened lamps or tubes replaced
31. Prevent slate blackboards from becoming gray and semipolished
32. Use high-grade white chalk, with a minimum of clay filter
33. Check the condition of all painted surfaces for the accumulation of dirt, particularly the ceiling, side walls, and front walls
34. Check the condition of desk tops so that the blond color is retained and not replaced by dirt, pencil marks, or paints used in class activities
35. Maintain high levels of artificial illumination in art and drafting rooms, home economics laboratories, science and music rooms, special education rooms, and libraries
36. Remove all curtains and all window decorations
37. Check height of desk-chair combinations so that the student receives the optimum light on the working surfaces
38. Develop in students a sense of responsibility for maintenance of good eye health
39. Stress the importance of proper illumination in home study as a part of health instruction
40. Participate in in-service education promoting good eye health
41. Stress the importance of good sitting posture during reading, writing, drawing, or other desk-top activities

## SCHOOL FURNITURE

Many types of school furniture are utilized in various parts of a school building. Desk-chair combinations may be found in classrooms. School libraries use tables and chairs. Auditorium seating differs from dressing or locker room benches. Furniture of special education classrooms has adjustments seldom found in lunchroom or cafeteria seating. The size of furniture for an elementary school classroom is considerably different from that of furniture for a high school classroom.

School furniture should have a variety of designs and sizes, be movable, and be adjustable. No single piece of school furniture is applicable to every teaching environment, nor can desk-chair combinations of the same size be used at all grade levels.

Desk-chair combinations should be movable. Noiseless gliders placed on the legs or supports of the combination will permit movement with the minimum of noise. Manufacturers of today's classroom furniture are using blond, straw, and other light-colored finishes on the desk-chair combination, and light-weight construction materials that a first-grader can push or an older child lift. Thus students can push the desk-chair combination into different seating arrangements to improve the quality of light on the working surface.

The adjustment of the desk-chair combination to the growth of the child is of paramount importance. For a long time educators have overlooked both the importance of posture and body mechanics as an essential part of the learning process, and the fact that the process of learning is physical as well as psychological. Eyestrain and body fatigue not only result in headache, irritability, and listlessness but also retard learning. A common fault of school personnel is purchasing nonadjustable desk-chair combinations in one size for each grade level. Varying sizes of desk-chair combinations should be used for every grade level. Numerous studies have shown that a large percentage of the traditional desk-chair combinations is oversized.

## Common Faults in Sitting Posture

Before the classroom teacher can adjust the desk-chair combination to the child's growth, she should be able to identify common postural faults in the pupils' sitting positions. A child who does the following illustrates some of these faults:

1. Sits in a slumped position. The chair is too small for him.
2. Has pressure under his knees. The chair seat is too deep from front to back; the front edge of the seat puts pressure under the child's knees.
3. Cannot touch the floor with the entire foot. The chair seat is too high.
4. Hunches over in poor posture. The chair is too small, and the desk top or chair arm is too low and too flat.
5. Overflows the chair. The chair is too small.
6. Leans to one side. The desk top or chair arm is too high.
7. Stretches his trunk muscles. The desk top is too high and does not have the correct slant for work.
8. Hunches over desk. The desk top is too low and too far away.
9. Sits on one foot. The desk top is too high.

These common postural faults may lead to scoliosis, kyphosis, forward head, and many other postural deviations.

## Guides for the Teacher

No two children have the same rate of body growth, and there are individual differences in sitting postures. At the beginning of the school year, the classroom teacher should allow each child to select an individual desk-chair combination. Following the selection, the teacher should tell the children that adjustments will be made in their desk-chair combinations so that they can be seated comfortably. Once the adjustments are made, each child keeps his own desk-chair combination. To be seated with acceptable posture, the child should be comfortable and avoid eyestrain and body fatigue. The child should *not* be seated in a tense, arched-back position, with his hips pushed back into the chair.

1. The seat must be low enough so that the child's feet can be placed flat on the floor and all pressure at the knees relieved.
2. There should be approximately the width of two or three fingers between the front edge of the seat and the calf, or the angle of the knee.
3. The desk top should be at the level of the elbows as the child sits in good posture at his desk.
4. The space between the underneath part of the desk and the child's knees must be adequate for comfort.
5. The space between the child's body and the top edge of the desk should be just the width of his hand.
6. Chair backs should support the small of the back at all times if the child is to maintain good sitting posture.
7. There should be a slight slope from the front edge of the seat toward the back edge.

Desk-chair combinations should be checked every three months by the classroom teacher, and necessary adjustments should be made. In intermediate grades, children can learn to make these adjustments as part of a health lesson on posture and body mechanics. Desk-chair combinations should be checked regularly in the primary grades because of children's rapid body growth.

In schools where students change rooms and seats throughout the day, or in classrooms where traditional furniture is used, students should be made aware of the different sizes of seats and different heights of desks in each room. Students should be aware of criteria for proper selection of desk-seat, tablet-arm chair, table-chair, or other combinations of school furniture. In classrooms having tablet-arm chairs, a few left-handed tablet-arm chairs should be provided.

## SAFETY

Accident prevention in the school environment can be promoted by school pedestrian safety patrols, school bus safety and patrols, traffic control on school grounds, bicycle safety patrols, and fire and disaster drills. Accident prevention procedures should be designed to take in the special problems of all classrooms, corridors and stairs, laboratories, special classrooms, shops, physical education facilities, auditoriums, and lunchrooms. Elementary schools and junior high or middle schools should have school pedestrian safety

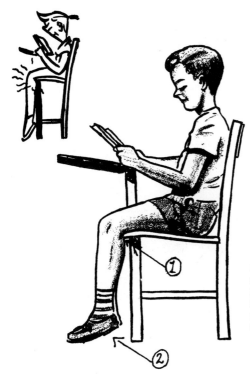

Figure 14. Arrow 1 indicates where front edge of seat is putting pressure under the knees. The chair seat is too deep from front to back. Second arrow indicates that the chair is too high. By permission from the Texas State Department of Health.

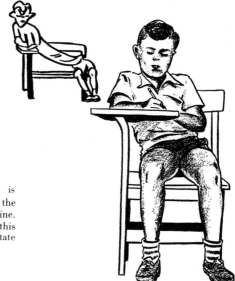

Figure 15. In this position, the child is leaning to one side and thus throwing the back into a lateral curvature of the spine. The arm of the chair is too high for this child. By permission from the Texas State Department of Health.

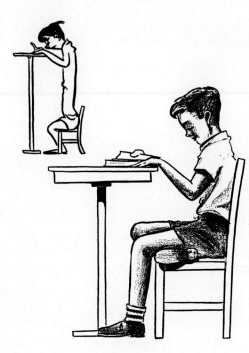

Figure 16. Very poor posture for study. No slant downward from front to back in the seat of the chair—the child feels as though he is slipping out of the chair. Desk is too far away and does not have correct slant for work. The most evident fault is that desk is too high. By permission from the Texas State Department of Health.

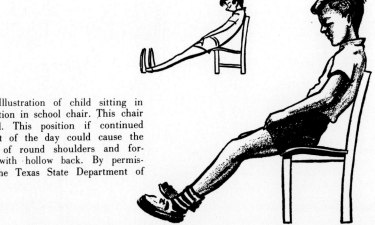

Figure 17. Illustration of child sitting in slumped position in school chair. This chair is too small. This position if continued through most of the day could cause the development of round shoulders and forward head with hollow back. By permission from the Texas State Department of Health.

patrols at street crossings within one block of the school. The school administration should realize the necessity of school bus safety patrols, traffic control on school grounds, bicycle safety patrols, and fire and disaster drills.

## Fire Drills

A school principal may delegate the responsibility of planning fire drills to a member of the faculty, but all procedures must have his approval. Before any planning is attempted, all hazards within the building that may cause fire should be eliminated as quickly as possible. However unlikely a fire, procedures to follow in the event of one must be planned. These procedures will involve:

1. Mapping *regular* and *alternate* routes of evacuation from every classroom, as well as from the auditorium, library, health service unit, and all other special purpose rooms to areas adjoining the school. *All* school personnel and pupils must be included. *All* situations of the school day must be considered, such as times of students changing classrooms, an auditorium program, and so forth. Evacuation of students who are in the shops, lunchroom, and locker and shower rooms must be considered.
2. Placing fire direction signs for evacuation in each classroom, in corridors and stairways, and in all other special purpose rooms.
3. Establishing first-aid centers, with proper supplies, off the school grounds with the school nurse or a faculty member in charge. Secondary school students who have had the American Red Cross First Aid course can assist the person in charge of this center. Each of these students should have designated duties.
4. Including procedures for congested and crowded areas, particularly the auditorium, lunchrooms, and physical education facilities.
5. Working out plans for summoning
   a. Fire-fighting equipment
   b. Police
   c. Community medical and nursing personnel
   d. Ambulance service.
6. Establishing fire signals that differ from disaster signals and checking to be sure that signals can be heard throughout the entire school.

7. Giving in-service education to school personnel concerning:
   a. Use of school fire-alarm boxes
   b. Methods of reporting fires within the school
   c. Recognizing fire signals for fire drills
   d. Evacuation routes for each teacher and her class
   e. Teacher and school personnel's responsibilities in:
      (1) Informing students at the beginning of each semester of the fire direction signs for that particular class or school activity
      (2) Appointing student leaders to assist teachers
      (3) Informing students to leave coats, books, and personal effects in the classroom from which they are being evacuated
      (4) Checking to be certain that all students leave the class by the designated routes in single file
      (5) Being calm, not hurried, and avoiding panic
      (6) Being the last person to leave the class
      (7) Realizing that some students may go to the first-aid center to assist in first-aid treatment
      (8) Reporting to the principal on arrival at the evacuation spot that all students and teacher are safe
      (9) Reporting serious and minor injuries, burns, and asphyxiation resulting from fire and evacuation.
8. Informing students through teachers of their responsibilities during a fire:
   a. Recognizing the fire signal for fire drill
   b. Reading fire direction signs in every part of the school
   c. Assisting teachers
   d. Leaving coats, books, and personal effects in classroom
   e. Leaving the particular class in a single file, not pushing, not shoving, walking quietly, walking in areas close to the building walls, and going directly to evacuation spot
   f. Realizing that some students will be assisting at the first-aid station
   g. Standing quietly at evacuation spot while the teacher checks class roll.
9. Informing parents, through bulletins, of school procedures during the fire and explaining to them about:
   a. Avoiding telephone calls to school
   b. Parking cars in designated areas so that the school building is accessible to fire-fighting equipment, physicians, nurses, and ambulance

c. Bringing coats and blankets and assisting teachers who have evacuated students from the building.

10. Establishing identification for all students and school personnel so that all persons can be quickly checked at evacuation spots.

11. Preparing school personnel in American Red Cross First Aid. At least three of every six school personnel should have had recent training in American Red Cross First Aid.

12. Having school personnel and students practice fire drills intermittently during the school year at hours and days differing from previously practiced drills.

13. Supervising the entire fire drill.

14. Evaluating each fire drill to identify procedures needing revision, addition, or elimination.

15. Informing school personnel and students of changes in procedures of fire drills and being certain that all personnel and students clearly understand the changes.

16. Practicing fire drills with the changed procedures.

17. Obtaining school personnel and students' opinions on means of improving fire drills.

## Self-Preservation in the Event of Natural Disaster

Natural disasters include tornadoes, floods, dust storms, hurricanes, earthquakes, blizzards, and other disasters that are caused by the forces within nature.

### Tornado

Tornadoes usually occur on hot, humid days with southerly winds and a threatening sky. An hour or two before a tornado, greenish-black clouds appear to be bulging downward. Rain and hail may precede the tornado with a heavy downpour after the tornado has passed.

When a funnel from the clouds touches the earth, the tornado has been formed. The funnel may be shaped like an elephant's trunk, column, or a coil of rope. The vortex, with a wind speed of 500 miles an hour, is the destructive part of the tornado.

The tornado's path is usually from 10 to 40 miles in length, and the average width of the tornado's path is about 400 yards; however, tornadoes have been reported to cut paths over a mile in width. Tornadoes travel about 25 to 40 miles per hour.

The National Weather Service issues *forecasts* when conditions in an area are such that a tornado may develop. When one or more local weather bureaus locate a cloud formation which may become a tornado, a tornado *alert* is issued. Tornado *warnings* are announcements that a tornado has been sighted. These warnings are for the purpose of advising persons in the path of the tornado to take immediate steps to protect themselves.

If a tornado warning is given when students are in a school building of reinforced steel construction, students should go to the lowest floor, along inside walls, and away from windows.

### Hurricane

Hurricanes are large revolving storms accompanied by violent destructive winds, heavy rains, high waves, and high tides. Hurricane winds have been reported as high as 150 miles per hour. The highest wind speeds are in the circular band beginning at the edge of the "eye" of the hurricane and extending out 20 to 30 miles or more. The "eye" is the calm center.

The area of destructive winds along the path of a hurricane may be from 25 to 500 miles wide. The forward movement of a hurricane is usually very slow, although occasionally the forward speed may reach 50 miles an hour or more.

Hurricane *advisories* provide forecasts of the hurricane's position over the next 24 hours, and give the time and source of the next advisory. A hurricane *watch* specifies an area which might be threatened. It indicates that the hurricane is near enough that everyone in the area should be ready to take safety measures. Hurricane *warnings* become part of the advisories when a hurricane is expected to strike within the next 24 hours. These warnings identify coastal areas where winds of at least 75 miles per hour are expected to occur.

If the hurricane strikes while students are in a school building, the students should remain indoors. If the school building is not on high ground, the students should go to designated shelter. Drinking water needs to be stored; foods which can be eaten without cooking should be available.

Procedures which may protect the lives of students and school personnel in any disaster include:

1. Mapping *regular* and *alternate* routes of evacuation to dispersal and shelter areas. In some disasters, students and school personnel will remain within the school building, such as in corridors. In other disasters, such as earthquakes, students and school personnel will be evacuated from the school building. The construction of the school building and its corridors will determine the evacuation. All classrooms and special purpose areas should be included on these routes. All pupils, school personnel, and situations must be considered.

2. Planning for identification of all students and school personnel, including name and address of the nearest of kin to notify, and the blood type.

3. Placing direction signs for procedures during disaster in all classrooms and special purpose areas.

4. Training school personnel in American Red Cross First Aid.

5. Appointing trained school personnel to different first-aid centers.

6. Establishing first-aid centers within the school building and at shelter areas. Secondary school students who have had the American Red Cross Standard First Aid course can assist at the first-aid center.

   Procedures should be established for:
   a. Classification of victims, that is: casualties needing immediate life-saving first aid, casualties for which speed is important but not as urgent as for the first group, and those having serious injuries but who can wait until the first two groups are treated
   b. Classification of types of injuries: burns, wounds, internal injuries, fractures, eye injuries, and so forth
   c. Labeling of casualties.

7. Including procedures for congested and crowded areas, such as the auditorium, lunchrooms, and physical education facilities.

8. Coordinating all school procedures with community disaster plans.

9. Establishing school disaster signals that differ from fire signals but correspond to community disaster signals.

10. Giving in-service education to all faculty and school personnel regarding:
    a. Community disaster signals
    b. School practice disaster signals
    c. Procedures for each teacher and his class to follow when practice disaster signals occur
    d. Teacher and school personnel's responsibilities in:
       (1) Informing students at the beginning of each semester about routes and procedures for that particular class or building area
       (2) Appointing student leaders to assist teachers
       (3) Instructing students to leave coats, books, and personal effects in the building
       (4) Checking to be certain that all students leave the particular building area and proceed to designated shelter areas
       (5) Being calm and unhurried, and avoiding panic
       (6) Being the last person to leave the particular building area
       (7) Reporting to principal on arrival at the shelter area so that all students and teacher are known to be safe
       (8) Reporting serious injuries, burns, asphyxiation, sickness, and wounds from disaster.

11. Informing students through teachers of their responsibilities during disaster:
    a. Recognizing the disaster practice signal
    b. Reading direction signs in each part of the building area
    c. Assisting teachers
    d. Leaving coats, books, and personal effects in classroom
    e. Going to designated shelter areas in single file, not pushing or shoving, walking quietly, and walking close to building walls
    f. Standing quietly at shelter area while teacher checks roll.

12. Informing parents through bulletins of all school procedures and coordination with community disaster plans.

13. Informing parents to:
    a. Avoid telephoning school
    b. Follow community procedures when children are sent home during "alert."

14. Establishing procedures for children not reaching their homes during an "alert" of community disaster.

15. Coordinating school procedures with community centers for victims of disaster.

16. Giving in-service education to school personnel in self-preservation during a disaster so that school personnel can pass the information and procedures along to pupils and parents:
    a. At home, as in taking precautions to avoid flying glass; turning off electricity, gas, water outlets; avoidance of food contamination and polluted water; disposal of garbage and sewage; self-preservation procedures from falling building structures, fires, and explosions; and care of small children and old persons

b. On the street

c. In a car, bus, or train

d. In a building other than home or school.

17. Having school personnel and students practice disaster drills at hours and days differing from previous disaster practice drills.

18. Supervising entire disaster practice drill.

19. Evaluating each drill to identify procedures needing revision, addition, or elimination.

20. Informing school personnel and students of changes in procedures of disaster practice drills and being certain that all personnel and students clearly understand the changes.

21. Practicing disaster drills using the changed procedures.

22. Obtaining school personnel and students' opinions on means of improving disaster drills.

These fire and disaster procedures may vary, depending on community, school, and community disaster planning. A wise school superintendent and alert principals will devise fire and disaster procedures and will practice these procedures regularly, because the lives of pupils and school personnel are involved.

## IMPLICATIONS FOR HEALTH EDUCATION

Environmental factors in a school building can have implications for three areas of health education: "Care of All Parts of the Human Body," "Community Health," and "Safety Education." Suggested units from these areas are:

| Environmental factors | Area of Health Education | Suggested units |
| --- | --- | --- |
| Water supply | Community Health | Water pollution, water-borne diseases, and water purification |
| Sewage | Community Health | Sewage treatment and sewage-borne diseases |
| Solid waste | Community Health | Solid wastes and proper disposal |
| Noise | Safety Education | Occupational safety |
| School Furniture | Care of All Parts of the Human Body | Seated posture and school furniture |
| Fire Drills | Safety Education | Fire drills in schools |
| Tornado | Safety Education | Self-preservation in the event of a tornado |
| Hurricane | Safety Education | Self-preservation in the event of a hurricane |

Other units possibly might include other natural disasters and man-made disasters. Civil riots could be considered in the area of Safety Education and air pollution in the area of Community Health.

## References for Further Study

American Association of School Administrators: *Schools for America.* Washington, D.C.: National Education Association, 1967.

American Society of Heating, Refrigerating, and Air Conditioning Engineers: *Handbook of Fundamentals, 1967.* New York: The Society, 1967.

Hopkins, E., and Bean, E.: *Water Purification Control.* 4th ed. Baltimore: The Williams & Wilkins Company, 1966.

Kilbourne, E. D., and Smillie, W. G.: *Human Ecology and Public Health.* 4th ed. New York: The Macmillan Company, 1969.

National Education Association, National Commission on Safety Education: *A School Safety Education Program.* Washington, D.C.: The Commission, 1966.

————: *School Safety Education Checklist: Administration, Instruction, Protection.* rev. ed. Washington, D.C.: The Commission, 1967.

————: *A Realistic Approach to Civil Defense: A Handbook for School Administrators.* Washington, D.C.: The Commission, 1966.

National Safety Council, Elementary School Section: *The Total Safety Program in Schools and Colleges— A Technique.* Chicago: The Council, 1966.

National Society for the Prevention of Blindness, Inc.: *Classroom Lighting.* New York: The Society, 1963.

Sartwell, P., ed.: *Maxcy-Rosenau Preventive Medicine and Public Health.* 9th ed. New York: Appleton-Century-Crofts, 1965.

School Environments Research: *SER 2: Environmental Evaluations.* Ann Arbor, Mich.: Architectural Research Laboratory, University of Michigan, 1965.

# Chapter 10

# *SCHOOL NUTRITION*

## AN INCIDENT

As the results of nutrition studies are being published, elementary school classroom teachers, teachers of health education in the secondary schools, and home economics teachers are asking questions concerning the lunch served in the school lunchroom and special milk program. Questions are being raised as to whether the lunch is a Type A lunch, the foods served fall within the Essential Four Food Groups and meet the Recommended Daily Dietary Allowances, and the signs of dietary deficiencies found among the students are indications of poor diets.

In 1946, Congress approved Public Law 396, the National School Lunch Act, under which the National School Lunch Program operates through the Food and Nutrition Service of the Department of Agriculture. The National School Lunch Program provides

financial assistance to public and nonprofit private schools of high school grade or under operating nonprofit school lunch programs. These funds are provided to schools on the basis of their need for assistance, and the number of meals served, with emphasis on those served free or at reduced prices to children from needy families. Participating schools also receive foods bought specifically to help them meet meal standards, and are eligible for foods distributed through the Commodity Distribution Program.[1]

The Child Nutrition Act of 1966 established the School Breakfast Program which provides cash grants to State educational agencies to assist schools in operating nonprofit breakfast programs meeting established nutritional standards. First preference is given to schools in low-income areas and to schools where children travel long distances to attend. In cases of severe need, the grant may provide up to 80 percent of the cost of operating a breakfast program. Participating schools are also eligible for food distributed through the Commodity Distribution Program.[2]

To initiate or expand school food service is provided by the Equipment Program under the Child Nutrition Act of 1966. This program is designed "to assist the States to supply schools in low-income areas with equipment for the storage, preparation, transportation, and serving of food to children."[3]

The Special Milk Program was established under the Agricultural Act of 1954. It is "designed to increase the consumption of fluid milk by children in nonprofit schools of high school grade and under."[4]

As a result of the White House Conference on Food, Nutrition and Health, Public Law 91-248, was approved. The law amends the National School Lunch Act and the Child Nutrition Act. It encourages the states to extend the school lunch program to every school within the state. The law establishes national standards of minimum income eligibility for free and reduced-price school lunches, which should be available to all eligible children in schools participating in lunch programs. The law strives to improve nutrition education in schools and school lunchrooms.

---

[1] *United States Government Organization Manual— 1971/1972.* p. 252.

[2] *Ibid.*
[3] *Ibid.*
[4] *Ibid.*

## NUTRITION STUDIES

In the past few years, there have been countless nutrition studies by nutritional authorities, nutrition agencies, and national research groups. The National Dairy Council reported in one study that a large proportion of adolescents have poor food habits and consume diets lacking the essential nutrients. Some of the influences on the food habits of adolescents were: (1) hunger and appetite; (2) family eating habits; (3) certain physiological, sociological, and psychological factors; (4) attitudes toward food; and (5) food selection and purchase. Hunger and appetite cannot be relied upon as a guide in food selection to meet specific needs of nutrients. Adolescent's food habits usually reflect those habits to which he has been exposed from early childhood. Unusually early or late maturation, social adjustment, and concern for overweight are some of the physiological, sociological, and psychological factors. The adolescent's attitude toward food reflects the manner in which he has been reared. Even though adolescents may have acquired knowledge of nutrition and have favorable attitudes concerning food habits, their food intake practices are not always influenced by their knowledge or attitudes. Finally, adolescents spend 25 to 33% of their money on lunches and snacks, a total of more than $11 billion annually.[5]

Previous to the 1969 White House Conference on Food, Nutrition, and Health, priorities in nutrition were reported by Mayer. In some states, the government food programs did not reach the majority of the very poor. In 1969, at least 600 counties had neither food distribution or food stamp systems, and only 1/4 to 1/3 of those eligible for the food programs were actually reached. One half to 2/3 of very poor children were not included in school lunch programs.[6]

In the first phase of the National Nutrition Survey, studies were made of low-income areas of ten states: Texas, Louisiana, New York (including a special survey of New York City), Kentucky, Michigan, California, Washington, South Carolina, West Virginia, and Massachusetts. The research techniques included use of clinical examinations, biochemical measurements, dietary assessments, dental examinations, and collecting data such as socioeconomic status, food sources, and level of education. Clinical examinations included medical examination, recent medical history, anthropometric studies, and bone x-ray measurements. Some of the findings of clinical examinations were: (1) nearly 4% of preschool children showed vitamin D deficiency; (2) 4 to 5% of the subjects showed winged scapula, pot-belly, or both, associated with protein-calorie malnutrition; (3) 5% of the subjects had enlarged goiter; and (4) several cases of Bitot's spots confirmed vitamin A deficiency. Some of the findings of dental examinations were: (1) 18% of all subjects aged ten and over reported difficulty and pain in biting and chewing food; and (2) 96% of the subjects had an average of ten teeth either decayed, missing, or filled. Findings of the study showed growth retardation: (1) height of children, ages one to three, fell below the average height reported for children in the United States; (2) three times the expected number of children fell below the sixteenth growth percentile; and (3) about 3.5% of children whose wrist bones were x-rayed had retarded growth. Some of the findings of the biochemical measurements were: (1) 33% of the children under six had blood hemoglobin levels in an unacceptable range; (2) 33% of children under six had serum vitamin A levels that were unacceptable; (3) serum vitamin C levels were less than acceptable in 12 to 16% of all age groups; (4) about 16% of the overall population had serum protein levels that were less than acceptable; and (5) levels of riboflavin and thiamine were unacceptable in 9 to 19% of the sample studied. Some of the findings of the dietary intake data were (1) large numbers of individuals from 10 to 16 years old consumed 50% (or less) of the amounts considered adequate for calories, iron, vitamin A and vitamin C; (2) iron intake was low in over 60% of young children; and (3) almost 40% of adolescents consumed less than half the desired amount of vitamin A.[7]

[5]Factors influencing adolescent food habits. *Dairy Council Digest 36* (January, February, 1965) :1-6.
[6]Jean Mayer: Priorities in nutrition. *Food and Nutrition News 41* (October, 1969) :1,4.

[7]Arnold E. Schaefer: Malnutrition in the U.S.A.? *Nutrition News 32* (December, 1969) :1,4.

Findings reported by other researchers indicate incidence of rickets in low-income areas. Even though vitamin D milk must have 400 U.S.P. units of vitamin D per quart by federal and state standards, recent investigations have disclosed that some diaries have not fortified fluid milk with vitamin D. However, milk companies selling 40% of the fluid milk in the United States indicate that all of their fluid whole milk sold was fortified with vitamin D to a level of 400 I.U. per quart.[8]

The Committee on Maternal Nutrition of the National Research Council has released a report, "Maternal Nutrition and Course of Pregnancy," which includes discussion of the dangers of adolescent pregnancy. Shank,[9] in his review of this report, indicated that anemia due to iron deficiency resulting from low iron intake is the most common complication of pregnancy. Most pregnant women need medically prescribed daily iron supplements during the last six months of pregnancy. The Committee on Maternal Nutrition pointed out that many biological risks for young mothers were connected with nutritional deficiency. Because adolescent girls are still growing, most pregnant girls under 17 years have greater nutritional requirements than otherwise comparable pregnant adult women. Large numbers of infants weighing less than 5.5 pounds are born to adolescents; death rates for both white and nonwhite babies born to mothers under 15 are much higher than those born to older women.[10]

Stare and Dwyer[11] have reported signs of beginning atherosclerosis in the coronary arteries of American men of the average age of 22. Some teenagers and children have the same signs. Fifteen-year-old boys may have serum cholesterol levels similar to those of men in their 40s and 50s. The rise in serum cholesterol levels in young persons in this country is avoidable since among those in similar age groups in other countries, the same rise in serum cholesterols does not occur.

## ESSENTIAL FOUR FOOD GROUPS

Nutritionists have grouped food into four groups and have determined the desirable daily amount of each:

*Breads and Cereals:*

Four servings daily of enriched, whole grain or restored breads and cereals; other baked foods with enriched or whole grain flour, enriched macaroni, spaghetti, and noodles, are included. A serving is one slice of enriched or whole grain bread, ½ to ¾ cup whole grain or restored cereal, 1 cup enriched macaroni products.[12]

*Milk and Milk Products:*

Three or more glasses of milk for children. Four or more glasses for teenagers. Two or more glasses for adults.[13]
1 slice (1 oz.) Cheddar-type cheese = ¾ cup whole milk
½ cup cottage cheese = ⅓ cup whole milk
2 tablespoons cream cheese = 1 tablespoon whole milk
½ cup vanilla ice cream = almost ⅓ cup whole milk.[14]

*Vegetables and Fruits:*

Four servings of vegetables and fruits daily. Source of vitamin C (citrus fruit, for example) every day; every other day a dark green or deep yellow vegetable for vitamin A. A serving is ½ cup of fresh, canned, or frozen fruit or vegetable.

*Meat and Other Protein Foods:*

Two servings daily of meat, fish, poultry, or eggs with beans, peas, lentils, nuts, or peanut butter as alternates. Include at least three to five eggs a week. The following are about equal in amount of protein provided: 1 ounce cooked lean meat, poultry, or fish; 1 egg; ½ cup cooked dried beans or peas; 2 tablespoons peanut butter.[15]

Recent developments in vitamin D. *Dairy Council Digest 41* (July, August, 1970) :19-24.
Robert E. Shank: The role of nutrition in the course of human pregnancy. *Nutrition News 33* (October, 1970) :1,4.
Dangers of adolescent pregnancies. *Public Health Reports 85* (November, 1970) :1031.
Frederick J. Stare and Johanna Dwyer: An eye to the future: healthy eating for teenagers. *J. School Health 39* (November, 1969) :595.

[12]Wheat Flour Institute: *Eat To Live.* Chicago: The Institute, 1969, p. 28.
[13]Busy day, balanced diet? Miniposter 3. Chicago: National Dairy Council, 1970.
[14]Ruth M. Leverton: *A Girl and Her Figure.* Chicago: National Dairy Council, 1970, p. 13.
[15]Wheat Flour Institute, *op. cit.,* p. 29.

## RECOMMENDED DAILY DIETARY ALLOWANCES, REVISED 1968

The Food and Nutrition Board, National Academy of Sciences—National Research Council has recommended the amounts of calories, protein, fat-soluble vitamins, water-soluble vitamins, and mineral elements needed by healthy persons of various ages. These amounts are given in the accompanying table.

## OBESITY IN CHILDREN AND ADOLESCENTS

Obese adults usually had difficulty in losing fat and maintaining fat loss when they were children and teenagers. Some researchers indicate that the prevention of obesity in adulthood lies with changing children's eating patterns. In one study of 3444 preschool children, a significant number of these children ate too much and benefited too little from what they ate. These children had too few fruits and vegetables, too little vitamin A and C, and too much candy and soft drinks. More than 75% of the children were not hungry at mealtime, causing worry among the majority of mothers. Only 4.9% of the mothers worried if the children ate too much. Food was used as a reward for good behavior; desserts were the top rewards—75%.

Among studies of factors influencing adolescent food habits, foods which elicited praise from parents and other adults were vegetables, milk, meat, and fruits. The "scold" foods were candy, pastry, ice cream, and carbonated beverages.[16]

Some studies find that the obese teenager may not consume as many calories in the day as the nonobese teenager. The intake of the obese averaged about 2600 calories while those of average weight had 3200 calories. Girls of normal weight averaged about 2000 calories per day while obese girls averaged about 1700 calories daily. Caloric intake varied between persons, from day to day, and from week to week. For boys, the variations ranged from 635 to 4700 calories; for girls, the variations ranged from 650 to 6000 calories. Week-to-week variations were 900 calories per day for boys and 700 calories per day for girls.

Snacking is popular among teenagers, and they may eat as often as five times a day. The obese teenager tends to eat less frequently, omitting breakfast and lunch more often than the nonobese. The obese ate fewer fruits and vegetables and drank less milk than nonobese.[17]

Vigorous physical exercise, dietary education, and psychological support introduced into a public school system can assist students, ages 8 through 14, to lose weight.[18] Vigorous exercise in special physical activity classes can be planned for the obese on the days on which regular school physical education is not scheduled. The obese children are not placed on low calorie diets but receive instruction concerning proper food intake. Encouragement and providing motivation are the forms of psychological support.

## TYPE A LUNCH

One third of the Recommended Daily Dietary Allowances (see table) should be provided by a Type A lunch. The local board of education makes the decision to participate in the National School Lunch Program. The program is administered by the state educational agency, which must enter into a written agreement with the United States Department of Agriculture. The local board of education must sign an agreement with the state educational agency to (1) provide the minimum nutritional standards for a Type A lunch; (2) comply with the state and local sanitation standards; and (3) supply lunches free or at reduced cost, without discrimination, to children who cannot pay the full cost of the lunch. Pupils receiving lunch free or reduced cost are designated by local school authorities. In 1968, the Department of Agriculture (1) clarified the responsibilities of the state educational agency administering the program; (2) provided means of establishing eligibility criteria for reduced-cost lunches; and (3) warned against singling

---

[16]Factors influencing adolescent food habits. *op. cit.*, p. 4.

[17]Ruth L. Huenemann: Consideration of adolescent obesity as a public health problem. *Public Health Reports 83* (June, 1968) :491-495.

[18]Carl C. Seltzer and Jean Mayer: An effective weight control program in a public school system. *Ame J. Public Health 60* (April, 1970):679.

## Table 2
### Recommended Daily Dietary Allowances[1]
**Designed for the maintenance of good nutrition of practically all healthy people in the U.S.A.**

| | Age[2] Years From–Up to | Weight Kg (lbs) | | Height cm (in.) | | Kcal | Protein gm | Fat Soluble Vitamins | | | Water Soluble Vitamins | | | | | | | Minerals | | | | |
|---|---|---|---|---|---|---|---|---|---|---|---|---|---|---|---|---|---|---|---|---|---|---|
| | | | | | | | | Vitamin A Activity I.U. | Vitamin D I.U. | Vitamin E Activity I.U. | Ascorbic Acid mg | Folacin[3] mg | Niacin mg equiv.[4] | Riboflavin mg | Thiamine mg | Vitamin $B_6$ mg | Vitamin $B_{12}$ μg | Calcium gm | Phosphorus gm | Iodine μg | Iron mg | Magnesium mg |
| **Infants** | 0 – 1/6 | 4 | 9 | 55 | 22 | kg × 120 | kg × 2.2[5] | 1500 | 400 | 5 | 35 | 0.05 | 5 | 0.4 | 0.2 | 0.2 | 1.0 | 0.4 | 0.2 | 25 | 6 | 40 |
| | 1/6 – 1/2 | 7 | 15 | 63 | 25 | kg × 110 | kg × 2.0[5] | 1500 | 400 | 5 | 35 | 0.05 | 7 | 0.5 | 0.4 | 0.3 | 1.5 | 0.5 | 0.4 | 40 | 10 | 60 |
| | 1/2 – 1 | 9 | 20 | 72 | 28 | kg × 100 | kg × 1.8[5] | 1500 | 400 | 5 | 35 | 0.1 | 8 | 0.6 | 0.5 | 0.4 | 2.0 | 0.6 | 0.5 | 45 | 15 | 70 |
| **Children** | 1 – 2 | 12 | 26 | 81 | 32 | 1100 | 25 | 2000 | 400 | 10 | 40 | 0.1 | 8 | 0.6 | 0.6 | 0.5 | 2.0 | 0.7 | 0.7 | 55 | 15 | 100 |
| | 2 – 3 | 14 | 31 | 91 | 36 | 1250 | 25 | 2000 | 400 | 10 | 40 | 0.2 | 8 | 0.7 | 0.6 | 0.6 | 2.5 | 0.8 | 0.8 | 60 | 15 | 150 |
| | 3 – 4 | 16 | 35 | 100 | 39 | 1400 | 30 | 2500 | 400 | 10 | 40 | 0.2 | 9 | 0.8 | 0.7 | 0.7 | 3 | 0.8 | 0.8 | 70 | 10 | 200 |
| | 4 – 6 | 19 | 42 | 110 | 43 | 1600 | 30 | 2500 | 400 | 10 | 40 | 0.2 | 11 | 0.9 | 0.8 | 0.9 | 4 | 0.8 | 0.8 | 80 | 10 | 200 |
| | 6 – 8 | 23 | 51 | 121 | 48 | 2000 | 35 | 3500 | 400 | 15 | 40 | 0.2 | 13 | 1.1 | 1.0 | 1.0 | 4 | 0.9 | 0.9 | 100 | 10 | 250 |
| | 8 – 10 | 28 | 62 | 131 | 52 | 2200 | 40 | 3500 | 400 | 15 | 40 | 0.3 | 15 | 1.2 | 1.1 | 1.2 | 5 | 1.0 | 1.0 | 110 | 10 | 250 |
| **Males** | 10 – 12 | 35 | 77 | 140 | 55 | 2500 | 45 | 4500 | 400 | 20 | 40 | 0.4 | 17 | 1.3 | 1.3 | 1.4 | 5 | 1.2 | 1.2 | 125 | 10 | 300 |
| | 12 – 14 | 43 | 95 | 151 | 59 | 2700 | 50 | 5000 | 400 | 20 | 45 | 0.4 | 18 | 1.4 | 1.4 | 1.6 | 5 | 1.4 | 1.4 | 135 | 18 | 350 |
| | 14 – 18 | 59 | 130 | 170 | 67 | 3000 | 60 | 5000 | 400 | 25 | 55 | 0.4 | 20 | 1.5 | 1.5 | 1.8 | 5 | 1.4 | 1.4 | 150 | 18 | 400 |
| | 18 – 22 | 67 | 147 | 175 | 69 | 2800 | 60 | 5000 | 400 | 30 | 60 | 0.4 | 18 | 1.6 | 1.4 | 2.0 | 5 | 0.8 | 0.8 | 140 | 10 | 400 |
| | 22 – 35 | 70 | 154 | 175 | 69 | 2800 | 65 | 5000 | -- | 30 | 60 | 0.4 | 18 | 1.7 | 1.4 | 2.0 | 5 | 0.8 | 0.8 | 140 | 10 | 350 |
| | 35 – 55 | 70 | 154 | 173 | 68 | 2600 | 65 | 5000 | — | 30 | 60 | 0.4 | 17 | 1.7 | 1.3 | 2.0 | 5 | 0.8 | 0.8 | 125 | 10 | 350 |
| | 55 – 75+ | 70 | 154 | 171 | 67 | 2400 | 65 | 5000 | -- | 30 | 60 | 0.4 | 14 | 1.7 | 1.2 | 2.0 | 6 | 0.8 | 0.8 | 110 | 10 | 350 |
| **Females** | 10 – 12 | 35 | 77 | 142 | 56 | 2250 | 50 | 4500 | 400 | 20 | 40 | 0.4 | 15 | 1.3 | 1.1 | 1.4 | 5 | 1.2 | 1.2 | 110 | 18 | 300 |
| | 12 – 14 | 44 | 97 | 154 | 61 | 2300 | 50 | 5000 | 400 | 20 | 45 | 0.4 | 15 | 1.4 | 1.2 | 1.6 | 5 | 1.3 | 1.3 | 115 | 18 | 350 |
| | 14 – 16 | 52 | 114 | 157 | 62 | 2400 | 55 | 5000 | 400 | 25 | 50 | 0.4 | 16 | 1.4 | 1.2 | 1.8 | 5 | 1.3 | 1.3 | 120 | 18 | 350 |
| | 16 – 18 | 54 | 119 | 160 | 63 | 2300 | 55 | 5000 | 400 | 25 | 50 | 0.4 | 15 | 1.5 | 1.2 | 2.0 | 5 | 1.3 | 1.3 | 115 | 18 | 350 |
| | 18 – 22 | 58 | 128 | 163 | 64 | 2000 | 55 | 5000 | 400 | 25 | 55 | 0.4 | 13 | 1.5 | 1.0 | 2.0 | 5 | 0.8 | 0.8 | 100 | 18 | 350 |
| | 22 – 35 | 58 | 128 | 163 | 64 | 2000 | 55 | 5000 | -- | 25 | 55 | 0.4 | 13 | 1.5 | 1.0 | 2.0 | 5 | 0.8 | 0.8 | 100 | 18 | 300 |
| | 35 – 55 | 58 | 128 | 160 | 63 | 1850 | 55 | 5000 | -- | 25 | 55 | 0.4 | 13 | 1.5 | 1.0 | 2.0 | 5 | 0.8 | 0.8 | 90 | 18 | 300 |
| | 55 – 75+ | 58 | 128 | 157 | 62 | 1700 | 55 | 5000 | -- | 25 | 55 | 0.4 | 13 | 1.5 | 1.0 | 2.0 | 6 | 0.8 | 0.8 | 80 | 10 | 300 |
| **Pregnancy** | | | | | | +200 | 65 | 6000 | 400 | 30 | 60 | 0.8 | 15 | 1.8 | +0.1 | 2.5 | 8 | +0.4 | +0.4 | 125 | 18 | 450 |
| **Lactation** | | | | | | +1000 | 75 | 8000 | 400 | 30 | 60 | 0.5 | 20 | 2.0 | +0.5 | 2.5 | 6 | +0.5 | +0.5 | 150 | 18 | 450 |

1. The allowance levels are intended to cover individual variations among most normal persons as they live in the United States under usual environmental stresses. The recommended allowances can be attained with a variety of common foods, providing other nutrients for which human requirements have been less well defined. See text for more detailed discussion of allowances and of nutrients not tabulated.

2. Entries on lines for age range 22-35 years represent the reference man and woman at age 22. All other entries represent allowances for the midpoint of the specified age range.

3. The folacin allowances refer to dietary sources as determined by *Lactobacillus casei* assay. Pure forms of folacin may be effective in doses less than ¼ of the RDA.

4. Niacin equivalents include dietary sources of the vitamin itself plus 1 mg equivalent for each 60 mg of dietary tryptophan.

5. Assumes protein equivalent to human milk. For proteins not 100 percent utilized factors should be increased proportionately.

[1]Food and Nutrition Board, National Academy of Sciences—National Research Council, 1968.

out and embarrassing children who receive reduced-cost lunches.[19]

The Type A lunch pattern is reviewed periodically. From a nationwide study of nutrient content of Type A lunches by the Department of Agriculture and changes in the Recommended Daily Dietary Allowances, the 1969 recommendation for The Type A lunch must contain as a minimum:

1. *Milk*—½ pint of fluid whole milk as a beverage.
2. *Meat or Meat Substitute*—lean meat, fish, or poultry (edible portion as served)—two ounces; cheese—two ounces; egg—one whole egg or its equivalent in whole dried eggs; dried beans or peas—½ cup cooked measure; peanut butter—4 tablespoons or ¼ cup; or an equivalent quantity of any combination of the above foods. To be counted in meeting this requirement, these foods must be served in a main dish or in a main dish and one other menu item.
3. *Vegetables and/or Fruit*—¾ cup. This requirement should be met by two or more servings of vegetables or fruits, or broth. Fruits and vegetables in salads and desserts contribute toward this requirement. Full-strength vegetable or fruit juice may be counted to meet not more than one-fourth cup of this requirement. Fruits or vegetables rich in vitamin C and vitamin A should be served several times a week.
4. *Bread*—one slice of whole-grain or enriched bread; or a serving of cornbread, biscuits, rolls, muffins, etc., made of whole-grain or enriched meal or flour. Crackers do not meet the bread requirement; therefore, when they are served, they should be served in addition to an enriched bread.
5. *Butter or Fortified Margarine*—1 teaspoon. Butter may be served separately, may be spread on bread, or preferably may be used in cooking.[20]

The Agricultural Research Service also suggests that foods with vitamin A be served once a day and several foods high in iron be served daily. In addition, larger or second servings of some of the Type A foods and other foods are often needed.

Older boys and girls need more of most foods in the Type A lunch than do younger children.[21]

In the Atlanta, Georgia, high schools, the students enjoy choices of lunches within the Type A pattern, termed "Hot Line" or "Express Line." Hot Line main dishes may be oven-fried chicken or meat loaf. The Express Line's main dishes may feature hamburgers, hot dogs, pizza, chili, or jumbo sandwiches served with other Type A foods. A low-calorie salad bowl with a minimum of two ounces of protein (egg, cheese, cold meat, or tuna) is popular, with extra bread and butter available.[22]

## CALORIC INTAKE

The daily and weekly caloric intake of the school lunch should be considered. If the child eats a complete meal at school each day, the meal will represent approximately one-third of his daily food intake. If the child eats a complete meal at school five days of the week, the five meals represent one-fourth of his total food intake for the week. Nutritionists give these statements on the assumption that the other two meals consumed each day are supplying their share of the child's nutritional needs. In some instances, if the child is not eating adequate amounts and varieties of foods at the other two daily meals, it may be desirable to supply more than one-third of the child's daily food requirement at the school lunch.

Small schools having no cafeteria or lunchroom facilities may provide one hot dish to be supplemented by packed lunches brought from home. If milk is served to drink, the supplementary dish need not contain milk. Some examples of hot dishes are creamed meat, fish, or eggs with a baked potato; escalloped macaroni with cheese; cheese fondue; meat and vegetable loaf; scrambled eggs with a vegetable; vegetable stew; and escalloped vegetables. Soups are also very popular. Orange juice might supplement the home-packed lunch in addition to milk.

[19]Phyllis Agran: The National School Lunch Program. *J. School Health 39* (September, 1969) :440.
[20]Consumer and Marketing Services, United States Department of Agriculture: The Type A lunch pattern. Washington, D.C.: Agricultural Research Service, Department of Agriculture, 1969.

[21]*Ibid.*
[22]Sara Sloan: "Turned on" school lunch program. *Nutrition News 32* (April, 1969) :7.

Schools that do not provide a hot dish or milk should work closely with parents to encourage them to make the home-packed lunch appetizing and nutritious. Foods in lunch boxes are often left uneaten or are thrown away for a number of reasons. The contents of the box may be unappetizing or untidy; there may be too much food; menus sometimes become monotonous; leftover foods may have been used; and the lunch box may be too cumbersome to carry. Through adult health education, parents can be given suggestions for lunch-box menus that will satisfy hungry boys and girls.

## SUPPLEMENTARY FEEDING

Supplementary "snacks" can be supplied in the midmorning and/or the midafternoon. These snacks provide additional food to the child who had an inadequate breakfast, or had a very early breakfast in order to reach school in time, or has a long bus trip home, or has been discovered to have nutritional problems by his family physician, or has recovered from a long siege of illness, or has a poor appetite. Young children and adolescents can profit most from these snack periods. This additional feeding usually consists of milk, orange juice, fruit, crackers, or sandwiches. These snacks should be small in quantity and should not take on the proportions of extra meals. Genuine fruit juices are appetizing, promote digestion, and are sources of vitamins and mineral elements. Milk is an excellent supplementary food, as it contains many of the needed vitamins, mineral elements, carbohydrates, fats, proteins, and water. Fruits are our most delicious natural food product. They stimulate appetite and digestion, assist in intestinal movements and prevent constipation, act as body alkalizers, and promote general health. If many children come to school without breakfast, a breakfast may be served. The breakfast may consist of ready-to-eat cereal, milk, and fruit.

## SCHOOL LUNCH

At least 19 million American elementary and secondary school students eat lunch at school each school day. They consume more than 4750 tons of milk; eighty-two carloads of ground beef for hamburgers; and nineteen million buns. More than a billion dollars worth of food is used in a year.[23]

A home-packed lunch supplemented by a hot dish, a plate lunch, and a cafeteria-style lunch are the three common types of noonday school meals. Soup or hot milk beverage often supplement the home-packed lunch. With the plate lunch, all foods are served on one plate except the half pint of milk. Schools with small enrollments prefer to serve the plate lunch because there is no need for extensive kitchen equipment and facilities and large staffs of lunchroom workers. The cafeteria-style lunch permits the student to select his own food. Varieties of food are prepared in cafeteria kitchens. Lunchroom workers place selected foods on plates, or students pick up their choice of foods.

### Supervision

Regardless of the type of noonday meal, supervision is essential. The kind of supervision will depend on the (1) size of the school and/or the school system; (2) availability of a dietitian as the director; (3) recruitment of community personnel serving as workers, and in many schools as lunch managers; (4) type of lunch served and method of service; and (5) length of the serving period.

The lunch manager is responsible for planning, preparing, and serving the noonday meal. The manager must train cooks, helpers, attendants, and other workers. The manager must plan daily menus, purchase food, provide adequate food storage, fulfill all sanitary measures, maintain cleanliness in food preparation and eating areas, comply with local health regulations, keep records, and handle finances.

Menus should be planned not less than one week nor more than two weeks in advance. A school lunch should be planned primarily for its nutritional values. Variety

[23]Ruth M. Leverton: The world's biggest lunch counter. *Food and Nutrition News 38* (March, 1967) :1.

in menus can be maintained from day to day by combining the same foods in different types of dishes. Using a different menu pattern each day will ensure variety. Texture and consistency of foods are important factors. There should be variety in texture of foods served together, and repetition of color should be avoided. Contrasting food flavors make meals more appetizing, but more common food likes and dislikes should be considered when flavors are combined. Popular foods should accompany foods not too well liked. Younger children like plain and unmixed foods, easy-to-eat foods, and moist—not soupy—foods. They object to strong flavors and highly seasoned foods.

## Food Preparation and Serving

The manager must devise plans for food preparation and serving. Care must be given to every detail of the noonday meal. Food preparation requires careful handling of food and proper methods of cooking. School meals must be balanced not only for nutritional values but also for attractiveness and palatability. Pupils will eat foods which are appetizingly prepared. Food served should consist of "whole" meals. Desserts should be the last item served. New foods should be served at intervals, and every effort should be made to persuade students to accept new foods. School menus should be adapted to seasons of the year, including festive touches for holidays and special school events. Foods should be carefully separated in suitable dishes. Trays of proper size for carrying complete meals should be provided.

The school lunch may be served by food workers at a counter, by service at tables, or by service in the classroom. Pupils pass in a line before a counter and either select their food or receive plates with prepared foods. The plate may be filled as pupils pass along the counter or may be filled before the pupils arrive. Milk, straws, napkins, and silverware are dispensed at the counter. Table service is most easily provided by placing the served plates on lunchroom tables before the pupils come to the lunch room. Service in the classroom may be provided when the school has no dining area. Food is prepared in the school kitchen (or a centrally located kitchen within the school system) and is taken to individual classrooms on a steam table.

The serving of food requires careful planning. For each serving period, there should be adequate amounts of food; cooked foods should be served hot; extra food should be available for refills; and food handling should comply with health regulations. If the school has limited facilities, several serving periods will be necessary. Sufficient time should be allotted for serving, for eating, and for cleaning up, so that there is no sense of hurry. The efficiency of the serving period can be judged as the pupil progresses along the serving line and is quickly served without undue rush or needless waiting. Food workers serving elementary school children should be familiar with the proper size of the serving.

## Sanitary Measures

The manager is responsible for maintaining scrupulous cleanliness of dishes. Dishes must be sterilized by approved methods, as soiled dishes, silverware, and cooking utensils can spread disease.

The manager will be responsible for planning the daily and weekly cleaning schedule and assigning these tasks to different workers. Cooking utensils, serving tables, eating areas, work counters, and other areas of the lunchroom should be cleaned daily. Stoves, ovens, refrigerators, and dish-washing machines should be cleaned weekly. The removal of garbage and waste must also be a part of the daily cleaning schedule, and daily measures must be taken to eradicate flies, roaches, ants, and rats. Nothing can damage the reputation of the school lunch as easily as an outbreak of digestive disturbances because of contaminated food.

All school lunchrooms should adhere to the regulations for sanitation established by local and state departments of health. These regulations usually require medical examinations, chest x-rays, and laboratory tests of all food workers. In order to prevent food-borne diseases, the workers need to receive in-service training for the handling of food. A daily check list can be used for the inspection of floors, walls and ceilings, doors and windows, lighting, ventilation, toilet facilities, water supply cleanliness of utensils and equipment, storage and handling of utensils and equip ment, disposal of wastes, refrigeration, storage and serving of food and drink, and cleanliness of employees.

## LUNCHROOM OR CAFETERIA— TEACHING LABORATORY

Nutritionists have urged elementary teachers and school health educators to use the lunchroom or cafeteria as a teaching laboratory. Nutrition education is more meaningful when the pupil is actually eating. Table etiquette can be practiced during his snack periods as well as during the lunch hour. Sitting posture when eating is an important part of social behavior. Rather than discuss foods, table etiquette, and posture, the teacher has a laboratory in which the pupil can practice proper health habits and social behavior. As the pupil eats his food, he can learn to identify the Essential Four Food Groups and give the reasons for his food selection. The pupil's use of silverware can be observed. The preparation of food and the sanitizing of dishes can be observed by pupils. Social behavior can be corrected and improved at the midmorning snack and noonday meal. With teacher supervision, pupils can prepare some foods in the lunchroom or cafeteria at hours when food workers have completed their daily tasks. Lunchroom tables can be used for table settings. The disposal of garbage from lunchrooms and cafeterias can be demonstrated to explain methods of preventing insect- and rodent-borne diseases. There are unlimited opportunities available to elementary teachers and school health educators in the use of the lunchroom or cafeteria as teaching laboratories.

## IMPLICATIONS FOR HEALTH EDUCATION

One of the most important areas of health education is the science of the basic nutrients and the improvement of daily dietary habits to ensure a wise selection and use of foods. In the area of "Nutrition," some suggested units are these:

1. Essential Four Food Groups
2. Carbohydrates and daily caloric intake
3. Proteins
4. Fats
5. Water and fiber
6. Mineral elements
7. Water-soluble vitamins
8. Fat-soluble vitamins
9. Daily diet based on a wise selection of nutrients
10. Obesity
11. Underweight
12. Influences upon our dietary habits
13. Nutrition quackery
14. Food fallacies
15. Misuse of coffee, tea, and sweetened soft drinks
16. School lunch
17. Milk and milk products
18. Meat and meat products
19. Fruits and vegetables
20. Breads and cereals
21. Food-, meat-, and milk-borne diseases
22. Table etiquette
23. Importance of nutrition in treatment of diseases, diabetes, and pregnancy

Other units in this area, Nutrition, are "Breakfast," "Foods for Snacking," "Picnic Foods," and "Caloric Expenditures for Different Activities." Every preteen and teenager should be aware of the number of calories needed to perform daily activities and strenuous physical exercise per minute so that he can control his weight.

## References for Further Study

Bogert, L. J., Briggs, G. M., and Calloway, D. H.: *Nutrition and Physical Fitness.* 9th ed. Philadelphia: W. B. Saunders Company, 1972.

Chaney, M. S.: *Nutrition.* 8th ed. Boston: Houghton-Mifflin Company, 1966.

Cooper, L. F., Barber, E. M., Mitchell, H. S., and Rynbergen, H. J.: *Nutrition in Health and Disease.* 15th ed. Philadelphia: J. B. Lippincott Company, 1968.

Guthrie, H. A.: *Introductory Nutrition.* St. Louis: C. V. Mosby Company, 1971.

Martin, E.: *Nutrition Education in Action.* 3rd ed. New York: Holt, Rinehart and Winston, Inc., 1971.

Mayer, J.: *Overweight.* Englewood Cliffs, N.J.: Prentice-Hall, Inc., 1968.

McWilliams, M.: *Nutrition for the Growing Years.* New York: John Wiley and Sons, Inc., 1967.

Nutrition Foundation, Inc.: *Present Knowledge in Nutrition.* New York: The Foundation, 1968.

Proudfit, F. T., and Robinson, C. H.: *Normal and Therapeutic Nutrition.* 13th ed. New York: The Macmillan Company, 1968.

Sherman, H., and Lanford, C.: *Essentials of Nutrition.* 4th ed. New York: The Macmillan Company, 1968.

United States Public Health Service: *Obesity and Health.* 1966.

Wayler, T., and Klein, R.: *Applied Nutrition.* New York: The Macmillan Company, 1965.

West, R.: *The Teen-age Diet Book.* New York: Julian Messner, 1969.

Wilson, E., Fisher, K. H., and Faqua, M. E.: *Principles of Nutrition.* New York: John Wiley and Sons, Inc., 1965.

Wohl, M. G., and Goodhart, R. S.: *Modern Nutrition in Health and Disease.* 4th ed. Philadelphia: Lea & Febiger, 1968.

# Chapter 11

# THE SCHOOL DAY AND ITS RELATION TO THE PUPIL'S TOTAL HEALTH

## AN INCIDENT

Teachers and school administrators ask how the pupil's total health will be affected by the number of hours each day the pupil is in school, the number of days in a year he attends school, the number of classmates the pupil has, and the characteristics of the teacher. Also, teachers and school administrators question how higher standards of intellectual achievement will affect the pupil's total health.

The length of the school day, daily program, teacher-pupil relations, and characteristics of the teacher may directly or indirectly affect the pupil's physical and mental health. The relation between the school day and the pupil's total health has been recognized for a long time.

In the school health program, physical health should not be considered separate from mental health. In this chapter, mental health, rather than freedom from disease, physical defects, and injury, will be emphasized.

## TIME ALLOTMENT

The school day may be lengthened in the future, even though the National Education Association has reported that 74% of some 326 school systems with enrollments of 12,000 or more pupils had neither lengthened nor shortened the school day.[1] The addition of new subjects and activities to the curriculum, knowledge explosion, and pupil interest-centered activities such as

intramural athletics may be among the reasons for lengthening the school day.

Some schools operate on a double-session schedule each day. Pupils may leave home early in the morning or arrive home late in the afternoon. Other students may attend classes in the evening. Whether pupils attending a half-day session are receiving the types and amounts of educational experiences they need is questionable.

The necessity of the two- or three-month vacation during the summer is being questioned. After two months of school, teachers and school administrators admit that students show signs of fatigue and need a vacation. Teachers and administrators also show signs of fatigue and need a change of pace and activities. Many schools are opening schools earlier in September and closing late in June to allow time for longer Christmas and spring vacations.

The school year is lengthened by summer school. Many high school students use their summer vacations to attend summer school. Remedial work is offered not only in the high schools but also in the elementary and junior or middle schools. In addition, enrichment study may be available in English, science, mathematics, history, health education, music, and arts.

## PUPIL GROUPING

Several types of pupil grouping are used: self-contained classrooms, nongraded classes, multigraded classes, departmentalized programs, cooperative teaching, and special classes to meet needs of particular pupils. In the self-contained classroom, the children have one teacher and grow accustomed to that teacher's ways of

[1]Research Division, National Education Association: Length of school year and school day. *Research Bulletin 43* (December, 1965):103-105.

working. Most elementary school classroom teachers work in self-contained classrooms where the teacher may have the children in small or large groups or work with the children individually. However, not every teacher is skilled in all subjects of the curriculum, nor able to provide the quality of education desired. Thus, other forms of pupil grouping become necessary.

The trend toward nongraded classes is growing rapidly in the elementary schools. A nongraded school has no formal grade levels or labels but has a plan of continuous upward programs. A nongraded school has no promotion of pupils. Content and materials of instruction are geared to individual differences and the individual pupil.[2] Since children progress differently, each child is allowed to progress at his own rate without any association with failure. He begins each school year where he left off the year before. Materials of instruction are at his level of development, and the child has learning experiences which meet with success.

In the multigraded unit, there may be an equal number of first-, second-, and third-grade children. One third of the children move on to the next unit each year. Children are grouped across grade lines in subject matter and can advance at different speeds. The multigraded class provides for a wider range of pupil abilities than the self-contained classroom. Older children can help the younger children.

Secondary schools have had departmentalization of instruction for many years. The teacher is a specialist in one subject-matter field and has more pupils in a day than in a self-contained classroom. Departmentalized programs are found in subject-centered schools where the teacher must be well informed in depth and up-to-date in subject matter. New subject-matter fields, such as the new sciences, have encouraged specialization.

Cooperative teaching involves two or more teachers from self-contained classrooms who come together for planning and teaching. Often called "team teaching," the pupils are assigned to two or more teachers

and then are divided into small or large groups or individualized study. There may be a master teacher, regular teacher, student teacher, and aides all working together. The school health educator (Chapter 19) can be a valuable asset to team teaching because he can contribute specific, up-to-date subject matter of health education.

Special classes to meet the needs of particular pupils may be organized for the gifted, mentally retarded, and the physically handicapped. One type of special class mentioned in Chapter 2 is physical education for the handicapped. Also included are the special education classes for the partially sighted, deaf, orthopedically handicapped, or for children with cerebral palsy or other chronic health problems.

## DAILY PROGRAM

Principals and teachers are responsible for the divisions of the school day, including time allotment for classes, lunch, physical education, and maintenance of a balance between morning and afternoon activities. Within these divisions, the pupil with a chronic health condition will need greater attention than will other pupils; for example, he will need more time to move from a classroom to the lunchroom, playground, or auditorium.

The elementary school classroom teachers and the principal work together in planning the daily program. There should be ample time for lunch so that the children do not feel they must rush through the meal. Physical education should be planned in such a manner that the children have time to wash off dirt and perspiration even when showers are not provided. Health education must be included in the instructional program, not as a part of science or social studies, but as a subject field dealing with pupil health problems.

In the secondary school, the principal is responsible for scheduling health education, art, physical education, industrial arts, home economics, music, and business education, in addition to the basic courses. If these are scheduled last, their objectives, class size, facilities, instructional materials, and teaching methods may be disregarded. Health education classes may be located in a room other than a health teaching laboratory.

[2] John Goodlad: Cooperative teaching in educational reform. *National Elementary Principal* 14 (January, 1965):10.

Many principals try to attain some degree of balance between the morning and afternoon sessions, if possible. The balance between the morning and afternoon may depend on the type of instructional program in the school. Facilities, number of instructional personnel, student class load, availability of instructional materials, and a city-wide course of study may force a principal to accept a routine pattern in scheduling secondary school classes. In the secondary school, the principal may schedule the basic courses interspersed with health education, art, physical education, music, and other curricular offerings.

With consolidation of schools, more pupils ride school buses. The length of time required to ride to and from school and bus service for students engaged in afterschool activities should be considered.

## PUPIL DIFFERENCES

Teachers should be aware of the range of pupil differences. Health coordinators and educators will hear teachers discuss pupils' academic achievements, intellectual capacities, group relations, and behavior. Little comment, though, may be made about signs of pupil emotional health disturbances, skin infections, nutritional deficiencies, posture conditions, communicable diseases, dental health problems, and vision and hearing difficulties. The health coordinator or educator may ask these questions of teachers: "Does Ruth complain of pain and swelling in her throat?" "Does Sally ask to have questions repeated in class?" "What are Mary's dietary habits at lunch?" "Does Bill have indications of a possible visual difficulty?" "What signs of emotional health problems are there in Joe's behavior?"

The concept of the "whole child" includes both physical and mental health. It may be necessary for the health coordinator or educator to inform teachers of the possible range of pupil health differences. Teachers should understand that academic progress, intellectual capacity, group relations, and individual behavior can indicate certain pupil differences. Other characteristics may be displayed in activities not found within the classroom; for example, indications of desirable mental health may be found in athletic contests. These characteristics may be of such a nature that the

teacher with limited understanding of pupil differences may never notice them.

This range of pupil differences should include many concepts of the whole child and should not be limited by academic grades and group behavior. Wide variations should be accepted as the concepts of the whole child are considered. Differences may be found in pupil achievements, aptitudes, personalities, social tendencies, capacities, interests, motor abilities, behavior, physical growth, mental health, remediable and chronic physical health conditions, and other pupil characteristics.

How does the teacher become aware of these pupil differences? Teacher observation is the most likely method. This observation is not casual, hurried, or without purpose, but is continuous, systematic, and informative. Skill in observing pupil differences naturally varies with teachers. Some teachers have been known to notice pupil behavior, conditions, characteristics, and skills unknown to the parent and physician.

When recognizing pupil differences, the teacher must accept the role that the gifted child plays among his classmates. He should be aware of the gifted child's range of aptitudes and behavior as well as his potentialities in acquiring knowledge and skills. His awareness of the gifted child's potentialities can open unlimited opportunities of learning to the child. Rapport between the child and teacher should be well developed. The gifted child should feel secure, enthusiastic, and confident of some degree of success as he forges ahead into new learning experiences. Individual conferences with the teacher can be used to encourage him to have learning experiences not available to other class members. Sometimes the gifted child may continue working on a project that the majority of the class members can no longer continue because of their lack of capacities and skills. Among the possibilities in helping the gifted child are enrichment of the regular curriculum, elective courses, rapid advancement, and a wide variety of activities in addition to regular classwork. The gifted child will need encouragement, kindness, patience, recognition for his achievements, and individual attention. The teacher can assist him by being aware of his potentialities, by guiding him continuously, and by providing him with new learning experiences.

## PUPIL-PUPIL RELATIONS

Among the most important experiences of the pupil during the school day are his relations with other pupils. These relations may influence behavior patterns that remain with the pupil the rest of his life. A teacher might use sociograms, storytelling, role playing and sociodrama, and written self-descriptions by pupils to discover isolated pupils, leaders among pupils, and pupils who have made inadequate adjustments in their relations with other pupils. Many opportunities are available to the teacher to foster better pupil-pupil relations. First, the teacher might use the term "we" to encourage group cohesion. Second, the teacher should consider many possible ways to handle conflicts between pupils. Third, there are some situations that the pupils can handle better than the teacher. Fourth, the teacher should accept the fact that there are times when the teacher is a source of guidance but not the leader. Fifth, the teacher must be alert to the formation of pupil cliques. Sixth, the teacher should be aware of pupils who are scapegoats or "loners," and he should try to prevent the formation of adverse group opinion about them.

## TEACHER-PUPIL RELATIONS

Teacher-pupil relations will be strengthened when the teacher understands the proper balance between the student's feelings, attitudes, values, and beliefs, on the one hand, and his acquisition of knowledge and skills, on the other. The student's behavior may be a translation of his feelings and values gained in the process of acquiring knowledge and skills. The student should realize that his opinions and feelings are important and that they can be expressed in a permissible emotional and social manner.

Self-improvement and acceptance of everyday realities are strengthened when desirable teacher-pupil relations are strongly entrenched. Criticism is acceptable as a means of self-improvement, whether the criticism is of the teacher or pupil. Failures are viewed by the teacher and pupils as opportunities to work together constructively to improve those situations creating the failures. Realities of everyday experiences are faced squarely. Some problems arising from these realities may need the help of parents. In facing realities, the student should accept the consequences when he breaks the rules of the group, misbehaves, or attempts to set himself above others.

When desirable teacher-pupil relations exist, teachers and pupils have an urge to be creative. In a healthful emotional climate, individuality and creative self-expression go hand in hand. The teacher, recognizing a pupil's desire to be creative, can encourage and guide his efforts into many possible outlets. Students who are encouraged and guided by the teacher will notice the teacher's creative efforts and may provide the impetus for further creative work by the teacher.

## PUPIL CONDUCT

Procedures used by principals and teachers in handling pupil misbehavior will reflect their understanding of pupil differences as well as of the factors that influence pupil behavior. These procedures will also show the patience and objectivity of principals and teachers and their willingness to seek assistance from other school personnel. Many factors within and outside the school influence pupil behavior. The pupil's home life and social relations or the teacher's judgment of the pupil's actions can be underlying causes for pupil misbehavior. Many facts should be obtained and weighed before attempting to punish a student.

The effect of misbehavior on the pupil concerned, on other pupils, on the instructional personnel, and the daily program must be considered. A group of classmates may shun the pupil who misbehaves, so further punishment may not be necessary. In dispensing punishment, principals and teachers should also be aware of the interpretations of their actions by other school personnel, who may have information to assist them when they are faced with problems of pupil conduct.

## CHARACTERISTICS OF THE TEACHER

The teacher with a clear understanding of his capacities and limitations can have a stabilizing effect on pupils. A teacher of this sort will be able to plan his daily tasks in such a manner that there will be no sense of hurry, tension, or irritating pressure to finish a given task. He will face the unexpected, be elastic in the daily schedule, and, having foresight, be capable of long-term planning. A teacher who is aware of his limitations and capacities will take time to gather materials of instruction and to outline systematically each day's goals. He will give students adequate explanations regarding sources of references and subject matter. With such a teacher, students find stability.

The teacher's self-confidence can establish a sense of security among pupils. Self-confidence may be the result of acknowledgment of the teacher's achievement by others, his own satisfaction in accomplishing difficult assignments, and long-term planning. The teacher's self-confidence may encourage students to explore their capacities and to acquire new skills. Self-confidence can assist the teacher to be self-reliant and to face realities.

The teacher should be free from personal problems and pressures exerted by parents or other school personnel. He will then be more alert to the variations in pupil capacities and be aware of differences in the pupils' physical and mental health and in the range of their interests. Instead of being preoccupied with his own problems, he can focus his attention on the pupil. He may be able to observe pupil actions objectively and systematically, and with more deliberation collect evidence pointing to the causes of pupils' actions. A teacher with overwhelming personal problems may not be aware of the differences in pupils' mental health and the range of pupils' interests.

The teacher's ability to manage his personal life is reflected in his performance of school tasks and his ability to get along with pupils, parents, and other school and community personnel. When the teacher cannot budget his finances to pay monthly expenses, financial troubles worry him. When the teacher cannot choose desirable friends, town gossip may make his private life unbearable. When the teacher cannot abstain from overindulgence in alcohol and tobacco, efficiency of teaching performance is lost. The teacher may try to hide his inability to manage his personal life. These weaknesses soon become apparent.

The teacher's sense of humor, courtesy, tact, kindness, patience, understanding, and honesty are revealed during the school day. These characteristics can be foundation stones for building sound mental health among both teachers and pupils, and they can be assets in developing desirable social relations with all age groups. Most persons seek these characteristics in their friends, and the student expects to observe them in teachers. The student will realize the importance of these characteristics as he watches the teacher during the school day.

## PREPARATION OF INSTRUCTION

The teacher, gathering objective information on the pupils' needs and interests and as a guide to planning, emphasizes instruction focused on these needs and interests. When the student is aware that the teacher has taken considerable time to understand him as an individual, he realizes the need for emphasis on certain basic learnings.

The teacher who is well prepared for each assignment in the school day gives the student an opportunity to acquire and use new learning experiences. The student then has a sense of accomplishment. In addition to being well prepared, the teacher should be able to organize his teaching in such a way that every student can daily acquire some specific new information or skill.

Teachers strive to present subject matter logically and concisely, using many types of materials of instruction. For example, the teacher must complete many procedures in order to have one visual aid ready at the exact moment in a demonstration. Today's teacher must explain not only by words but also by many other techniques. He should have a wide vocabulary so that all students understand the intent of the teaching, because with a limited vocabulary he will have difficulty in conveying the concepts and skills to be learned.

Teachers should be free to express their own ideas as well as the concepts of others; to create new concepts, skills, and materials; and to explore possibilities within learning experiences. Freedom of expression, creativity, and exploration are vital in developing better teaching as well as in stimulating students to widen their horizons of learning and to discover some of their capacities. Common sense and discretion are abandoned when teachers misuse this freedom. Similarly, students can abuse their freedom when their efforts are not continuously guided by teachers.

The creative efforts of teachers should be encouraged by administrative and supervisory personnel. The experienced teacher may fall into a pattern of daily performance with little variation, few opportunities to explore new concepts and teaching methods, and occasional spurts of creativity. Students who come into contact with teachers of this type have no desire to attempt skills or acquire knowledge beyond the class presentation.

There should be some opportunity during the school day for the teacher to witness a student's achievement. A student may be progressing slowly, his achievements may be unnoticed by others, his efforts may be clumsy, and he may acquire limited knowledge. However, the amount of observed student achievement is gratifying to the teacher. There should be an attempt not only to broaden the learning experiences of the gifted child but also to allow the slow learner some degree of success.

Preparation of instructional materials should provide the teacher with opportunities for daily self-evaluation. During the day, he listens to class discussion, student answers, and questions asked by students. He should question whether the subject matter was well presented, well explained, and meaningful. Continuous self-evaluation will encourage him to seek better teaching methods and new materials of instruction. Self-evaluation may be more critical than evaluation by administrators and other teachers. The teacher, continuously evaluating his daily school tasks and the results of these tasks on students, is aware of his shortcomings. As he seeks ways to overcome these shortcomings, self-evaluation becomes a means of self-improvement. As the teacher's self-improvement continues over the years, students benefit.

## TEACHER'S ORGANIZATION OF THE SCHOOL DAY

Even though a tentative hourly guide and weekly schedule may be accessible to the teacher, the organization of the pupil's daily activities is the responsibility of the teacher. This organization may affect the pupil's total physical and mental health.

### Changes of Class Activities

An elementary school pupil, seated at a desk-chair combination, has been seated for a half hour. What signs of pupil fatigue might be observed by the teacher? Some of these signs might be the pupil's squirming, stretching, placing his head on the desk top, slumped posture, dangling of feet, resting of his head on the back of the chair, inattentiveness, and moving from the desk-chair combination to the floor. A high school student has studied at a library desk for 2 hours without arising. What signs of fatigue might he show? He might rub his eyes, rest his forehead on the palm of one hand, stretch, yawn, assume many sitting postures, and repeat movements such as foot stamping and nail biting. A junior high or middle school student with some preseason athletic conditioning is practicing basketball free-throws. What signs of fatigue might be observed by his physical education teacher as the student attempts his twentieth try? The physical education teacher might observe loss of motor coordination, inaccurate placement of the basketball on the backboard, tendency toward erratic performance, loss of timing, and gradual reduction in the number of completed baskets. These examples all show the effects of fatigue on mental concentration and muscular work.

After the teacher has recognized signs of fatigue, what can be done? Children and teenagers should be aware of the onset of fatigue and should practice health habits that replace fatigue with energy. If they pay no attention to warning signals pointing to fatigue, chronic and nervous fatigue may become habitual. Such pupils can be accident prone as well as emotionally unstable and physically ill. They require continuous teacher supervision and should be taught the importance of rest. As for teacher supervision, a change of pupil activities might involve changes from sitting to standing to walking. Participation in group work is a change from individual seated activities. Pupil science experiments can be substituted for arithmetic problems, and big-muscle activities might replace the fine coordinated hand movements required in art projects. There are many ways the teacher can vary classroom activities.

Visual and hearing difficulties, the onset of communicable diseases, emotional health problems, nutritional deficiencies, dental health problems, and posture difficulties can contribute to fatigue. Every teacher should be aware that physical and mental health deficiencies create an extra burden on the pupil. The pupil with a health difficulty must supply more energy to the afflicted areas of his body or to other areas that are attempting to compensate for the difficulty. Teachers may have observed the student with a hearing difficulty lean forward tensely in order to hear only a small percentage of what is said.

### Placement of Classroom Activities

In order to combat rising fatigue levels during the school day, the scheduling of classroom activities must be considered. Teachers should be aware of the pupils' energy patterns and fatigue levels, as they vary from one pupil to another. Age, bodily growth, sex, nutritional status, endocrine functions, and mental and physical health status will create variations not only among pupils of one age level but also among pupils of different age levels.

Physiologists have given data on how the rise and fall of human fatigue depends on periods of rest and the replacement of fatigue with energy. When should certain classroom activities be included within the school day? Because individual students vary, it is usually necessary to consider the fatigue levels of the majority of students in a classroom. We shall assume that they have had ample sleep during the preceding night, sufficient food for breakfast and the preceding evening meal, no needless scampering for the morning school bus, no undue excitement, adequate fulfillment of all before-school health habits, reasonably few mental and physical health deficiencies, and are within normal patterns of bodily growth for their ages and sex. We might assume that these students' fatigue levels are rather low at early morning school hours. Therefore curricular offerings requiring muscular work in combination with mental concentration could be placed in the early morning school hours.

Human fatigue increases during the day, but periods of rest diminish the production rate of fatigue. School personnel have tended to place curricular offerings requiring mental concentration in the early morning and have delegated the afternoon to activities combining muscular activities with mental concentration.

### Rest and Relaxation

Periods of rest and relaxation should be included in the pupil's daily schedule. These periods might occur during the change of classroom activities. Some elementary teachers allow their pupils to take a short afternoon nap after the noonday meal. The pupils stretch out on light, easily folded rubber mattresses. Other elementary school teachers provide a quiet relaxing period through a "listening hour" of recorded classical music or short dramatizations. It is not uncommon to find children of elementary school age resting their heads on the tops of the desk-chair combinations, following the noonday meal. Some physical education classes conclude activities with relaxation. All students lie flat on their abdomens, arms resting on the floor above their heads, and heads turned to one side. Shoes are removed, and the eyes are closed. This relaxation can be accompanied by quiet music.

Rest must be provided in the school day for students who have recovered from rheumatic fever and for pupils who have undergone a seizure of grand mal epilepsy. Rest is vital to the health of a pupil returning to school after prolonged illness or recent surgery. Pupils with emotional health problems will also profit from daily rest periods.

At the secondary school level, periods of rest and relaxation are necessary during the surging rush of class activities. Clubs, study halls, library browsing, and lunch periods provide some of this needed rest and relaxation. The student should have opportunities during scheduled class activities to replace fatigue with energy.

### METHODS OF SUPERVISION

The principal's supervisory practices can affect the pupil's total health. Working cooperatively with teachers, the principal can develop a friendly, positive, and constructive school atmosphere that is felt by all pupils. When democratic supervision is apparent, pupil differences are recognized. Cooperative action by the teacher and principal solves pupil problems and promotes the pupil's total health.

The principal's concepts of supervision will be evident in his treatment of school personnel. When the principal stresses democratic supervision, he will respect the opinions of school personnel, delegate authority, and encourage leadership, and acknowledge meritorious service. In addition to the principal's supervision, there is supervision by the curriculum consultants or supervisors. These consultants can assist teachers by formal and informal visits and by arranging a conference with teachers as soon as possible after the visit. Consultants and principals can keep cumulative records on all teachers and share the information on these records with teachers. Consultants can encourage creativity among teachers and serve as resource persons. Interclass and school visitations, demonstrations, and workshops afford opportunities for teachers to share their special skills with other teachers.

How do these democratic supervisory practices affect the pupil's total health? A teacher whose supervisors promote self-growth and security will exert every effort to do the best possible teaching job. The teacher will have a "sense of belonging," display leadership, attempt the best in teaching methods, be prepared for daily teaching, recognize pupil differences, and give pupils opportunities to explore their potentialities.

## IMPLICATIONS FOR HEALTH EDUCATION

Even though the relation between the school day and the pupil's total health has been recognized, there are units of instruction from the area "Mental Health" which can be included in health education. These units grow out of teacher-pupil relations, characteristics of the teacher, teacher's organization of the school day, and pupil-pupil relations. Some of these units from this area are:

1. Adjustment to school life
2. Control of emotions
3. Respect for others and self
4. Courtesy and thoughtfulness
5. Cooperation and sharing
6. Honesty
7. Friends and getting along with others
8. Rights and property of others
9. Self-discipline
10. Tolerance
11. Scheduling work and play
12. Fatigue
13. Rest, relaxation, and sleep
14. Member of a group

In the secondary schools, some of the teenage emotional problems of insecurity, lack of self-control, lack of self-acceptance, fear and worry, lack of respect for property of others, and suicide might be considered. Many of the frustrations of teenagers are due to prior pupil-pupil relations, teacher-pupil relations, and chronic fatigue.

## References for Further Study

American School Health Association, Committee on Mental Health in the Classroom: *Mental Health in the Classroom.* Kent, Ohio: The Association, 1968.

Anderson, R. H.: *Teaching in a World of Change.* New York: Harcourt, Brace, and World, 1966.

Arkoff, A.: *Adjustment and Mental Health.* New York: McGraw-Hill Book Company, 1968.

Association for Supervision and Curriculum Development: *Learning and Mental Health in Schools.* Washington, D.C.: National Education Association, 1966.

Association of State and Territorial Health Officers, The Association of State and Territorial Mental Health Authorities, and The Council of Chief State School Officers: *Mental Health in the Schools.* Washington, D.C.: Council of Chief State School Officers, 1966.

Crow, L. D.: *Psychology of Human Adjustment.* New York: Alfred A. Knopf, Inc., 1967.

DeSalvo, C., and Cox, C.: *Faces People Wear.* New York: Hawthorn Books, Inc., 1968.

*Facts About Mental Illness.* New York: National Association for Mental Health: 1969.

Joint Committee on Health Problems in Education of the National Education Association and the American Medical Association: *Mental Health and School Health Services.* Washington, D.C.: National Education Association, 1966.

Lazarus, R. S.: *Patterns of Adjustment and Human Effectiveness.* New York: McGraw-Hill Book Company, 1969.

London, P., and Rosenhan, D., eds.: *Foundations of Abnormal Psychology.* New York: Holt, Rinehart and Winston, Inc., 1968.

Martin, L. E.: *Mental Health/Mental Illness: Revolution in Progress.* New York: McGraw-Hill Book Company, 1970.

Noar, G.: *The Teacher and Integration.* Washington, D.C.: National Education Association, 1966.

Smith, H. C.: *Personality Development.* New York: McGraw-Hill Book Company, 1968.

Swenson, G., and Keys, D.: *Providing for Flexibility in Scheduling and Instruction.* Englewood Cliffs, N.J.: Prentice-Hall, 1966.

Westby-Gobson, D.: *Grouping Students for Instruction.* Englewood Cliffs, N.J.: Prentice-Hall, 1966.

# Part III

## *HEALTH EDUCATION*

# Chapter 12

# HEALTH EDUCATION IN THE ELEMENTARY AND SECONDARY SCHOOLS

## AN INCIDENT

Members of state legislatures, discovering the lack of health education, particularly drug abuse education, in schools and colleges, have passed legislation making health education mandatory in the public elementary and secondary schools, for freshmen in state-supported colleges and universities, and for undergraduates and graduates being prepared for teaching and administrative positions in public schools. Some public school and college faculties have interpreted health education as instruction in anatomy and physiology, physical conditioning and other activities, and pharmacy.

The goal of health education is to "help *each* individual view health as *a way of life* that will help to attain individual goals and utilize one's highest potential for the betterment of self, family, and community. Every individual, regardless of a chosen profession or occupation, will be confronted with health decisions every day of his life."[1] Thus, health education must provide valid information which can be easily understood by and be available to all people. In this way, everyone, either as an individual or as a member of a family, community, or nation, can understand his health problems, make decisions to take action, and solve his problems. It is apparent from the following data that the American people have not received adequate health education.

There are 17 million mentally or emotionally disturbed Americans in need of psychiatric treatment.
Suicide has become one of the leading causes of death among young adults.
Accidents are among the major causes of death and disability to the school-age population.
Almost 1 million Americans cannot read newsprint even with the aid of glasses.
Probably about 3 million Americans have major hearing defects.
Cigarette smoking is the most important cause of chronic bronchitis, emphysema, and lung cancer.
Alcoholism among employees costs American industry and business approximately $2 billion a year. Even though the exact number of alcoholics is not known, the number is increasing.
Some authorities believe that 24 million Americans have used marijuana at least once in their lives.
At least half of the supply of amphetamines available in this country enters illegal channels in a year.
There are 10 million overweight teenagers.
Adequate amounts of vitamins D, A, and C; iron; and iodine are lacking in the diets of many Americans.
Americans have an estimated 800 million dental cavities in need of treatment.
More than 2 million persons under 25 years of age are infected with the tubercle bacilli.
At least 1500 young adults become infected with venereal diseases each day.
About 17 million Americans have high blood pressure or hypertension.
The public water supplies of over 19 thousand communities, serving 58 million people, do not meet U.S. Public Health Service standards of quality.
Communities in the United States produce over 3.5 billion tons of solid wastes each day.

School Health Education Study: *Health Education—A Conceptual Approach to Curriculum Design*. Washington, D. C.: The Study, 1967. p. 11.

At least 150 million tons of pollutants are discharged into America's air every year.

More than 2 million people in the United States have food-, meat-, and milk-borne diseases each year.

At least $2 billion a year are spent on medical quackery, including more than $100 million spent on ineffective drugs and devices for weight reduction.

As data concerning health problems become evident to the American public, demands will grow for health education in the schools. Parents, state legislators, and health professionals are asking what is being done in health education for the elementary school child and secondary school youth. *Health education* is defined as those "experiences favorably influencing understandings, attitudes, and practices relating to individual, family, and community health."[2]

We might ask these questions: Is the content (subject matter) directed to broad concepts of individual, family, and community health? Are many possible types of understandings, attitudes, and practices included? Does the content involve the student to such an extent that it becomes a personal matter? Does the student take action to improve his health, the health of his family, and health of his community? Is the student helped to reach the stage of optimal physical and mental health by the content of health education courses? Does the student question, re-examine, and reappraise previously learned practices, beliefs, and information? Is the content relevant to the health problems of our daily and future lives?

## PURPOSES OF HEALTH EDUCATION

Often students ask why they should study health education? Or why should they not study the parts and functions of the human body? What has health education to offer that cannot be found in social studies, biology, or physical education? Health education helps the individual to

1. Recognize his health problems and those of his family and community

2. Reach decisions concerning his and others' health behaviors, attitudes, and knowledge
3. Solve his health problems and those of other individuals, his family, and community
4. Develop attitudes and practices which promote healthful living
5. Eradicate misinformation surrounding his health problems and those of his family and community
6. Become aware that these are many health problems which may be unsolved
7. Recognize that health problems are highly individual
8. Accept the fact that health problems can only be solved by the teamwork of many persons in the health professions
9. Accept the fact that some health issues will always be controversial for political, religious, economic, or social reasons
10. Prevent and control diseases occurring to man and animals and to eradicate diseases which are insect-borne
11. Accept chronic health conditions
12. Promote accident prevention
13. Recognize that hazards causing disability or death threaten everyone throughout his lifetime
14. Recognize that mental illness can affect anyone
15. Promote his nutritional status and that of his family, while at the same time recognizing that obesity and undernutrition are common nutritional problems
16. Accept the challenges of overpopulation and strive to reverse man's pollution of his environment
17. Accept his role in community programs to reduce air and water pollution, to dispose of solid waste properly, and to convert sewage into usable water
18. Evaluate health products and services as a consumer
19. Recognize the many types of quackery
20. Accept his responsibilities in sexual behavior when dating, during engagement, and throughout marriage
21. Accept that the problems of drug abuse, alcoholism, and smoking not only include education about the facts but also demand changing the attitudes of those involved in drug abuse, alcoholism, and smoking. In addition, these problems involve social mores, statutes and methods of law enforcement, and medical assistance
22. Develop a broad understanding of the health problems in other countries

[2]Health education terminology. *J. Health, Physical Education and Recreation* 33 (November, 1962):21-22.

These are a few of the many purposes of health education.

## HEALTH EDUCATION AS A PART OF THE SCHOOL HEALTH PROGRAM

The third part of the total school health program, health education is the most important. The main purpose of our elementary and secondary schools is to provide constructive teaching that changes the individual, not only intellectually, but also socially, morally, physically, and emotionally. As a teacher of a single subject-matter field, the school health educator can measure, to some degree, changes in the pupil's health practices, attitudes, knowledge, and status. Particularly is this possible in secondary schools, where health education is regularly scheduled, meeting five class periods a week. Not only can the school health educator discover the pupil health practices, attitudes, and knowledge at the beginning of the semester, but he can also observe changes during the course and determine the new health practices, attitudes, and knowledge at the close of the semester. It is health education that provides the "why," "what," and "how," and changes to the pupil—intellectually, socially, morally, physically, and emotionally.

## PRINCIPLES OF HEALTH EDUCATION

There are six basic principles of health education. First, health education is concerned with *everyday living* as it affects the individual, his family, and his community. For many years, health education was based on learning the life stories of Edward Jenner, Marie Curie, Robert Koch, Louis Pasteur, and others who contributed to man's well-being. More recently, the content of health education has been placed in social studies with topics unrelated to health education. Many pupils reading these life stories and learning about unrelated topics had significant health problems; yet teachers emphasized the irrelevant curriculum. They ignored health information that could have been used to solve the pupil's problems. Health education must deal not only with the health problems of the individual but also

with those of the family and with those of the community and the nation as well. These problems are not of the past but of the present and future.

Second, health education deals in *specific facts* and not simply in theory. These facts are the results of experimentation, research, and well-founded conclusions of professionals of many fields—school health education, medicine, dentistry, public health, nursing, related biological and sociological sciences, engineering, nutrition, and pharmacy. The purpose of health education is to interpret the experimentations, research, and conclusions so that the facts can be easily understood by all students. False information, misleading and ambiguous statements, and disorganized and meaningless subject matter have no place in health education. Desirable health behavior is acquired through continuous practice with an acceptance of the reasons for the behavior. Students' attitudes are favorably influenced by scientifically accurate facts, compiled and evaluated without bias.

Third, health education is *positive in its approach*. Elementary and secondary school students want and need guidance to direct them into healthful effective living. Health education does not moralize or coerce but provides reliable factual evidence so that the student can form positive opinions to guide his actions. For example, the unit about smoking, taught in the fifth or sixth grade, can include the evidence of the increased incidence of respiratory infections among smokers. In those school systems having continuous anti-smoking instruction, a decline in smoking among students may well have already taken place. In a 1968 nationwide survey of teenagers, 91% believed that smoking was harmful to health. Smoking had decreased as much as 9 to 10% in some age groups. More than 34% of the teenagers said they definitely did not expect to become smokers.[3] If smoking can be reduced by inclusion of specific facts concerning smoking at the elementary school and middle school level,

[3]National Clearinghouse for Smoking and Health: *What We Know About Children and Smoking.* 1968.

is it not possible that additional facts can reduce the probability of smoking when peer-group habits influence high school students? Most school health educators are aware that cigarette advertising is directed toward persons who have not become regular smokers, many of whom are in the secondary schools. Valid health information that is positive in its approach may redirect a developing nonbeneficial health behavior into one that is beneficial.

Fourth, health education has a *five-pronged attack*. It attempts to improve the pupil's physical and mental health status, expose the false information, eliminate attitudes retarding improvement of the pupil's health status, promote health practices that benefit him, and stimulate continuous interest in health education. Specific and valid health facts are necessary. These facts applied to everyday living can strengthen the individual's health practices, attitudes, and interests so that health becomes a "state of complete physical, mental, and social well-being and not merely the absence of disease or infirmity."[4] As an example, second-graders may permanently reduce their dental health problems by learning to use correct tooth-brushing procedures after eating, to eat a daily diet that omits highly fermentable carbohydrates, and to visit their family dentist regularly.

Fifth, health education depends on the *teacher's enthusiasm and interest*. There are elementary and secondary school teachers who consider health education of no significant value; they believe it to be less important than traditional subjects. The School Health Education Study indicated a lack of enthusiasm for and interest in health education on the part of elementary school teachers. At the secondary school level, there was evidence of weak preparation in health education when the same teacher was responsible for both health education and physical education. School administrators and others indicated that there was not only inadequate professional preparation but also disinterest on the part of some teachers assigned to

health education.[5] A teacher's lack of enthusiasm and interest may be caused by several factors. First, many elementary school classroom teachers and those assigned to teach health education in secondary schools have very little acquaintance with the subject matter. Second, the teacher then feels extremely inadequate and insecure when faced with areas and units of health education. Third, the teacher receives little or no assistance because supervisors or consultants with major preparation are *seldom* found in the elementary and secondary schools. Fourth, many of these teachers may feel that health education warrants no time allotment in the schools, because, to their knowledge, it has no subject matter. Fifth, subject matter in health education may be offensive to some teachers because they cannot accept the fact that health problems exist among individuals, families, and communities. Lastly, some teachers consider all health problems the sole concern of physicians, local health departments, or federal agencies. If the teacher is disinterested and apathetic, health education has no opportunity to accomplish its purposes.

Sixth, health education is based on *objective information* about the individual pupil's physical and mental health status and his health practices, attitudes, interests, and knowledge. How this objective information is gathered, how it is used, why it is necessary for health education, and by whom and when it is compiled will be discussed in Chapter 13. To be meaningful to the pupil, health education must satisfy his many health needs and interests. A course of study, a single textbook on health, and a committee of teachers totally unaware of pupil health needs and interests cannot provide meaningful health education. The life story of Robert Koch undoubtedly has very little meaning to fourth-graders of whom one third have measles and are absent from school. The integumentary system of the human body has little significance to high school students who are wondering whether they

[4]Constitution of the World Health Organization. p. 3. *Chronicle of the World Health Organization* 1(1947): 29-43.

[5]School Health Education Study: *A Summary Report of a Nationwide Study of Health Instruction in the Public Schools, 1961-1963*, Washington, D.C.: The Study, pp. 11, 41-42.

should use or not use alcoholic beverages. There is statistical evidence of serious dental health problems among school-age children. Does not this evidence emphasize the need for dental health units in the elementary and secondary schools? Studies of growth and development indicate age levels at which to teach about menstrual hygiene, boy-girl relations, dating, problems of engagement, and the birth of a baby. Pupil health records show an increasing need for inclusion of units on posture, skin infections, and weight control. Local health departments indicate the increase of venereal diseases among secondary school youth, clearly revealing a need for more education about the subject. School health educators must use objective information to improve continuously the content and the relevance of health education.

## GROWTH AND DEVELOPMENTAL PATTERNS

Certain physical characteristics, behaviors, and interests appear among boys and girls as they progress through different stages of growth and development. Some of these should be considered in determining the specific content of health education courses at the time the changes take place in the pupil's growth and development.

Between the ages of 11 and 14, the girl reaches her menarche—the first menstrual period; thus a unit on menstrual hygiene would be most appropriate. Acne is often reported among teenagers; a unit on skin infections would assist those suffering from acne, especially because acne not only mars the facial appearance but also changes the teenager's personality. The shedding of the deciduous teeth and eruption of the permanent teeth can create innumerable dental health problems when there is little or no professional dental care. A dental health unit on mixed dentition would help the child. The rapid growth of the adolescent boy presents many health problems that relate to his health practices and to his relations with girls. A unit on boy-girl relations in health education has significant meaning to the boy. Many health practices associated with good grooming need to be developed in pre-teenagers, because after boys and girls leave childhood they must accept responsibility for their personal appearance.

Other units related to the pupil's growth and development are these:

| | | |
|---|---|---|
| Primary grades | Area: Mental Health | Unit: Adjustment to school life |
| Intermediate grades | Area: Nutrition | Unit: Calories and weight |
| Grade 7 | Area: Drug abuse, narcotic addiction, smoking, and misuse of of alcoholic beverages | Unit: To smoke or not to smoke |
| Grade 9 | Area: Family life and sex education | Unit: Dating |
| Grade 11 | Area: Safety education | Unit: Occupational safety |

School health educators should consider the different stages of the pupil's growth and development when they select specific health education units.

## ELEMENTARY SCHOOL HEALTH EDUCATION—PRIMARY GRADES

The supervisor or consultant in health education is often asked, "Why is health education important in the primary grades?" Health education has many *purposes* at these age levels. Health education continues the parental instruction about desirable health and safety practices, and it introduces beneficial health and safety practices not taught by parents. It fosters understanding of the basic health and safety practices, and it tries to eradicate undesirable practices. It emphasizes that desirable practices are necessary for future well-being. It encourages the child to accept some of his responsibilities for healthful and safe living. It reveals to the child that other children have both desirable and undesirable health and safety practices. It stresses health problems and accident hazards so that the child learns to protect himself. It encourages acceptance of family physicians, dentists, and other professional health workers coming into contact with the child. It attempts to eradicate some of the fears instilled into the child by parental misconceptions about health.

The *competencies* resulting from health education are numerous. In ten of the 13 areas of health education, the following competencies can be developed:

1. Having a daily bath, shower, or sponge bath
2. Keeping the hair combed
3. Dressing appropriately according to the weather
4. Cleaning the fingernails and washing the face and hands throughout the day
5. Having clean, pressed clothes each day
6. Using toilet facilities properly
7. Brushing the teeth correctly
8. Having adequate sleep
9. Knowing how to relax during the day
10. Measuring height and weight
11. Sitting and standing correctly
12. Taking proper care of toothbrush, brush and comb, and glasses
13. Preventing colds and sore throats
14. Receiving adequate vaccinations
15. Preventing the spread of diseases
16. Using handkerchiefs properly when sneezing or coughing
17. Blowing the nose correctly
18. Accepting health problems of others
19. Learning to understand health habits
20. Controlling nosebleeds
21. Providing American Red Cross First Aid for simple emergencies
22. Crossing streets and intersections correctly
23. Getting on and off school buses without accidents
24. Preventing accidents in the classroom
25. Practicing the basic self-preservation procedures in the event of disaster
26. Preventing accidents on the school playground
27. Practicing safe fire drills
28. Adjusting to school life
29. Controlling emotions
30. Being a member of a group
31. Taking turns
32. Sharing and cooperating with others
33. Assuming certain responsibilities
34. Being courteous and thoughtful
35. Choosing foods from the Essential Four Food Groups
36. Participating in school noonday meals
37. Practicing desirable table etiquette
38. Selecting a well-balanced meal
39. Reducing amounts of candy and other sweet foods
40. Accepting the family physician, dentist, and other professional health workers
41. Drinking purified water
42. Understanding the directions on the labels of some foods, drugs, and medicines
43. Accepting new brothers and sisters in the family
44. Understanding the birth of chicks and other small animals
45. Understanding how new trees and plants develop

With these competencies as a guide, what subject matter in health education might be included for the primary grades? Subject matter for units mentioned in this chapter can be found throughout this text.

1. Area: Care of All Parts of the Human Body
   Unit: Cleanliness
   Unit: Six-year molars and care of the new teeth
   Unit: Types of teeth and injuries to the teeth
   Unit: Sleep and rest
   Unit: Sitting and standing posture
   Unit: Clothes for daily weather and special activities
2. Area: Prevention of Diseases to All Parts of the Human Body
   Unit: Colds
   Unit: Spread and prevention of diseases
   Unit: Vaccinations
   Unit: Sore throats and what they mean
3. Area: Chronic Health Conditions
   Unit: Health problems of classmates or other friends
4. Area: American Red Cross First Aid
   Unit: Nosebleeds
   Unit: First Aid for simple emergencies
5. Area: Safety Education
   Unit: Pedestrian safety
   Unit: School safety
   Unit: School bus safety

Unit: Fire drills at school
Unit: Disaster drills at school
Unit: Playground safety

6. Area: Mental Health
   Unit: Adjustment to school life
   Unit: Control of emotions
   Unit: Respect for others
   Unit: Cooperation and sharing with others
   Unit: Responsibilities at school
   Unit: Courtesy and thoughtfulness

7. Area: Nutrition
   Unit: Essential Four Food Groups
   Unit: Table etiquette
   Unit: School noonday meals
   Unit: Well-balanced meals
   Unit: Fruits and vegetables

8. Area: Community Health Problems
   Unit: Community helpers in health
   Unit: Purified drinking water

9. Area: Consumer Health
   Unit: Labels on foods, drugs, medicines

10. Area: Family Life and Sex Education
    Unit: New brothers and sisters
    Unit: Reproduction in pets
    Unit: Pollenization in common plants

How much time should be allotted to health education during the primary school day? For many years, educators and physicians have recommended that health education be allotted the same amount of time as that given to other major fields of learning to strengthen health and safety practices that are fundamental to the child's well-being now and in the future. Also, direct health education has proved to be far more effective than incidental teaching on a "hit-or-miss" basis. Thus the teacher in the primary grades needs to set aside specific time in each school day for health education.

## ELEMENTARY SCHOOL HEALTH EDUCATION— INTERMEDIATE GRADES

Health education can be challenging and realistic in the intermediate grades if the *purposes* of health education are accepted. Health education strengthens desirable health and safety practices and develops new health attitudes and knowledge. It answers the child's questions of "why." It reveals to the child why parents and teachers stress desirable health and safety practices. It recognizes that the child has individual health problems. It accepts that some girls reach puberty early and that boys have specific personal health problems. It encourages the boy and girl to become aware of the individual differences in children's health problems. It reveals accident hazards and community health problems that previously were of little concern to the boy and girl. It stimulates the desire for more valid health information. It promotes the assuming of responsibility for certain health practices that formerly were considered largely the concern of parents and the teacher.

The *competencies* resulting from health education in the intermediate grades are numerous. In 11 of the 13 areas of health education, many competencies may result:

1. Developing acceptable posture in walking, lying, and working
2. Providing proper care of the feet
3. Choosing correct socks and shoes
4. Preventing dental caries
5. Developing good habits of personal cleanliness
6. Learning to relax
7. Avoiding fatigue caused by overexertion
8. Preventing pimples, boils, and blackheads
9. Taking proper care of the hair
10. Providing proper care of the nails
11. Preventing eye injuries and diseases
12. Avoiding ear injuries and infections
13. Understanding the causative agents of diseases
14. Preventing measles
15. Preventing chicken pox and mumps
16. Preventing whooping cough
17. Having tuberculin tests
18. Accepting cancers in children
19. Accepting and assisting the epileptic, diabetic, palsied, cardiac involved, dystrophic, speech-defective, crippled child, and the child who is defective in vision or hearing
20. Giving proper care to wounds
21. Providing proper care for shock
22. Recognizing poisonous snakes and providing first aid for snake bites
23. Giving first aid for household poisoning
24. Giving artificial respiration
25. Assembling a first-aid kit
26. Recognizing poisonous insects and providing first aid for insect bites
27. Avoiding community accident hazards
28. Practicing bicycle safety at all times
29. Preventing accidents caused by improper handling of guns
30. Promoting accident prevention while on vacation

31. Promoting accident prevention during all types of camping
32. Preventing drowning by common safety procedures while boating, surfing, and water skiing
33. Preventing fires at home
34. Preventing accidents in the home
35. Getting along with others
36. Being honest
37. Respecting parents and teachers
38. Respecting rights and property of others
39. Developing self-control and self-discipline
40. Controlling anger
41. Assuming responsibilities at home
42. Planning ahead and having daily time schedules
43. Developing courage
44. Controlling weight
45. Planning and preparing simple meals with assistance
46. Preparing a ready-to-eat breakfast
47. Choosing foods with a wide variety of nutrients
48. Avoiding being underweight
49. Preventing nutritional deficiencies
50. Liking milk and milk products
51. Avoiding misuse of coffee, tea, and sweetened soft drinks
52. Trying new foods
53. Avoiding polluted water
54. Preventing the spread of diseases by solid wastes
55. Preventing rabies in human beings and animals
56. Being aware of the need for adequate sewage treatment
57. Appreciating and supporting the functions of the local health department
58. Avoiding self-medication
59. Recognizing prescription and over-the-counter drugs
60. Accepting responsibilities at parties
61. Developing social etiquette
62. Accepting responsibilities for menstrual hygiene
63. Accepting responsibilities for personal hygiene for young boys
64. Accepting a role in the family
65. Avoiding strangers who invite boys and girls into their cars
66. Recognizing marijuana, heroin, bromides, and barbiturates
67. Avoiding inhalants used in "sniffing" and other agents
68. Reporting persons attempting to give or sell narcotics

To develop these competencies, what subject matter might be included for the intermediate grades? Eleven of the 13 areas of health education are used.

1. Area: Care of All Parts of the Human body
   Unit: Walking, working, and lying posture
   Unit: Dental caries
   Unit: Malocclusion and effects of diet on the teeth
   Unit: Care of the feet
   Unit: Relaxation and fatigue
   Unit: Pimples, boils, and blackheads
   Unit: Eye defects, infections, and injuries
   Unit: Ear injuries and infections
2. Area: Prevention of Diseases to All Parts of the Human Body
   Unit: Causative agents of diseases
   Unit: Measles (rubeola and rubella)
   Unit: Chicken pox and mumps
   Unit: Whooping cough and tetanus
   Unit: Tuberculin tests
3. Area: Chronic Health Conditions
   Unit: Common chronic health conditions
4. Area: American Red Cross First Aid
   Unit: Wounds
   Unit: Shock
   Unit: Poisonous snakes and first aid
   Unit: Poisonous insects and first aid
   Unit: Artificial respiration
   Unit: Household poisoning and first aid
   Unit: First-aid kits
5. Area: Safety Education
   Unit: Bicycle safety
   Unit: Gun safety
   Unit: Vacation safety
   Unit: Camping safety
   Unit: Common safety procedures for boating, surfing, and water skiing
   Unit: Fire prevention in the home
   Unit: Accidents in the home
6. Area: Mental Health
   Unit: Friends and getting along with others
   Unit: Honesty
   Unit: Courage
   Unit: Rights and property of others
   Unit: Self-control and self-discipline
   Unit: Respect for parents and teachers
   Unit: Tolerance
   Unit: Responsibilities at home
   Unit: Daily time schedules and planning ahead
7. Area: Nutrition
   Unit: Nutrients in the daily diet
   Unit: Nutritional deficiencies
   Unit: Calories and desirable weight
   Unit: Menu planning

Unit: Breakfast
Unit: Milk and milk products
Unit: Coffee, tea, and sweetened soft drinks
8. Area: Community Health Problems
Unit: Water and water-borne diseases
Unit: Sewage treatment and garbage disposal
Unit: Rabies
Unit: Local health department
9. Area: Consumer Health
Unit: Self-medication and nostrums
Unit: Common health fallacies
10. Area: Family Life and Sex Education
Unit: Social etiquette at parties
Unit: Menstrual hygiene for girls
Unit: Personal hygiene for boys
Unit: The family
11. Area: Drug Abuse, Narcotic Addiction, Smoking, and Misuse of Alcoholic Beverages
Unit: Narcotics, stimulants, and depressants
Unit: "Sniffing" and misuse of other agents

There has been for many years an acceptance of the practice of setting time aside in each school day for health education. Health education should *not* be taught along with science, social studies, physical education, or some other subject in the curriculum. Recommendations for a specific time allotment have come from the American Association of School Administrators, Joint Committee on Health Problems in Education of the NEA and the AMA, and the National Committee on School Health Policies of the NEA and the AMA.[6]

## JUNIOR OR MIDDLE HIGH SCHOOL HEALTH EDUCATION

Sometimes health education, as a single regularly scheduled subject-matter field, may be completely missing in the junior or middle high school curriculum. Increased emphasis on the biological sciences, mathematics, and foreign languages is partly the cause of this omission. In other instances, physical education may be considered health education, although health education is a subject-matter field completely separate from physical education. A unit

[6]National Committee on School Health Policies of the NEA and the AMA: *Suggested School Health Policies* 4th ed. Washington, D.C.: National Education Association, 1966, p. 9.

on tuberculosis which takes three health education class meetings to present thoroughly has no relation to volleyball, square dancing, or archery. So-called "health" on a rainy day when physical education classes cannot use outdoor facilities, incidental health teaching on a hit-or-miss basis, and curriculum juggling of two periods of "health" and three periods of physical education a week—all these practices reveal disregard for the junior high school student's need for health education.

In the junior or middle high school, regularly scheduled health education courses should be taught by teachers of health education or school health educators. These professionals have studied a specialized curriculum including preparation in a number of subjects: school health program; mental health; content in health education for secondary schools; community health; nutrition; American Red Cross First Aid and safety education; family life and sex education; drug abuse, narcotic addiction; smoking and misuse of alcoholic beverages; disease prevention and chronic health conditions; and methods and materials of health education. With graduate studies, the professional has studied consumer health; international health; current health problems of various ethnic, economic, and age groups; and other research and content areas. Many of those assigned to teach health education are professionally prepared in physical education, science, social studies, or coaching, but not in health education. Occasionally, a school nurse with none of the requirements for the secondary school teaching certificate attempts to teach health education. These nurses and teachers may have little or no preparation in the subject matter or content of health education. It is inconceivable that unqualified school personnel should be permitted to continue to teach health education, with its controversial and comprehensive content, to impressionable junior or middle high school students. The situation can be rectified only with employment of professionally prepared teachers of health education.

The *purposes* of health education in the junior or middle high school are related to the basic needs of adolescents. Health education strengthens the student's desirable health practices, attitudes, and knowledge and develops additional health practices, attitudes, and knowledge that promote effective healthful living. It involves the student in a personal manner and encourages the student to take action to solve some of his own health problems, with appropriate parental and teacher guidance. It fosters a careful examination by the student of the health practices and attitudes of other adolescents and adults. It includes discussion of everyday health problems of the adolescent and does not exclude problems that may be unfamiliar to the student or unpopular with certain parental groups. It stimulates the student to seek valid health information, and it probes into basic facts so that the student begins to realize the scope of health education. It forces him to accept and evaluate situations that are controversial and reveals sources of information needed in the evaluation of controversial health problems. It discloses community and national health problems that were unfamiliar to the student.

Numerous *competencies* result from health education in the junior or middle high school. If we use 12 of the 13 areas of health education in developing units, some of these competencies are the following:

1. Preventing acne, impetigo, and ringworm
2. Having acceptable posture in sitting, standing, walking, lying, and working
3. Preventing eye and ear infections and injuries
4. Having appropriate personal grooming
5. Preventing periodontal diseases
6. Making arrangements for medical and dental appointments
7. Preventing influenza and pneumonia
8. Using measures to eradicate tuberculosis
9. Understanding some of the scientific evidence about chronic bronchitis and smoking
10. Preventing rheumatic fever
11. Avoiding exposure to syphilis and gonorrhea
12. Understanding heart diseases
13. Eradicating fears and misconceptions about diabetes, epilepsy, and cerebral palsy
14. Completing satisfactorily Junior and Standard American Red Cross First Aid courses

15. Practicing self-preservation procedures in the event of natural disasters
16. Practicing accident prevention in school activities
17. Promoting accident prevention at home
18. Practicing recreational safety
19. Promoting accident prevention on farms and ranches
20. Preventing accidents from motor bikes and at home pools
21. Practicing self-preservation procedures in community disasters
22. Scheduling time so that there is adequate time for work and recreation
23. Being aware of many adolescent emotional health problems
24. Knowing from whom assistance can be obtained for emotional health problems
25. Selecting foods that satisfy the daily dietary needs
26. Preventing obesity through regulated caloric intake, exercise, and medical care
27. Avoiding dietary habits leading to malnutrition
28. Avoiding food fads
29. Evaluating food fallacies
30. Selecting foods that are not carriers of diseases
31. Being aware of influences on daily dietary habits
32. Understanding the problems associated with food allergies
33. Selecting food, milk, and meat that have been inspected
34. Understanding the importance of environmental sanitation procedures
35. Accepting the significance of purified water
36. Avoiding insect-borne diseases
37. Cooperating in the control of communicable diseases
38. Evaluating advertising of health products
39. Avoiding health fads and cults
40. Disproving health fallacies
41. Selecting health services wisely
42. Recognizing and avoiding all forms of quackery
43. Being aware of the many types of health careers
44. Utilizing official health and consumer protection agencies
45. Having daily exercise to promote physical well-being
46. Understanding the health problems of the arthritic
47. Understanding the problems associated with glaucoma

48. Having satisfactory, wholesome boy-girl relations
49. Dating rather than going steady with one person
50. Accepting the growth changes that occur to boys
51. Having worthy home membership
52. Avoiding stimulants and depressants such as bromides and tranquilizing drugs
53. Avoiding the use of marijuana, amphetamines, and barbiturates
54. Avoiding the use of tobacco
55. Compiling factual information on alcoholism
56. Avoiding use of "hard" narcotics
57. Understanding the health problems of Canada and Central and South America

It is possible that some of the competencies mentioned for the intermediate elementary school-age boy or girl might be added to the competencies in the junior or middle high school. This may be necessary when the health needs and interests of pupils of 10, 11, and 12 years of age have been overlooked. What subject matter might be included for the junior or middle high school student? All of the 13 areas of health education will be used:

1. Area: Care of All Parts of the Human Body
   Unit: Acne, impetigo, and ringworm
   Unit: Acceptable or poor posture
   Unit: Personal grooming
   Unit: Periodontal diseases
   Unit: Health responsibilities
2. Area: Prevention of Diseases to All Parts of the Human Body
   Unit: Influenza and pneumonia
   Unit: Tuberculosis
   Unit: Lung cancer and smoking
   Unit: Rheumatic fever
   Unit: Syphilis and gonorrhea
   Unit: Medical care of the patient with heart disease
3. Area: Chronic Health Conditions
   Unit: Diabetes
   Unit: Epilepsy
   Unit: Cerebral palsy
4. Area: American Red Cross First Aid
   Unit: Junior American Red Cross First Aid
   Unit: Standard American Red Cross First Aid
5. Area: Safety Education
   Unit: Community disasters
   Unit: Natural disasters
   Unit: School safety
   Unit: Home safety
   Unit: Recreation safety
   Unit: Farm and ranch safety
   Unit: Motorcycle and home pool safety
6. Area: Mental Health
   Unit: Adequate time for work and play
   Unit: Adolescent emotional problems
   Unit: Sources of assistance for emotional health problems
7. Area: Nutrition
   Unit: Selection of foods for daily dietary needs
   Unit: Obesity and weight control
   Unit: Malnutrition
   Unit: Food fallacies
   Unit: Food allergies
8. Area: Community Health Problems
   Unit: Environmental sanitation
   Unit: Insect-borne diseases
   Unit: Rodents and rat-borne diseases
   Unit: Pollution of water supplies
9. Area: Consumer Health
   Unit: Advertising of health products
   Unit: Health fads and cults
   Unit: Health fallacies
   Unit: Quackery
   Unit: Health careers
   Unit: Official health agencies
   Unit: Consumer protection agencies
10. Area: Adult Health Problems
    Unit: Exercise and health
    Unit: Arthritis
    Unit: Glaucoma
11. Area: Family Life and Sex Education
    Unit: Adolescent and the parent
    Unit: Boy to young man
    Unit: Boy-girl relations
    Unit: Dating or going steady
12. Area: Drug Abuse, Narcotic Addiction, Smoking, and Misuse of Alcoholic Beverages
    Unit: Marijuana
    Unit: "Uppers" and "downers"
    Unit: To smoke or not to smoke
    Unit: Alcoholism
    Unit: "Hard" narcotics
13. Area: International Health
    Unit: Health problems of Canada and Central and South America

As for time allotment in the junior or middle high school, the National Committee on School Health Policies of the NEA and the AMA stated

health teaching should be in keeping with that scheduled for other academic areas. Recommended time allotment for the health education or health science course is one semester at the seventh grade and one semester at the ninth grade, or a year course at the eighth grade, or an equivalent plan.[7]

## SENIOR HIGH SCHOOL HEALTH EDUCATION

Health education in the high school can be provocative and highly significant if its content is directed at the health needs and interests of young adults. In addition, health education should be taught in regularly scheduled health education courses meeting five periods a week for designated semesters. As in the junior or middle high school, health education should be taught by professionally prepared teachers of health education or school health educators.

The *purposes* of health education in the high school are different from those of the junior or middle high school. Health education in the senior high school motivates the student to evaluate his own health attitudes, practices, and knowledge and those of his adult associates. It forces the student to reach definite decisions about his health habits. It stimulates the student to take action for the promotion and protection of his health. It seeks to develop informed adults who can cope with present and future health problems. It deals specifically with the health problems of the student's future occupation, marriage, and family. It encourages the student to take action regarding his family's health problems. It stimulates the student to do research and to be critical of contemporary health problems. It forces the student to accept his role in community, national, and international health. It makes the student aware that health education is a continuous process of learning throughout life. It provides opportunities for an enriched curriculum in health education.

*Competencies* resulting from high school health education are numerous. It is possible that some of the competencies mentioned at the junior or middle high school level may need to be added to the senior high school competencies. If regularly scheduled health education courses had been omitted at the junior or middle high school level, the high school student will not have acquired the competencies listed earlier. In the 13 areas of health education, the competencies are these:

1. Evaluating and improving individual health practices, attitudes, and knowledge related to personal health
2. Seeking correction of dental health problems
3. Taking action to promote family health
4. Preventing infectious hepatitis
5. Being aware of the complications resulting from infectious mononucleosis
6. Recognizing the seven warning signals of cancers
7. Evaluating advertising and quackery related to cancer
8. Assuming responsibilities for early detection of cancer and for further cancer education
9. Avoiding exposure to all venereal diseases
10. Understanding the problems of multiple sclerosis, muscular dystrophy, cystic fibrosis, and myasthenia gravis
11. Understanding the problems associated with heart disease
12. Completing satisfactorily the Advanced American Red Cross First Aid course
13. Understanding the effects of man-made national disaster
14. Being aware of accident rates in various occupations
15. Practicing accident prevention in occupations held while attending school and during school vacations
16. Eradicating fears and misconceptions concerning mental illness
17. Understanding suicide and accepting responsibilities for preventing suicides
18. Being aware of the agencies and services for the mentally ill
19. Understanding the significance of nutrition in the treatment of diseases and alcoholism, to pregnancy, and to other health problems
20. Practicing adequate sanitation in the preparation of meals
21. Seeking reliable information about cholesterol, diets, and other nutrition topics
22. Avoiding crash diets and diets of food faddists
23. Cooperating with local community efforts to control air pollution
24. Understanding the problems related to radiation control
25. Supporting the functions of the state health departments and the United States Public Health Service
26. Being aware of the services of nonofficial health agencies
27. Being aware of the need for professionally prepared personnel in the numerous health professions

28. Acquainting associates with school health education
29. Selecting hospital, medical-surgical, and disability insurance that satisfies individual and family needs
30. Selecting a family physician and dentist, medical and dental specialists, nurses, and a hospital
31. Buying health products wisely
32. Assuming responsibilities for medical examinations and immunizations
33. Avoiding obesity
34. Exercising daily and promoting the health of the cardiovascular system
35. Accepting responsibilities during the period of engagement
36. Realizing that promiscuous sexual relations do not promote a happy marriage
37. Understanding the development of the unborn child during pregnancy and the birth of the baby
38. Accepting obligations in marriage
39. Understanding the problems of newly wedded young couples
40. Being aware of the importance of family planning
41. Understanding the many problems of sexual behavior
42. Being aware of the physical, social, economic, and psychological factors involved with alcoholism
43. Understanding the problems associated with the treatment of alcoholics
44. Avoiding the misuse of alcoholic beverages
45. Avoiding the use of hallucinogens
46. Understanding the problems involved with drug abuse
47. Being aware of the criminal aspects associated with narcotic addiction
48. Recognizing the need for international malaria eradication
49. Being aware of the scope and diversity of international health problems
50. Accepting health problems encountered by space travel
51. Understanding the need for comprehensive health planning
52. Accepting health education as a continuous process of learning

Units from the 13 areas of health education for the subject matter concerned with the above-mentioned competencies are as follows:

1. Area: Care of All Parts of the Human Body
   Unit: Improvement of personal health
   Unit: Adult dental health problems
   Unit: Fluoridation of drinking water supplies
   Unit: Promotion of the family's health
2. Area: Prevention of Diseases to All Parts of the Human Body
   Unit: Infectious hepatitis and infectious mononucleosis
   Unit: Cancers
   Unit: Venereal diseases
3. Area: Chronic Health Conditions
   Unit: Multiple sclerosis, muscular dystrophy, cystic fibrosis, and myasthenia gravis
   Unit: Coronary thrombosis and other heart conditions
4. Area: American Red Cross First Aid
   Unit: Advanced American Red Cross First Aid course
5. Area: Safety Education
   Unit: Man-made national disasters
   Unit: Occupational safety
6. Area: Mental Health
   Unit: Mental illness
   Unit: Agencies and services for the mentally ill
7. Area: Nutrition
   Unit: Nutrition as related to the treatment of diseases, to alcoholism, to pregnancy, and to other health problems
   Unit: Sanitation in meal preparation
   Unit: Controversial nutrition topics
   Unit: Crash diets and food fads
8. Area: Community Health Problems
   Unit: Air pollution
   Unit: Radiation control
   Unit: Food-, meat-, and milk-borne diseases and methods of control
   Unit: State health departments and the United States Public Health Service
   Unit: Nonofficial health agencies
9. Area: Consumer Health
   Unit: Health insurance
   Unit: Selection of a physician, dentist, nurse, and hospital
   Unit: Wise purchasing of health products
10. Area: Adult Health Problems
    Unit: Medical examinations and immunizations
    Unit: Obesity and exercise
11. Area: Family Life and Sex Education
    Unit: Engagement and its significance
    Unit: Marriage and its obligations
    Unit: Pregnancy and birth of the baby
    Unit: Problems of newly wedded couples
    Unit: Family planning
    Unit: Problems in sexual behaviors
12. Area: Drug Abuse, Narcotic Addiction,

Smoking, and Misuse of Alcoholic Beverages
Unit: Hallucinogens
Unit: Problems of drug abuse
Unit: Alcoholic beverages and alcoholism
13. Area: International Health
Unit: Malaria
Unit: Significant international health problems
Unit: Health in space travel
Unit: Comprehensive health planning

As for time allotment in the senior high school, the National Committee on School Health Policies of the NEA and the AMA indicated that health education "should be equal to that of other academic areas. A recommended plan is providing a semester course at the tenth grade . . . and a semester course at the eleventh or twelfth grade."[8]

A 1970 study found that 22 states have certification requirements for teachers of health education in the secondary schools. The mean required number of semester hours was 25.4 in health education. Teachers of health education have received certification for their own specialized preparation separate from physical education, health and physical education, and the biological sciences.[9]

## TEACHER RESPONSIBILITIES

Every elementary school classroom teacher and school health educator should be acquainted with his responsibilities for health instruction. The teacher should show evidence of:

1. Building student-teacher rapport
2. Respecting student opinions
3. Being sensitive to youth's problems
4. Being positive and direct in guiding student opinions
5. Having courage to teach specific facts and to face the realities of student problems
6. Having an "air of understanding" so that students will feel free to ask for teacher-pupil conferences

7. Being honest
8. Omitting intimidation and sarcasm
9. Admitting that there are student questions the teacher desires parents to answer
10. Admitting that the teacher may not have all the specific facts but will be willing to gather further information
11. Keeping detailed notes on specific facts
12. Keeping a record of student questions regarding controversial topics
13. Remaining as the discussion leader
14. Avoiding sensational statements and false information

Other teacher responsibilities will be discussed in Chapter 13, including orientation procedures to be completed before actual teaching and the teacher's precautionary procedures.

## References for Further Study

Anderson, C. L.: *School Health Practice.* 5th ed. St. Louis: The C. V. Mosby Company, 1972.
Cornacchia, H., Staton, W. M., and Irwin, L. W.: *Health in Elementary Schools.* 3rd ed. St. Louis: The C. V. Mosby Company, 1970.
Fodor, J. T., and Dalis, G. T.: *Health Instruction: Theory and Application.* Philadelphia: Lea & Febiger, 1966.
Grout, R. E.: *Health Teaching in Schools.* 5th ed. Philadelphia: W. B. Saunders Company, 1968.
Joint Committee on Health Problems in Education of the NEA and the AMA: *Health Education.* 5th ed. Washington, D. C.: National Education Association, 1961.
Kilander, H.: *School Health Education.* 2nd ed. New York: The Macmillan Company, 1968.
Mayshark, C., and Irwin, L. W.: *Health Education in the Secondary Schools.* 2nd ed. St. Louis: The C. V. Mosby Company, 1968.
Oberteuffer, D., Harrelson, O., and Pollock, M.: *School Health Education.* 5th ed. New York: Harper & Row, 1972.
Smolensky, J., and Bonvechio, L. R.: *Principles of School Health.* Boston: D. C. Heath and Company, 1966.
Turner, C. E., Randall, H. B., and Smith, S. L: *School Health and Health Education.* 6th ed. St. Louis: The C. V. Mosby Company, 1970.
Willgoose, C. E.: *Health Education in the Elementary School.* 3rd ed. Philadelphia: W. B. Saunders Company, 1969.
_____ : *Health Teaching in Secondary Schools.* Philadelphia: W. B. Saunders Company, 1972.

[8]*Ibid.*
[9]Jessie Helen Haag: Comparisons of the preparation of health education teachers in the United States: 1949-1970. *Inter. J. Health Education* 13 (1970 #4):163-168.

# Chapter 13

# *DISCOVERY OF THE PUPIL AND THE COMMUNITY'S HEALTH PROBLEMS*

## AN INCIDENT

A school health educator was asked to evaluate curriculum guides in health education for medium-sized school system's elementary schools, junior high schools, and high schools. Before attempting his evaluation, the school health educator compiled extensive data on the pupils' physical and mental health status, health practices, health attitudes, health interests, and health knowledge. Also, the school health educator gathered information on the community's health problems. When this compilation of pupil health needs and interests and community health problems were compared to the curriculum guides, there was little evidence that those who contrived the curriculum guides considered the pupils' health needs and interests and community health problems.

Six principles of health education were discussed in the last chapter. The sixth

principle dealt with objective information about the individual pupil's physical and mental health status, his health practices, attitudes, interests, and knowledge. Why should the teacher determine this information? In order to influence the pupil beneficially as well as to improve his health status, the teacher must discover the pupil's *existing* health status, practices, attitudes, interests, and knowledge.

Much of this objective information comes from the *school health program.* How can the teacher discover the pupil's physical and mental health status from school health services? How can the teacher determine the pupil's health practices from school health services and health education? What parts of the school health program can the teacher use to discover the pupil's health attitudes and interests? How can the teacher determine the pupil's health knowledge from health education?

In Table *3* are listed the sources of information about pupil's specific health needs and interests.

*Table 3*

*Some Sources of Information about the Pupil's Health Needs and Interests*

| Part of the School Health Program | Where Discovered | Type of Information |
|---|---|---|
| **PHYSICAL AND MENTAL HEALTH STATUS** | | |
| SCHOOL HEALTH SERVICES | 1. School personnel's systematic and continuous observations | Signs of visual difficulties, hearing difficulties, emotional health problems, communicable diseases, skin infections, nutritional deficiencies, posture conditions, dental health problems, chronic conditions, other health conditions and diseases |

| Part of the School Health Program | Where Discovered | Type of Information |
|---|---|---|
| | 2. Health record<br>  a. History | History of diseases, habits, illnesses, operations, emotional disturbances |
| | b. Results of medical examination | Chronic health conditions, diseases, emotional problems |
| | c. Results of dental examination | Dental defects and diseases |
| | d. Results of immunizations and disease detection procedures | Smallpox vaccination; immunization for diphtheria, rubeola and rubella, whooping cough, mumps, tetanus, polio; tuberculin tests |
| | e. Results of follow-through | Home visits by nurse; parental actions to seek correction of pupil's remediable health conditions |
| | f. Results of screening of vision, hearing, nutritional status, and posture | Visual and hearing difficulties, nutritional deficiencies, posture conditions |
| | 3. Emergency Care Record | Accidents and illnesses |
| HEALTHFUL SCHOOL LIVING<br>A. Environmental Factors | 1. Observations of accident hazards | Types of accidents, location of accidents, fire hazards |
| | 2. Observations of unsanitary school facilities | Possibility of food-, meat-, milk-, and water-borne diseases; skin infections; other communicable diseases |
| B. School Nutrition | Dietary habits at noonday school meals | Signs of nutritional deficiencies |
| HEALTH EDUCATION | 1. Teacher's observations | As given in school health services |

## HEALTH PRACTICES

| | | |
|---|---|---|
| SCHOOL HEALTH SERVICES | 1. Teacher's observations | Pupil's actions regarding visual difficulties, hearing difficulties, emotional health problems, nutritional deficiencies, posture conditions, dental health problems, skin infections, chronic conditions, other health conditions and diseases |
| | 2. Follow-through | Pupil's and parents' actions in home during pupil's illness and convalescence; seeking correction of remediable health conditions |
| | 3. Immunization Record | Parental and pupil actions regarding type and frequency of immunization |
| | 4. Emergency Care Record | Accident proneness and types of illnesses |

| Part of the School Health Program | Where Discovered | Type of Information |
|---|---|---|
| **HEALTHFUL SCHOOL LIVING**<br>A. Environmental Factors | Teacher's observations | Accident proneness, actions during fire and disaster drills, housekeeping and sanitation procedures |
| B. School Nutrition | Teacher's observations | Dietary habits, posture while seated, tooth brushing, hand washing, table manners |
| C. School Day | Daily school activities | Actions during pupil's relations with other pupils, particularly emotional health problems |
| **HEALTH EDUCATION** | 1. Teacher's observations | Care of all parts of the human body, prevention of diseases and injuries, dietary habits, boy-girl relations, disaster procedures |
| | 2. Pupil demonstrations | As above |
| | 3. Pupil surveys | As above |
| | 4. Pupil rating scales | As above |
| | 5. Pupil checklists | As above |
| | 6. Parent-teacher conferences | Pupil health habits regarding sleep, exercise, dietary habits, etc. |
| | 7. A.R.C. First Aid and safety skills | Correct or incorrect procedures |
| | 8. Published health practices measuring devices (Chapter 22) | As No. 1 |

## HEALTH ATTITUDES

| Part of the School Health Program | Where Discovered | Type of Information |
|---|---|---|
| **SCHOOL HEALTH SERVICES** | 1. Teacher-pupil conferences | Pupil's response when encouraged to seek correction of remediable health conditions |
| | 2. Teacher-parent conferences | Parent's willingness to seek correction of remediable health conditions |
| | 3. Follow-through | As Nos. 1, 2 |
| | 4. Health counseling | As above |
| | 5. Screening procedures | As above |
| **HEALTHFUL SCHOOL LIVING**<br>A. School Day | 1. Teacher listening to pupil conversations | Pupil's opinions, superstitions, fears, misconceptions |
| | 2. Sociodrama | As above |
| **HEALTH EDUCATION** | 1. Teacher-guided discussions | Pupil's opinions, superstitions, fears, misconceptions |
| | 2. Questions to teacher | As above |
| | 3. Questionnaires | As above |
| | 4. Attitude rating scale | As above |
| | 5. Panels | As above |
| | 6. Debates | As above |
| | 7. Published health attitude measuring devices (Chapter 22) | As above |

| Part of the School Health Program | Where Discovered | Type of Information |
|---|---|---|
| **HEALTH INTERESTS** | | |
| HEALTHFUL SCHOOL LIVING<br>A. School Day | 1. Choices of health education reading materials | Areas of health education (Chapter 14) |
| | 2. Written work in health education | As above |
| | 3. Teacher listening to pupil conversations | As above |
| HEALTH EDUCATION | 1. Interest inventories | Areas of health education (Chapter 14) |
| | 2. Questions directed to teacher | As above |
| | 3. Teacher-guided class discussions | As above |
| | 4. Experiments | As above |
| | 5. Pupil-made surveys, checklists, questionnaires | As above |
| | 6. Opinion polls | As above |
| **HEALTH KNOWLEDGE** | | |
| HEALTH EDUCATION | 1. Teacher-made objective and subjective tests | Pupil's incorrect, ambiguous, out-of-date health information |
| | 2. Published health knowledge tests (Chapter 22) | As above |
| | 3. Teacher-guided discussions | Pupil's fund of information |
| | 4. Oral response to teacher's questions | As above |
| | 5. Panels and debates | As above |

## RESULTS OF COMPILED PUPIL INFORMATION

The results of compiled objective information gathered from pupil's physical and mental health status (What is he like?), his health practices (What does he do?), his health attitudes (What does he believe or fear?), his health interests (What does he want to know?), and his health knowledge (What does he know?)—all indicate *what the teacher is to teach.* How can the compiled information be used to determine the health education course content?

As the elementary teacher and school health educator utilize the sources, a compilation of positive and negative findings for each pupil appears. When these findings for all pupils in a class are listed, some will appear with greater frequency. Positive findings, repeatedly occurring, should indicate health education units needing less emphasis; that is, if nearly all pupils have good dental health, little classtime is needed. Negative findings with many frequencies should reveal health education units taking top priority in the instruction. These units indicate the *content or subject matter.*

When the top-priority units include controversial subject matter, the elementary teacher and school health educator should present other noncontroversial top-priority units at the beginning of the school semester or year. The controversial top-priority units can be taught later in the school semester or year when the teacher has the principal's approval for including the controversial units and the teacher is better acquainted with students.

The information gathered from records and observations about the pupil's physical and mental health status, his health practices, his health attitudes, and his health knowledge indicates the real health needs. Pupil's health *interests* are not the same as pupil's real health *needs.* Often teachers believe that the pupil's health interests should be satisfied before the pupil's real health needs. The teacher's compilation of the negative findings of the pupil's real health needs discloses the subject matter necessary to satisfy the pupil's health needs. Once this very important content is determined, the pupil's health interests can be considered to supplement the other content of health education.

## COMMUNITY HEALTH PROBLEMS

Local and state health departments, state divisions of nonofficial health agencies, the United States Public Health Service, the Food and Drug Administration, and other governmental agencies have a wealth of information about community health problems. This information may be in the form of vital statistics, demographic data, morbidity rates, accident reports of industries, records of local sanitarians, records of incidence of illness and disability from diseases and chronic health conditions from nonofficial health agencies, spot maps indicating locations of garbage dumps and industrial air pollution, charts, graphs, bulletins, certificates of live birth, and many other forms. It may be necessary for the school health educator to interpret some of this information to other teachers.

## CONTROVERSIAL TOPICS

There are many topics or units of health education which may be controversial because they are misunderstood and not accepted. These units are those dealing with alcoholic beverages and alcoholism, smoking, drug abuse, mental illness, suicide, venereal diseases, immunization, quackery, health insurance, chiropractic, and fluoridation of drinking water. Many units in family life and sex education are also controversial, such as those concerned with dating, boy-girl relations, engagement, marriage, pregnancy, and birth of the baby, as well as contraception, abortion, and sexual deviations. The following procedures may minimize controversy:

1. Orientation procedures to be completed before actual teaching
   a. Teacher's responsibilities to school officials and parents
      (1) Accept that parents share responsibilities in familiarizing the student with some of these topics
      (2) Attend in-service health education or graduate courses which include these units
      (3) Prepare a tentative but detailed outline of subject matter
      (4) Present outline to principal
      (5) Have approval of principal
      (6) Present approved outline to parent-teacher groups whose sons and daughters will receive the instruction
      (7) Inform parent-teacher groups that some questions might be better answered in the home
      (8) Invite parents to visit health education classes
      (9) Present films and other audio-visual aids, to be used with outline, to parent-teacher groups
      (10) Have approval of parent-teacher groups on outline and instructional materials
   b. Teacher's precautionary procedures
      (1) Accept, that in some systems, boys may be separated from girls for these units
      (2) Include controversial units after the sixth week of the school year after becoming acquainted with students
      (3) Be aware of the students' community, family, religious, and social backgrounds
      (4) Use correct terminology, developing a vocabulary list
      (5) Evaluate carefully all audio-visual instruction aids
      (6) Present the unit in conjunction with a special lecturer or independently
      (7) Be objective
      (8) Be aware that some questions may be better answered in a teacher-pupil conference or by parents
      (9) Keep notes on students' questions
      (10) Have an "air of understanding" student problems
      (11) Gain the students' confidence
      (12) Be positive in the teaching

2. Students' responsibilities
   a. Discuss all questions openly

b. Seek a conference with the teacher if there is hesistancy about asking a question

c. Use correct terminology when discussing these topics

d. Use periodicals, pamphlets, and books recommended by the teacher and librarian.

Accepting the teacher responsibilities and following the precautionary procedures before teaching any controversial unit will allay some of the bitter opposition to these units. Parents, if informed, are usually willing to listen to reasons for teaching these controversial units.

### Teach Us What We Want To Know

Are controversial units high on the lists of students' health interests? More than 5000 students from kindergarten through twelfth grade throughout Connecticut were involved in the Student Health Concerns Project during 1967 and 1968. The purposes of the study were (1) to gather data on health interests of boys and girls, K through 12th grade; and (2) to explore techniques to elicit the data so that these techniques would be valuable to the classroom teacher. The methods used were discussions, observations, life situations, free and anonymous writing, incomplete story, dramatization, role playing, and tape recordings. Controversial units were among the health interests of elementary and secondary school students. In kindergarten through grade two, there were questions raised about the differences in sex roles and about babies. In grades three and four, questions about babies, mental health, drug abuse, smoking, and alcoholic beverages and alcoholism were asked. Students in grades five and six raised questions about babies, mental health, social-emotional development, alcoholic beverages and alcoholism, drug abuse, and smoking. In grade seven, questions about mental illness, sex education, alcoholic beverages and alcoholism, drug abuse, and smoking were asked. In grade eight, dating, abortion, sexual deviations, venereal diseases, and drug abuse were among the interests. In grade nine, questions concerning sex education commanded high interest, vene-

real diseases, alcoholic beverages and alcoholism, drug abuse, and smoking were also mentioned frequently. In grade ten, sex education, smoking, alcoholic beverages and alcoholism, drug abuse, mental illness, abortion, marriage, venereal diseases, mental health, and birth control were listed as topics which tenth graders thought should be included in health education. In the eleventh grade, questions were raised about pre-marital sexual intercourse, birth control, alcoholic beverages and alcoholism, venereal diseases, and drug abuse. In the twelfth grade, students listed the following units to be included in health education: mental health, venereal diseases, vaccinations, sex education, birth control, abortion, alcoholic beverages and alcohol, smoking, and drug abuse.[1]

## References for Further Study

Anderson, C. L.: *School Health Practice.* 5th ed. St. Louis: The C. V. Mosby Company, 1972.

Cornacchia, H., Staton, W. M., and Irwin, L. W.: *Health in Elementary Schools.* 3rd ed. St. Louis: The C. V. Mosby Company, 1970.

Fodor, J. T., and Dalis, G. T.: *Health Instruction: Theory and Application.* Philadelphia: Lea & Febiger, 1966.

Grout, R. E.: *Health Teaching in Schools.* 5th ed. Philadelphia: W. B. Saunders Company, 1968.

Joint Committee on Health Problems in Education of the NEA and AMA: *Health Education.* 5th ed. Washington, D.C.: National Education Association, 1961.

Kilander, H. F.: *School Health Education.* 2nd ed. New York: The Macmillan Company, 1968.

Mayshark, C., and Irwin, L. W.: *Health Education in the Secondary Schools.* 2nd ed. St. Louis: The C. V. Mosby Company, 1968.

Oberteuffer, D., Harrelson, O., and Pollock, M.: *School Health Education.* 5th ed. New York: Harper & Row, 1972.

Smolensky, J., and Bonvechio, L. R.: *Principles of School Health.* Boston: D. C. Heath and Comapny, 1966.

Turner, C. E., Randall, H. B., and Smith, S. L.: *School Health and Health Education.* 6th ed. St. Louis: The C. V. Mosby Company, 1970.

Willgoose, C. W.: *Health Education in the Elementary School.* 3rd ed. Philadelphia: W. B. Saunders Company, 1969.

————: *Health Teaching in Secondary Schools.* Philadelphia: W. B. Saunders Company, 1972.

[1]Ruth Byler, Gertrude M. Lewis, and Ruth J. Totman: *Teach Use What We Want To Know.* New York: Mental Health Materials Center, Inc., 1969, pp. iii-111.

# Chapter 14

## *CONTENT WITHIN HEALTH EDUCATION AREAS AND UNITS*

### AN INCIDENT

Parents have demanded that more foreign languages, science, and mathematics be added to an already crowded curriculum. Also, parents have asked that "health" be eliminated in the elementary and secondary schools since the parts and functions of the human body are taught in science. The superintendent of schools has requested elementary school teachers and school health educators to explain the subject matter of health education, particularly emphasizing that content which includes individual, family, and community health problems.

In the previous chapter, sources of information about pupil health needs and interests were discussed. From these sources the elementary school teacher and the school health educator can determine the health education content to be taught. This content should be outlined for every unit and lesson so that it becomes meaningful to the student. In order to outline the content, the teacher should understand the areas of health education, the units within each area, and the lessons within a unit. In this chapter, areas and units will be discussed, and in the following chapter, specific lessons will be presented.

### AREAS OF HEALTH EDUCATION

An *area* is a specific phase of health education. It is broad in content and has many divisions called "units." Some areas, as may be expected, are more appropriate for courses in the secondary school than in the elementary school. There are 13 areas of health education.

1. Care of all parts of the human body
2. Prevention of diseases to all parts of the human body
3. Chronic health conditions
4. American Red Cross First Aid
5. Safety education
6. Mental health
7. Nutrition
8. Community health problems
9. Consumer health
10. Adult health problems
11. Family life and sex education
12. Drug abuse, narcotic addiction, smoking, and misuse of alcoholic beverages
13. International health

The titles of some of the areas may need explanation:

Chronic health conditions—Recognition and acceptance of conditions caused by malfunctions or defects that are not remediable

Safety education—Recognition and avoidance of hazards causing disability or death

Nutrition—Science of the basic nutrients and improvement of daily dietary habits to insure wise selection and use of food

Community health—Environmental sanitation and services of agencies promoting health

Consumer health—Wise selection of health products and services, agencies concerned with the control of these products and services, evaluation of quackery and health misconceptions, health careers, and health insurance

Family life and sex education—Problems associated with the student's sex adjustment during his growth and development and ranging from simple matters of personal health to the complicated physical, social, psychological, and moral factors promoting successful marriage and family relations

## SUGGESTED UNITS WITHIN NUTRITION

The area of "Nutrition" might contain the following units. Each unit includes many specific items of information related to the central topic. There is no attempt to include all the possible units of Nutrition, and no particular unit is outlined completely. In a later section of this chapter, more nearly complete outlines of subject matter are given.

### AREA: NUTRITION

Unit I     Essential Four Food Groups

Unit II    Carbohydrates
  A. Sources of carbohydrates
  B. Carbohydrate-rich foods
  C. Effects of diets deficient in carbohydrates
  D. Carbohydrates in the daily diet
  E. Daily caloric intake

Unit III   Proteins
  A. Conditions determining the amount of proteins
  B. Sources of proteins
  C. Amino acids
  D. Complete and incomplete proteins
  E. Effects of diets deficient in proteins

Unit IV   Fats
  A. Essential fatty acids
  B. Sources of fats
  C. Functions of fats in diet

Unit V    Water and Fiber
  A. Water losses and replacements
  B. Importance of water as a body regulator and as a tissue-building material
  C. Fiber and its importance
  D. Foods containing fiber

Unit VI   Mineral Elements
  A. Necessity of mineral salts in the regulation of body processes
  B. Mineral elements
    1. Amounts needed in daily diet
    2. Sources of mineral elements
    3. Effects of diets deficient in mineral elements
      a. Calcium
      b. Phosphorus
      c. Iron
      d. Iodine
  C. Mineral supplements—are they needed?

Unit VII   Vitamins
  A. Importance of vitamins in daily diet
  B. Vitamin C—ascorbic acid
    1. Foods containing vitamin C
    2. Importance of vitamin C
    3. Effects of diets lacking vitamin C
    4. Water-soluble vitamin C
  C. Water-soluble vitamins
    1. Thiamine
      a. Importance of thiamine in daily diet
      b. Foods containing thiamine
    2. Riboflavin
      a. Effects of diets lacking riboflavin
      b. Foods containing riboflavin
    3. Niacin
      a. Importance of niacin in daily diet
      b. Foods containing niacin
    4. Other B-complex vitamins and their importance
  D. Fat-soluble vitamins
    1. Vitamin A
      a. Foods containing vitamin A
      b. Effects of diets deficient in vitamin A
    2. Vitamin D
      a. Foods containing vitamin D
      b. Effects of diets deficient in vitamin D
    3. Vitamin E
    4. Vitamin K

Unit VIII   Daily Diet Based on Wise Selection of Nutrients

Unit IX   Obesity
  A. Factors influencing weight
  B. Caloric requirements
  C. Causes
  D. Disadvantages
  E. Family physician and treatment of obesity
  F. Crash diets, reducing fads, and quackery

Unit X    Underweight
  A. Characteristics
  B. Causes
  C. Disadvantages
  D. Diet prescribed by physician

Unit XI    Influences upon Dietary Habits
   A. Improvement of staple foods
   B. Variety in menu planning
   C. Proper cooking methods and conservation of certain nutrients
   D. Trends in American dietary habits
Unit XII    Nutrition Quackery
Unit XIII    Food Fallacies
   A Fallacies concerning nutrients
   B. Fallacies concerning milk, eggs, butter, oleomargarine, fruits, vegetables, meat, breads, and cereals
   C. Fallacies concerning food processing
Unit XIV    Misuse of Coffee, Tea, and Sweetened Soft Drinks
   A. Caloric value
   B. Effects on dental health
   C. Effects as diuretics
Unit XV    Importance of Nutrition
   A. Signs of possible nutritional deficiencies
   B. Prenatal and postnatal care
   C. Care of the diabetic
   D. Treatment of the tuberculous patient
   E. Therapy for the alcoholic
Unit XVI    Food-borne Diseases
Unit XVII    Milk and Milk Products
   A. Nutrients in milk
   B. Types of milk and milk products
   C. Milk in menu planning
   D. Milk grading and labeling
   E. Inspection of dairy farms and milk plants
   F. Examination of milk and milk products
   G. Pasteurization
   H. Milk-borne diseases
   I. Milk-like beverages
      a. filled milk
      b. imitation milk
Unit XVIII    Meat
   A. Types of meat
   B. Nutrients in meat
   C. Meat in menu planning
   D. Meat inspection
   E. Meat-borne diseases
Unit XIX    Fruits and Vegetables
Unit XX    Breads and Cereals
Unit XXI    Sanitation in the Preparation and Serving of Foods
Unit XXII    Food Allergies
Unit XXIII    School Lunch

In addition to these 23 units, there are other possible units, such as "Foods for Snacks," "Controversial Topics in Nutri-tion," and "Calories Needed for Work and Play." Among the units of particular interest to high school students are those dealing with (1) weight loss and dieting; (2) proper foods for a well-balanced diet; and (3) effects of deficiencies and excesses of nutrients.

## OUTLINES OF UNITS OF HEALTH EDUCATION

A health education *unit* is a series of lessons built around a central topic. Before the lessons can be planned with methods and materials of instruction, the entire unit can be outlined by the teacher, teacher and pupils, or pupils, depending upon the unit and age level of the class. In this way, much of the specific information meaningful to the pupils' health needs and interests can be included within the unit.

The following health education units may be used at the elementary or secondary school levels. The pupils' health needs and interests will determine the amount of content within each unit. The following units are outlined to indicate some of the specific information included.

### Dental Health (Chapter 5)

Concept: Proper dental health practices and professional dental care maintain healthy permanent teeth.

Area of health education—Care of All Parts of the Human Body

1. Prevalence of dental health problems among pupils in elementary and secondary schools
2. Diet during pregnancy and its relation to the future child's dental health status
3. Deciduous teeth: number, location, structure, age when the teeth appear
4. Care of the deciduous teeth by the child, parent, and dentist
5. Six-year molars
6. Mixed dentition
7. Permanent teeth: number, location, structure, age when the teeth appear
8. Functions of teeth
9. Tooth brushing
10. Care of the permanent teeth
11. Dental caries
12. Common dental health problems
    a. Periodontal diseases

      (1) Gingivitis
      (2) Pyorrhea
      (3) Vincent's infection
    b. Malocclusion
    c. Impacted teeth
13. Signs of dental health problems
14. Family dentist and his services
15. Topical fluoride applications
16. Dental specialists and their services
17. Choosing a dentist
18. Dental hygienist and her services
19. Fluoridation of drinking-water supplies
20. Nutrition and its significance to dental health
21. False advertising of dental products
22. Misconceptions about dental health
23. Adult dental health problems
24. American Dental Association

## Eye Infections, Injuries, and Defects

Concept: Prevention of eye infection, injuries, and aggravated defects ensures better vision.

Area of health education—Care of All Parts of the Human Body

1. Incidence of eye infections, injuries, and defects among pupils in elementary and secondary schools
2. The parts of the eyeball and the physiology of vision
3. Loss of vision and what it means
4. Eye infections and diseases (Chapter 2)
    a. Blepharitis
    b. Conjunctivitis
    c. Sty
    d. Trachoma
5. Eye injuries
    a. Blows
    b. Chemical burns
    c. Careless play
    d. Hunting accidents
    e. Occupational hazards
6. Eye defects (Chapter 2)
    a. Amblyopia
    b. Astigmatism
    c. Cataract
    d. Color blindness
    e. Diplopia
    f. Glaucoma
    g. Hyperopia
    h. Myopia
    i. Nystagmus
    j. Strabismus

7. Vision screening procedures (Chapter 2)
8. Ophthalmologist, optometrist, orthoptist, and optician
9. Quality of light and avoidance of glare (Chapter 9)
10. Vision and sitting posture
11. Protecting vision: daily dietary practices, sleep, avoidance of foreign objects in the eye, and effects of alcohol and tobacco on vision
12. Signs of possible visual difficulties (Chapter 2)
13. Corrective lenses: purposes, care, and types
14. Contact lenses
15. Quackery in products and services related to vision
16. National Society for the Prevention of Blindness

## Self-Preservation in the Event of a Tornado

Concept: Awareness of procedures for self-preservation in the event of a tornado helps victims to survive.

Area of health education—Safety Education

1. National Weather Service
    a. Local storm forecast centers
    b. Local stations and their functions coordinated with storm forecast centers
    c. Forecasting of possible tornadoes
    d. Notification of possible tornadoes
    e. Notification of tornadoes in progress
2. Tornadoes
    a. Occurrence
    b. Weather associated with tornadoes
    c. Types of funnel-shaped clouds
    d. Speed of travel and wind speed in its vortex
    e. Path of destruction
    f. Destructive force
3. Self-preservation procedures in schools
    a. Coordination of school procedures with community disaster plans
    b. Parental responsibilities
    c. School shelters and routes to them
    d. School practice signals and drills

e. Self-preservation techniques
f. Care of younger children
g. Fire protection
h. American Red Cross First Aid stations and personnel functions
i. Postdisaster procedures
4. Self-preservation procedures in homes
  a. Planning before disaster strikes
  b. Community signals
  c. Radio and television forecasts and notifications
  d. Turning off utilities
  e. Shelter area in home
  f. Care of young children, persons who are ill, and the elderly
5. Self-preservation procedures in cities and towns
6. Self-preservation procedures in industrial plants
7. Self-preservation procedures in open country

**Drug Abuse—** ...

Concept: H...
iological and p...
Area of he...
Narcotic Addi...
Alcoholic Bev...

1. Term...
  a. S...
  b. D...
  c. A...
  d. T...
  e. ...
  f. ...
2. De...
3. Ge...
4. Pa...
5. Ma...
  a.
  b.

  c.

    10) Dangers of marijuana abuse
6. LSD—(D-lysergic acid diethylamide tartrate 25)
  a. Jargon of the user
  b. Motivations of the user
  c. Chemistry
  d. Potency
  e. Amount needed
  f. Price
  g. How taken by user
  h. Physiological effects
  i. Psychological effects
  j. Significance of LSD state
  k. Dangers of LSD use
  l. Treatment of user
  m. Black-market sale
  n. Fallacies connected with LSD
7. Mescaline
  a. Extracted from peyote cactus
  b. Stimulant
  c. Physiological effects
  d. Psychological effects
8. Psilocybin
  a. *Psilocybe mexicana* mushroom
  b. Psychological effects
  ... STP (4-methyl-2,5-dimethoxy-a-phenethylamine)
  ... ncy
  ... gers
  ... (Dimethyltryptamine)
  ... (Diethyltryptamine)
  ... ion for prevention of drug

  ... unity response to drug abuse
  ... controls of drug abuse

... verages—Their Use, Nonuse
Each person has responsibilities
ivior and attitudes about alco-
ges whether he uses them or

health education—Drug Abuse, ddiction, Smoking, and Misuse Beverages
coholic beverages
Types of alcoholic beverages
  1) Fermented juices containing natural sugar
  2) Fermented malt beverages
  3) Distilled liquors
. Fermentation
. Distillation
. Percentage of alcohol, by volume, in "sweet" and "dry" wines

e. Percentage of alcohol, by volume, in beer and ale
f. Percentage of alcohol, by volume, in distilled liquors
g. "Proof" of liquor
2. Popular names of alcoholic beverages
3. Caloric content
4. Factors that influence effects of alcoholic beverages
   a. Body weight of user
   b. Amount of alcohol taken by the user
   c. Amount of non-alcoholic chemicals in alcoholic beverages
   d. Presence of food in stomach
   e. Rapidity of consumption
   f. Conditions affecting the emptying time of the stomach
5. Physiological effects upon the human body
   a. Absorption in the stomach
   b. Distribution of alcohol
   c. Oxidation rate
   d. Central nervous system
      1) Depressant
      2) Reaction time
   e. Habituation and dependency
   f. Digestive fluids
   g. Small blood vessels in the skin
   h. Nutritional deficiencies
   i. Kidneys, liver, cardiovascular system, water balance
   j. Intoxication
   k. Hangover
6. Social and economic effects
   a. Prevalence of use of alcoholic beverages
   b. Federal and state taxes
   c. Traffic accidents
   d. Costs to industry—loss of manpower, replacements, inefficiency, and training expenses
   e. Arrests for drunkenness
   f. Costs of fire protection
   g. Costs of automobile insurance
7. Reasons for use and nonuse
8. Drinking among young adults
9. Adult attitudes toward teenage drinking
10. Responsibilities of the young adult who decides to use alcoholic beverages
11. Responsibilities of the young adult who decides not to use alcoholic beverages

12. Impact of the use of alcoholic beverages
    a. Antialcohol bias
    b. Views on intoxication
    c. Viewpoints of religious groups
    d. Morality of use of alcoholic beverages
       1) Conflict of state laws
       2) Disagreement as to teaching about alcoholic beverages—their use, abuse, and nonuse—in secondary schools.
       3) Hostility and defiance of adolescents toward adult authority over use of alcoholic beverages
       4) Parental attitudes of use, abuse, and nonuse
       5) Beliefs that alcoholic beverages are the direct causes of racial strife, juvenile delinquency, civil disobedience, riots, poverty, divorce, and antisocial behavior of adults
13. Type of drinking practices
    a. Moderate drinking
    b. Social drinking
    c. Problem drinking
       1) Personal aspects
       2) Social aspects
14. Alcoholism
    a. Steps leading toward alcoholism
    b. Prevalence
    c. Signs of alcoholism
    d. Possible causes of alcoholism
       1) Physiological factors
       2) Psychological factors
       3) Sociological factors
    e. Treatment
    f. Rehabilitation
15. Prevention of the abuse of alcoholic beverages
16. National Council on Alcoholism

**Quackery**

Concept: Evaluation of quackery provides the individual with a wise selection of health services and products.
Area of health education—Consumer Health

1. Definition of quackery
2. Costs of quackery
3. Means of recognizing the quack
   a. Advertisements
   b. "Unique" treatments and cures

c. House-to-house "doctor"
d. "Expert" or "authority" on every disease, chronic health condition, illness, or injury
e. Claims of persecution by the American Medical Association, Food and Drug Administration, and National Institutes of Health
f. Mail-order practice
g. No consultation with licensed medical doctor
h. No contact with accredited and licensed hospitals
i. Lack of license in accredited health professions
j. Fees charged without evidence of usual clinical and laboratory tests
k. Distortion of statements from valid research by professional groups
l. Contact with customer: free series of lectures, books or pamphlets written by quack, free samples of products sold, testimonials and claims, products offered on money-back guarantee, special "clinics," and sales on radio and television
4. Types of persons buying products or services
5. Why quackery exists
6. Results of quackery: fraud, theft, and death
7. Cancer quackery
   a. Money spent each year
   b. "Cure-alls" sold
   c. Services offered
   d. Use of electrical machinery
   e. Results to cancer victim
   f. Actions taken to combat cancer quackery by official and nonofficial health and consumer agencies
8. Arthritis quackery
   a. Money spent each year
   b. Nostrums, gadgets, and "cure-alls" sold
   c. Services offered
   d. Period of remission occurring to arthritis victim used by quack
   e. Results to arthritis victim
   f. Actions taken to combat arthritis quackery by official and nonofficial health and consumer agencies

9. Nutrition quackery
   a. Money spent each year
   b. Myths and fallacies promoted
   c. Products sold
   d. Types of sales promotion
   e. Claims made for products sold
   f. Actions taken to combat nutrition quackery by official and nonofficial health and consumer agencies
10. Weight-reducing quackery
    a. Money spent each year
    b. Products sold
    c. Services offered: special massage, mechanical devices, diets, pills, etc.
    d. Results to consumer
    e. Actions taken to combat weight-reducing quackery by official and nonofficial health and consumer agencies
11. Mechanical quackery
12. Psychoquackery
13. Occult fads
14. Scientology
15. National Health Federation
16. Spinal adjustment specialists, herbalists, naturopaths
17. Beauty quackery
18. Sexology
19. Other forms of quackery: Cures for baldness, diabetes, hearing loss, visual difficulties, dental problems, alcoholism, kidney diseases, hernia, constipation, sexual impotency, hemorrhoids, epilepsy, cerebral palsy, and heart disease
20. Roles of the Food and Drug Administration, Federal Trade Commission, Department of Agriculture, Post Office Department, United States Public Health Service, state and local health departments, American Medical Association, American Dental Association, American Dietetic Association, National Better Business Bureau, Consumers' Union, National Dairy Council, American Cancer Society, Arthritis Foundation, and American Heart Association, etc., in combating quackery
21. Responsibilities of the consumer

**Cancers**

Concept: Detection of early warning signals of cancer reduces the death rate from cancers of the human body.

Area of health education—Prevention of Disease

1. Successful treatments and cures of cancer
2. Normal cell growth
   a. Cell division
   b. Cell differentiation
3. Abnormal cell growth
   a. Benign
      1) Collection of localized abnormal cell growths
      2) Varieties
   b. Malignant
      1) Abnormal cell growth no longer localized
      2) Dedifferentiation
      3) Malignant growth spreads
         a) Infiltration
         b) Metastasis
      4) Types
         a) Carcinoma
         b) Sarcoma
      5) Thirty common types of human cancers
4. Cancers of the skin
   a. Rate of cure
   b. Principal factor in development
   c. Precancerous skin condition
      1) Keratosis
      2) Leukoplakia
   d. Skin malignancies
      1) Basal cell cancer
      2) Squamous cell cancer
      3) Malignant melanoma
      4) Treatment
5. Cancers of the mouth and respiratory system
   a. Mouth
      1) Contributing factors
      2) Leukoplakia
      3) Treatment
   b. Larynx
      1) Malignant tumor
      2) Keratosis
      3) Signs
      4) Treatment
   c. Lungs
      1) Cigarette smoking
      2) Primary type
      3) Secondary type
      4) Signs
      5) Detection
      6) Treatment

6. Cancer of the stomach
   a. Signs
   b. Detection
   c. Treatment
7. Cancers of the colon and rectum
   a. Polyps
   b. Signs
   c. Hemorrhoids
   d. Detection
   e. Treatment
8. Cancer of the breast
   a. Self-examination
   b. Annual medical examination
   c. Signs
   d. Treatment
9. Cancer of the uterus
   a. Importance of the "Pap" test
   b. Signs
   c. Detection
   d. Treatment
10. Cancer of the bladder
    a. Exposure to aniline dyes and cigarette smoking as agents
    b. Signs
    c. Treatment
11. Cancer of the prostate
    a. Benign tumors
    b. Signs
    c. Treatment
12. Cancers of the bone
    a. Benign tumors
    b. Malignant tumors
       1) Primary
       2) Secondary
    c. Signs
    d. Treatment
13. Leukemia
    a. Cancers of blood-forming tissues
    b. Acute leukemia
       1) Lymphocytic leukemia
       2) Myelocytic leukemia
       3) Signs of acute leukemia
       4) Treatment
    c. Chronic leukemia
       1) Lymphocytic leukemia
       2) Myelocytic leukemia
       3) Signs of chronic leukemia
       4) Treatment
14. Lymphoma
    a. Abnormal growth of cells making up the lymphoid tissue
    b. Signs
    c. Treatment
15. Seven warning signals of cancer
16. Responsibilities in cancer detection

17. American Cancer Society
18. National Cancer Institute

# UNITS OF HEALTH EDUCATION OUTLINED WITH DETAILED INFORMATION

## Rabies

Concept: Immunization of domestic animals against rabies reduces the incidence of rabies.

Area of health education Community Health Problems

1. Animals acquiring rabies
   a. Domestic animals: dogs, cats, pigs, and horses
   b. Rats and mice can be infected
   c. Wildlife: skunks, squirrels, rabbits, coyotes, bobcats, foxes, wolves, and raccoons
   d. Insectivorous rabid bats transmit rabies virus by biting and by contaminating the air in bat caves
      1) Rabies virus has been found in the kidneys of Mexican free-tailed bats and may be transmitted by urine
      2) Fallen bat should not be picked up with the hands; it should be brushed onto a shovel for disposal
2. Cause is a virus
   a. Virus is found in saliva of rabid animal
   b. Rabies virus is passed into an animal or human by a puncture wound made by the rabid animal's biting
   c. Virus cannot enter the skin unless there is a break in the skin
3. Bites on head, face, and neck are more dangerous than on arms and legs. Bites on exposed skin are more dangerous than bites through clothing
4. Virus affects central nervous system
5. Incubation period is three to six weeks
   a. In dogs, incubation period is shorter
   b. Cattle have longer incubation period
6. Signs in man
   a. Pain, irritation, and numbness occur at the bite area on skin
   b. Voice is husky
   c. Depression, irritability, and hypersensitivity are apparent
   d. Swallowing becomes difficult
   e. Saliva may appear on lips
   f. Fever
   g. Paralysis occurs in muscles of tongue and throat
   h. Bowel and bladder control is lost
   i. Death comes with heart failure or respiratory paralysis
7. Signs in animals
   a. Furious rabies
      1) Animal is easily irritated but may be more affectionate
      2) Animal may bite savagely when picked up
      3) Animal becomes excitable and restless
      4) Animal eats straw and sticks and may chew on wire cracking its teeth
      5) Animal's eye become glazed and wide open
      6) Animal has wobbly gait when paralysis starts to develop, ending with animal not able to stand
      7) Animal lives several days (up to 11 days), then dies
   b. Dumb rabies
      1) Animal is sad and sleepy and hides away by itself
      2) Paralysis occurs to the animal's tongue and throat muscles
      3) Saliva appears at sides and front of animal's mouth
      4) Animal submerges its head in water in order to quench thirst
      5) Animal seldom bites
      6) Animal lives for three days, then dies
   c. Rabid animal may not show any signs of furious or dumb rabies, then dies
8. Rabid animal bites man
   a. Wound should be cleansed thoroughly with soap and water and then bandaged
   b. Animal must be apprehended and observed for ten days. Positive evidence of rabies virus can be obtained by a laboratory ex-

amination of the nerve cells of the animal's brain

  c. Person bitten should go immediately to his family physician

    1) Rabies hyperimmune serum is infiltrated under bite wound by physician

    2) At first evidence of rabies in animal, the physician starts the full course of the vaccine

    3) If person has bites in the head, face, and neck, rabies hyperimmune serum is given followed by full course of vaccine

  9. Rabies vaccine

    a. Vaccine is injected under skin of abdomen for 14 consecutive days

    b. If person has multiple or severe bites, injections of vaccine are given for 21 or more days

  10. Pre-exposure rabies vaccine for man

    a. Farmers, veterinarians, operators of kennels, and other animal handlers can receive vaccine before bite

    b. Three injections will immunize the person

  11. Animals vaccinated against rabies

    a. Local ordinances, requiring yearly vaccine to protect animals, should be enforced

    b. Domestic animals should be protected

  12. If signs of rabies are observed in an animal, the police or local health department should be notified

## Menstrual Hygiene

Concept: Acceptance of responsibilities during menstruation is vital in becoming a woman.

Area of health education—Family Life and Sex Education

  1. Female reproductive organs

    a. External genitalia are the two pairs of labia, clitoris, mons pubis, vestibule, and hymen

    1) The labia (lips) surround the opening of the vagina. There is an outer and larger pair of labia, as well as an inner pair

    2) The clitoris is found above the opening of the urethra, at the junction of the outer labia; it is about the size of a pea

    3) The mons pubis is a fleshy prominence above the outer labia

    4) The vestibule is the space between the inner labia, into which the vagina opens

    5) The hymen is a membrane partially covering the opening of the vagina

    b. Internal organs

    1) The ovaries are the two glands, located in the lower part of the abdomen protected by the pelvis, that produce hormones and ova or egg cells

    2) The fallopian tubes are narrow tubelike passageways extending from the top of the uterus to each ovary

    a) Fallopian tubes have numerous fingerlike projections flaring open near each ovary

    b) The passageways opposite the fingerlike projections enter the right and left side of the uterus

    3) The uterus is a muscular, hollow, pear-shaped organ that contains the fetus of a pregnant woman

    a) The upper portion of the uterus is the corpus

    b) The necklike portion of the uterus extending into the vagina is the cervix

    c) The endometrium, the inner lining of the uterus, is heavily supplied with blood vessels

    4) The vagina is a short, muscular canal leading to the external genitalia. The walls of the vagina contain Bartholin's glands and mucus-producing glands

  2. Menstrual cycle

    a. Three hormones from the anterior pituitary gland and two hormones from the ovaries are necessary for the menstrual cycle

1) Estrogen and progesterone are the ovarian hormones
2) Increased production of hormones from the pituitary gland and maturation of the ovaries are the beginning of sexual maturity in the girl

b. Menarche is the first menstrual period

c. Menopause is the cessation of menstruation caused by the gradual reduction of estrogens to almost nothing. Ovaries cease to produce and expel ova

d. One ovum will mature during each menstrual cycle. About 400 mature ova will be produced during the woman's reproductive years

e. Ovulation is the ejection of the mature ovum from the ovary
   1) Ovum is expelled into the abdominal cavity
   2) Fingerlike projections of fallopian tube pick up the ovum
   3) Endometrium thickens in preparation for receiving the ovum

f. Ovum travels along the fallopian tube and into the uterus

g. Menstruation is the monthly flow of blood from the vagina
   1) Ovum disintegrates
   2) Endometrium is shed and passes from the uterus into the vagina
   3) Menstruation occurs every 28 to 30 days
      a) Between 1.5 and 5 ounces of blood leave the body
      b) Flow of blood may last from three to seven days

h. Purpose of menstruation is to prepare the uterus in the event that the ovum is fertilized
   1) Ovum disintegrates if ovum is not fertilized
   2) Endometrium is shed if ovum is not fertilized
   3) Each month another ovum matures and the endometrium thickens in the event that the ovum may be fertilized

3. Menstrual hygiene
a. During menstruation, the young woman has specific responsibilities
   1) Organs of menstruation should be free of infection and injury
   2) Dates of each period of menstruation should be kept on a calendar
   3) Protection to avoid soiling clothing
      a) External protection can be provided by the sanitary napkin made of absorbent, soft, cellucotton wadding
      b) Internal protection can be provided by the tampon of soft surgical cotton inserted into the vagina
   4) To dispose of the used sanitary napkin or tampon it should be wrapped in toilet tissue and placed in a waste container
   5) Daily shower and bath can be taken during menstruation
   6) Routine physical activities can be continued during menstruation, very strenuous activities for a long period of time should be avoided
   7) Additional sleep and rest are needed
   8) Extreme irregularities before, during, or after menstruation should be discussed with the family physician
      a) Dysmenorrhea (painful) menstruation) which creates incapacity to work needs the care of the physician
      b) Amenorrhea (absence of menstruation) should be called to the attention of the physician
   9) Breast self-examination should be completed after each menstrual period
   10) The numerous fallacies about menstruation and menstrual hygiene need to be disproved

The outlines of the representative units in this chapter have been presented to show the possible scope of information.

## SUGGESTED HEALTH EDUCATION UNITS, GRADES K-12

| Area | ELEMENTARY SCHOOL K-Primary | ELEMENTARY SCHOOL Intermediate | MIDDLE OR JUNIOR HIGH SCHOOL Grade 7 | MIDDLE OR JUNIOR HIGH SCHOOL Grade 9 | SENIOR HIGH SCHOOL Grade 11 |
|---|---|---|---|---|---|
| 1. CARE OF ALL PARTS OF THE HUMAN BODY | Cleanliness<br>Six-year molar<br>Types and care of the teeth<br>Sleep and rest<br>Sitting and standing posture<br>Clothes for daily weather and special activities | Walking, lying, and working posture<br>Care of the feet<br>Dental caries<br>Malocclusion<br>Relaxation and fatigue<br>Pimples, boils, and blackheads<br>Care of the hair<br>Care of the nails<br>Eye injuries, infections, and defects<br>Ear injuries, infections, and defects | Acceptable or poor posture<br>Good grooming | Acne, impetigo, and other skin diseases<br>Periodontal diseases<br>Health responsibilities | Improvement of personal health<br>Adult dental health problems<br>Fluoridation<br>Family health |
| 2. PREVENTION OF DISEASES | Colds<br>Spread and prevention of diseases<br>Vaccinations<br>Sore throats and what they mean | Causative agents of diseases<br>Measles<br>Chicken pox and mumps<br>Whooping cough and tetanus<br>Tuberculin tests<br>Cancer in children | Influenza and pneumonia<br>Tuberculosis<br>Rheumatic fever | Chronic bronchitis and smoking<br>Syphilis and gonorrhea<br>Heart disease | Infectious mononucleosis and infectious hepatitis<br>Cancers<br>Venereal diseases |
| 3. CHRONIC HEALTH CONDITIONS | Health problems of some friends or classmates | Common chronic health conditions | Diabetes | Epilepsy<br>Cerebral palsy | Multiple sclerosis, muscular dystrophy, cystic fibrosis, and myasthenia gravis<br>Coronary thrombosis and other conditions |

| | | | Junior American Red Cross First Aid | Standard American Red Cross First Aid | Advanced American Red Cross First Aid |
|---|---|---|---|---|---|
| 4. AMERICAN RED CROSS FIRST AID | Nosebleeds First aid for simple emergencies | Wounds Shock Poisonous snakes Insect bites Artificial respiration Household poisoning First-aid kits | | | |
| 5. SAFETY EDUCATION | Pedestrian School School bus Fire drills at school Playground | Bicycle Gun Vacation Camping Common safety procedures for boating, surfing, and water skiing Home fire prevention Accidents in the home | Natural disasters Recreation School Motorcycle and home pool | Community disasters Home Farm and ranch Note: Driver Education taught as separate course | Man-made national disasters Occupational |
| 6. MENTAL HEALTH | Adjustment to school life Control of emotions Respect for others Member of a group Responsibilities at school Courtesy and thoughtfulness Cooperation and sharing | Friends and getting along with others Honesty Rights and property of others Self-control and self-discipline Tolerance Responsibilities at home Daily time schedules Courage | Budgeting daily time | Adolescent emotional health problems Sources of assistance for emotional health problems | Mental illness Suicide Agencies and services for the mentally ill |
| 7. NUTRITION | Essential Four Food Groups Table etiquette School noonday meals | Calories and weight Menu planning Breakfast Nutrients | Selection of foods for daily dietary needs Malnutrition Food fallacies | Obesity and weight control Food allergies | Nutrition as related to treatment of diseases and alcoholism and to pregnancy |

SUGGESTED HEALTH EDUCATION UNITS, GRADES K-12—*Continued*

| Area | ELEMENTARY SCHOOL K-Primary | ELEMENTARY SCHOOL Intermediate | MIDDLE OR JUNIOR HIGH SCHOOL Grade 7 | MIDDLE OR JUNIOR HIGH SCHOOL Grade 9 | SENIOR HIGH SCHOOL Grade 11 |
|---|---|---|---|---|---|
| 7. NUTRITION— *Continued* | Well-balanced meals Fruits and vege- tables | Nutritional defi- ciencies Milk and milk products Coffee, tea, and sweetened soft drinks | | | Sanitation in meal preparation Controversial nutri- tion topics Crash diets and food fads |
| 8. COMMUNITY HEALTH PROBLEMS | Personnel promot- ing healthful community Purified drinking water | Water and water- borne diseases Sewage treatment Solid wastes Rabies Local health depart- ment | Pollution of water supplies Insect-borne dis- eases | Rodents and rat- borne diseases Environmental sani- tation | Air pollution Food-, meat-, and milk-borne dis- eases and meth- ods of control Radiation control State health depart- ments and United States Public Health Service Nonofficial health agencies |
| 9. CONSUMER HEALTH | Labels on foods, drugs, and medi- cines | Self-medication and nostrums Prescription and over-the-counter drugs | Health fads and cults Health careers Official health agencies | Health fallacies Quackery Advertising of health products Consumer protec- tion agencies | Health insurance Selection of a physi- cian, dentist, and hospital Wise purchasing of health products |

| | | | | |
|---|---|---|---|---|
| **10. ADULT HEALTH PROBLEMS** | | | Exercise and health | Arthritis<br>Glaucoma | Medical examination and immunizations<br>Obesity and exercise |
| **11. FAMILY LIFE AND SEX EDUCATION** | New brothers and sisters<br>Reproduction in pets<br>Reproduction in common plants | Social etiquette<br>Menstrual hygiene for girls<br>Personal hygiene for boys<br>The family | Adolescent and parents<br>Boy-girl relations | Boy to young man<br>Dating | Engagement<br>Marriage<br>Pregnancy and birth of baby<br>Newly wedded couples<br>Family planning<br>Problems in sexual behaviors |
| **12. DRUG ABUSE, NARCOTIC ADDICTION, SMOKING, AND MISUSE OF ALCOHOLIC BEVERAGES** | | Narcotics, stimulants, and depressants<br>"Sniffing" and misuse of other agents | To smoke or not to smoke<br>Alcoholism<br>Marijuana<br>"Uppers" and "Downers" | "Hard" narcotics<br>Bromides and tranquilizers | Hallucinogens<br>Problems of drug abuse<br>Alcoholic beverages and alcoholism |
| **13. INTERNATIONAL HEALTH** | | | | Health problems of Canada and Central and South America | Malaria<br>International health problems<br>Health in space travel<br>Comprehensive health planning |

## References for Further Study

American Cancer Society: *'71 Cancer Facts and Figures*. New York: The Society, 1970.

American Dental Association: *Answers to Criticism of Fluoridation*. Chicago: The Association, 1964.

Allen, H. F.: *Make Sure Your Child Has Two Good Eyes*. New York: National Society for the Prevention of Blindness, 1968.

American Medical Association: *Facts on Quacks: What You Should Know About Quackery*. Chicago: The Association, 1967.

American Public Health Association: *Control of Communicable Diseases in Man*. 11th ed. New York: The Association, 1970.

American School Health Association and Pharmaceutical Manufacturers Association: *Teaching About Drugs: A Curriculum Guide*. Kent, Ohio: American School Health Association, 1970.

Anderson, G., Arnstein, M., and Lester, M.: *Communicable Disease Control*. 4th ed. New York: The Macmillan Company, 1962.

Berland, T., and Seyler, A.: *Your Children's Teeth*. New York: Meredith Press, 1968.

Better Business Bureau: *Facts You Should Know About Health Quackery*. Boston: The Bureau, 1967.

Block, M.: *Alcohol and Alcoholism*. Belmont, Calif.: Wadsworth Publishing Company, 1970.

Burt, J., and Brower, L.: *Education for Sexuality: Comcepts and Programs for Teaching*. Philadelphia: W. B. Saunders Company, 1970.

California State Department of Education: *Drug Abuse: A Source Book and Guide for Teachers*. Sacramento: The Department, 1967.

Carroll, C.: *Alcohol: Use, Nonuse, and Abuse*. Dubuque, Iowa: Wm. C. Brown, 1970.

Cohen, S.: *The Drug Dilemma*. New York: McGraw-Hill Book Company, 1969.

Diehl, H.: *Tobacco and Your Health: The Smoking Controversy*. New York: McGraw-Hill Book Company, 1969.

*Drug Abuse: Escape To Nowhere*. rev. ed. Washington, D.C.: American Association for Health, Physical Education and Recreation, 1969.

Editors of Consumer Reports: *The Medicine Show*. rev. ed. Mount Vernon, N.Y.: Consumers Union, 1963.

Florio, A. E., and Stafford, G.: *Safety Education*. 3rd ed. New York: McGraw-Hill Book Company, 1969.

Haag, J. H.: *Teacher's Edition of Focusing on Health (High School)* and *Growing into Womanhood* and *into Manhood*. Austin, Texas: The Steck-Vaughn Company, 1972.

Kilander, H. F.: *Sex Education in the Schools*. New York: The Macmillan Company, 1970.

Magnuson, W., and Carper, J.: *The Dark Side of the Marketplace*. Englewood Cliffs, N.J.: Prentice-Hall, Inc., 1968.

National Society for the Prevention of Blindness: *Your Eyes: For a Life Time of Sight*. New York: The Society, 1968.

Sartwell, P.: *Maxcy-Rosenau Preventive Medicine and Public Health*. 9th ed. New York: Appleton-Century-Crofts, 1965.

Schulz, E., and Williams, S.: *Family Life and Sex Education: Curriculum and Instruction*. New York: Harcourt, Brace and World, Inc., 1969.

Shimkin, M.: *Science and Cancer*. rev. ed. Public Health Service Publication #1162, 1969.

Smith, R.: *At Your Risk: The Case Against Chiropractic*. New York: Pocket Books, 1969.

Stack, H., and Elkow, J. D.: *Education for Safe Living*. 4th ed. Englewood Cliffs, N.J.: Prentice-Hall, Inc., 1966.

Stoll, F., and Catherman, J.: *Dental Health Education*. 4th ed. Philadelphia: Lea & Febiger, 1972.

Top, F.: *Communicable and Infectious Diseases*. 6th ed. St. Louis: The C. V. Mosby Company, 1968.

United States Public Health Service: *The Health Consequences of Smoking*. 1971 Supplement. 1971.

————: *Research Explores Nutrition and Dental Health*. 1969.

# Chapter 15

# CONTENT WITHIN LESSONS OR DIVISIONS OF UNITS

## AN INCIDENT

Beginning teachers have asked their principals why the teachers must make lesson plans or even decide what to teach in health education. The teachers have reported that school nurses plan to teach dental health. A policeman has indicated that he will talk to students on safety and drug abuse. A representative from the local unit of the American Cancer Society will present some films on cancer. A member of the local health department has invited all students to the community's well-child clinic, water purification plant, and sewage treatment plant. A college professor opposed to sex education will give a series of lectures on the human reproductive system. A member of the counseling and guidance services will speak about mental health. The principal has informed the beginning teachers that the visitors to the classes only supplement the lesson and that the teachers need to prepare lesson plans.

Teachers who have units of health education content in outline form (with or without detailed information) can easily decide how many lessons shall be in each unit. The lessons are sections or divisions of the unit.

The objectives of the unit are the outcomes which the students should achieve. The objectives are written for the student. In some cases, the students might decide what the objectives should be. The objectives should improve the student's physical and mental health status, practices, attitudes, interests, and knowledge.

The teacher should indicate which lessons are in the unit. The lesson title can be written on the chalkboard, and students can decide what content should be found within the lesson. The first lesson always includes an introduction to the unit, and the last lesson summarizes the highlights of the unit.

The information within the unit is the content or subject matter. The content of each lesson is divided into three parts. The first part of each lesson is the *Review or Introduction*. Each lesson of a unit, except the first, begins with a summation of the past lesson or *Review*. In the first lesson of the unit, the *Introduction* takes the place of the *Review*. The second part of each lesson is the *New Content*, and the third part is the *Conclusion*. The main points of the *New Content* are emphasized in the *Conclusion*.

The methods are "how" the lesson is done. These methods include demonstration, question and answer, group discussion, panel, debate, and critical incident along with other methods. Methods will be explained in the next chapter. In some curriculum guides, methods are labeled "Learning Activities."

The materials of instruction are objects used by the teacher, pupils, or the teacher and pupils at the same time. In health education, these materials may be a drug identification kit, manikin, graphs, x-ray viewer and x-rays, reaction-time testing devices, prescription and over-the-counter drugs, and samples of food additives among the numerous materials of instruction. The next chapter will list the many materials of instruction available for health education. In some curriculum guides, materials of instruction are omitted so that the teacher relies on films as the only materials of instruction.

The first of the sample lessons is the fourth lesson of the unit "Keep Those New Teeth" for children who have their six-year molars and new permanent central incisors. This lesson will have a unit title; objectives of the unit; lessons of the unit; content divided into review, new content, and conclusion; methods; materials of instruction; and evaluation. Teacher's references will be given.

Name of the teacher
Age of student—7 or 8 years
Area of health education—Care of All Parts of the Human Body

Unit Title—Keep Those New Teeth
Objectives of the Unit
1. To brush my teeth correctly after eating
2. To understand the importance of my teeth
3. To appreciate the services of my family dentist
4. To choose foods which help my teeth
Lessons of the Unit
1. My teeth
2. My friend—the dentist
3. Foods helping my teeth
4. Tooth brushing after eating
5. Why I take care of my teeth

## TOOTH BRUSHING AFTER EATING

| Content | Methods | Materials of Instruction |
|---|---|---|
| *Review* <br> 1. Foods helping my teeth <br>  a. Which fruits help my teeth? <br>  b. How much milk should I have each day? <br><br>  c. Which vegetables should I eat? <br>  d. Which type of bread helps my teeth? <br> 2. Foods for breakfast <br><br> 3. Foods for lunch <br> 4. Foods for dinner | Question and answer <br> Children select fruits, milk, vegetables, and so forth, from assortment of food samples <br><br><br><br><br> Children select one food which they might have at breakfast, lunch, and dinner | Oranges, grapefruit, cantaloupe, apricots, raisins, peaches, etc. <br> Three or four cups of whole milk <br> Peppers, spinach, tomatoes, carrots <br> Whole wheat bread <br><br> Egg or meat <br> Whole-grain cereals <br> Cheese <br> Green, leafy vegetables <br> Cauliflower <br> Cabbage |
| *New Content* <br> A. Tooth brushing of upper and lower sets of teeth | 1. Teacher demonstration <br>  a. Preparation of toothbrush <br><br> 2. Start with outside surface of right upper six-year molar; proceed to left upper six-year molar <br> 3. Brush inside surface of right upper six-year molar; proceed to left upper six-year molar <br> 4. Pupils practice tooth brushing following second teacher demonstration of #2 and #3 <br> B. Pupils practice tooth brushing without teacher demonstration <br> C. Teacher demonstration <br> 1. Start with outside surface of right lower six-year | Model of upper and lower teeth <br> Toothbrush <br><br><br><br><br><br><br><br><br> Pupils' toothbrushes <br> Hand mirror <br> Paper towels for each desk |

## TOOTH BRUSHING AFTER EATING

| Content | Methods | Materials of Instruction |
|---|---|---|
| | molar; proceed to left lower six-year molar<br>2. Brush inside surface of right lower six-year molar; proceed to left lower six-year molar<br>3. Pupils practice tooth brushing following second teacher demonstration of C. #1 and #2<br>D. Pupils attempt tooth brushing without any teacher demonstration while teacher moves around class correcting pupils<br>E. Pupils alternate the brushing of the upper and lower sets of teeth<br>F. Teachers and pupils clean toothbrushes, place toothbrushes in containers, place mirrors in storage trays, and throw away paper towels | Pupils' toothbrushes |
| B. Tooth brushing after midmorning snack and noonday school meal | Demonstration | |
| *Conclusion*<br>A. Pupils practice tooth brushing at home after meals | Demonstration | |
| B. Pupils asked to give reasons for taking care of their teeth, next lesson | Group discussion | |

*Evaluation*

1. After midmorning snack and noonday meals, do children brush their teeth as they practiced in this lesson?
2. Has there been a reduction in dental caries among these children reported by parents at parent-teacher conferences?
3. Has there been a reduction in dental injuries among these children?
4. Has there been omission of candies and sweetened soft drinks in the children's daily diets?
5. Have the children developed a strong desire to maintain cleanliness of their mouths?
6. Do the children realize that dental caries can mean loss of their permanent teeth?

*Teacher References*

1. American Dental Association: *Teeth, Health, and Appearance.* 6th ed. Chicago: The Association, 1966.
2. Berland, T., and Seyler, A. E.: *Your Children's Teeth.* New York: Meredith Press, 1968.
3. Stoll, F., and Catherman, J.: *Dental Health Education.* 4th ed. Philadelphia: Lea & Febiger, 1972.
4. Division of Dental Health, Texas State Department of Health: *Texas Teachers' Handbook on Dental Health Education, Grades 1-6.* Austin: The Department, 1970.
5. United States Public Health Service: *Healthy Teeth.* Washington, D.C.: Government Printing Office, #405, 1966.

The second of these sample lessons is the second lesson of the unit "Drug Abuse" presented to fifth graders.

Name of teacher

Age of student—11 or 12 years

Area of health education—Drug Abuse, Narcotic Addiction, Smoking, and Misuse of Alcoholic Beverages

Unit Title—Drug Abuse

Objectives of the Unit

1. To recognize some dangerous drugs, narcotics, and hallucinogens

2. To be familiar with some signs of behavior of a boy or girl who has been "sniffing" or smoking "pot"

3. To know what to do if a friend has been "sniffing" or smoking "pot"

4. To take proper action if an adult or teenager offers me "pot"

Lessons of the Unit

1. Dangerous drugs, narcotics, and hallucinogens

2. "Sniffing" and "pot"

3. Ways to combat drug abuse

## "SNIFFING" AND "POT"

| Content | Methods | Materials of Instruction |
|---|---|---|
| *Review* | | |
| 1. Classification and characteristics of drugs, narcotics, and hallucinogens | Question and answer | Drug identification kit |
|   a. Dangerous drugs | | Chalkboard |
|     1) Amphetamines | | |
|     2) Barbiturates | | |
|   b. Narcotics | | |
|     1) Opium | | |
|        Morphine | | |
|        Heroin | | |
|   c. Hallucinogens | | |
|     1) Marijuana | | |
|     2) LSD | | |
| 2. Drug users' jargon | | Drug identification kit |
|   a. Amphetamines | | |
|     1) Crystals | | |
|     2) Bennies | | |
|     3) Dexies | | |
|   b. Barbiturates | Conceptual approach 3M Co., Sub-concept: "Discussing Why Certain Mood- and Behavior-Modifying Substances Are Used Rather Commonly and Others Only Under Special Circumstances," #4794, Level 2, 1968 | |
|     1) Yellowjackets | | |
|     2) Reds, red birds | | |
|     3) Blue heavens | | |
|   c. Heroin | | Transparencies |
|     1) Smack | | |
|     2) H | | |
|     3) Horse | | |
|   d. Marijuana | | |
|     1) Weed | | |
|     2) Joint | | |
|     3) Grass | | |
|   e. LSD | | |
|     1) Acid | | |
|     2) Trip | | |
|     3) Cube | | |
| *New Content* | | |
| 1. "Sniffing" | Panel of junior high school students | Gasoline |
|   a. Inhalants sniffed | | Paint thinner |
|   b. How inhaled | | |
|   c. Immediate effects after several long "drags" | Roleplaying by panel | |
|   d. Case histories of sniffers | | |

## "SNIFFING" AND "POT"

| Content | Methods | Materials of Instruction |
|---|---|---|
| 2. "Pot"<br>  a. How to recognize a "joint"<br>  b. How obtained<br>  c. Cost<br>  d. How smoked<br>  e. Immediate effects<br>3. Vocabulary list:<br>  marijuana<br>  cannabis<br>  inhalant<br>  sniffing<br>  hallucinogen<br>  depressant<br>  stimulant<br>*Conclusion*<br>1. Panel is asked questions by class<br>2. Incidents of "sniffing" and smoking "pot"<br>  a. Incidents recalled<br>  b. Recognition of signs of "sniffing" and smoking "pot"<br>  c. Procedures to be taken | Panel of four students from junior high school<br><br><br><br>Roleplaying by panel<br><br><br><br><br><br><br><br><br><br><br>Critical incident technique | Drug identification kit<br>Photographs of "joint"<br>Photographs of *Cannabis sativa* |

*Evaluation*

1. Do the class members know what substances are used in "sniffing"?
2. Are the class members able to tell if one of their friends has been "sniffing"?
3. Can the class members recognize a "joint" when compared to a cigarette of tobacco?
4. Are the class members able to tell how they could distinguish the odor of "pot" when smoked?
5. Is there evidence that the class members reject the use of inhalants and "pot"?

*Teacher References*

1. American School Health Association and Pharmaceutical Manufacturers Association: *Teaching About Drugs—A Curriculum Guide, K-12.* Kent, Ohio: American School Health Association, 1970.
2. California State Department of Education: *Drug Abuse—A Source Book and Guide for Teachers.* Sacramento: The Department, 1967.
3. Einstein, S.: *The Use and Misuse of Drugs: A Social Dilemma.* Belmont, Calif.: Wadsworth Publishing Company, Inc., 1970.
4. Kaplan, R.: *Drug Abuse: Perspectives on Drugs.* Dubuque, Iowa: William C. Brown Company, 1970.
5. Michigan Department of Education: *A Teacher Resource Guide for Drug Use and Abuse for Michigan's Schools.* Lansing: The Department, 1970.

The third of these sample lessons is the second lesson of a four-lesson unit, "To Smoke or Not To Smoke," presented to students in the sixth grade.

Name of teacher

Age of students—12 or 13 years

Area of health education—Drug Abuse, Narcotic Addiction, Smoking, and Misuse of Alcoholic Beverages

Unit Title—To Smoke or Not To Smoke

Objectives of the Unit

1. To be aware of some of the effects of smoking on the human body
2. To develop critical attitudes which influence the decision not to smoke

3. To take action that discourages parents from smoking

Lessons of the Unit
1. Cigarettes (plain or filtered), cigars, and pipe tobacco
2. Case against tobacco
3. Advertisements of cigarettes, cigars, and pipe tobacco
4. Smoking and effects on athletes

## CASE AGAINST TOBACCO

| Content | Methods | Materials of Instruction |
|---|---|---|
| *Review* | | |
| 1. What cigarettes have filters? | Questions read by designated students; questions were submitted at the close of the last lesson by students | Question box |
| 2. How much money is spent on tobacco each year? | | |
| 3. Why do people smoke? | | |
| 4. Does smoking increase one's popularity? | | |
| 5. Why does tobacco stain the fingers? | | |
| 6. How many people smoke pipes and cigars? | | |
| 7. Are there cigarettes with low amounts of nicotine? | | |
| 8. What is smokers' cough? | | |
| 9. Does smoking affect endurance? | | |
| 10. How much nicotine and tar are found in popular brands of cigarettes? | | |
| *New Content* | | |
| 1. Classification of students' questions: | Classification suggested by students | Chalkboard |
|   a. Facts concerning sales, brands, and tar and nicotine content | | |
|   b. Effects of smoking physiologically, economically, and socially | | |
| 2. Nicotine and tar content by brand and type of cigarettes | Report given by a student | "Tar and Nicotine Content of Cigarettes, National Clearinghouse for Smoking and Health |
| 3. Reasons why teenagers object to smoking cigarettes | Class discussion | Chalkboard |
| 4. Effects of cigarette smoking upon human body | Conceptual approach, 3M Co., Sub-Concept: "Comparing Potential Social and Psychological Values of Smoking with the Possible Detrimental Effects," #4892, Level 3, 1968 | Pamphlets: "What To Tell Your Parents About Smoking," American Heart Association; |
|   a. Sinusitis | | "100,000 Doctors Have Quit Smoking Cigarettes," American Cancer Society, 1969; |
|   b. Smoker's cough | | "Smoking and Illness," Public Health Service Publication #1662, 1969 |
|   c. Spitting of mucus | | |
|   d. Respiratory infections | | |
|   e. Diminished athletic performance | | |
| 5. Reasons why adults smoke | Report by four students | |
| 6. Vocabulary list: | | Transparencies, 3M Co. |
|   nicotine | | |
|   tar | | |
|   mucus | | |
|   respiratory | | |
|   sinusitis | | |

## CASE AGAINST TOBACCO

| Content | Methods | Materials of Instruction |
|---|---|---|
| *Conclusion:* | | |
| 1. Assignment: | | |
| a. Red team surveys 25 pupils in middle or junior high school and classifies them as non-smokers and smokers and tells what brands the smokers use. | Survey | Questionnaire |
| b. White team surveys 25 adults and classifies them as nonsmokers and smokers and tells what brands the smokers use. | Survey | Questionnaire |
| 2. Each student is to bring two advertisements for cigarettes, cigars, and pipe tobacco. | | Newspapers Magazines |

*Evaluation*

1. Do the students look critically at the nicotine and tar content by brand and type of cigarette?
2. Are the reasons why teenagers object to smoking related to their habits of healthful living?
3. Is there evidence that some of the students have tried to get their parents to quit smoking?
4. Are the effects of cigarette smoking upon the human body of importance to the students?
5. Is there a correlation between scholastic achievement or athletic performance and the degree of students' objections to smoking?

*Teacher References*

1. American Cancer Society: *Helping People To Stop Smoking Cigarettes.* New York: The Society, 1968.
2. Diehl, H. S.: *Tobacco and Your Health: The Smoking Controversy.* New York: McGraw-Hill Book Company, 1969.
3. National Interagency Council on Smoking and Health: *World Conference on Smoking and Health: A Sum-*

*mary of the Proceedings.* Arlington, Va.: The Council, 1967.
4. United States Public Health Service: *Smoking and Health Experiments, Demonstrations, and Exhibits* (1968); and *Health Consequences of Smoking* (1971 Supplement).

The fourth of these lessons is the third lesson of a three-lesson unit, "Purified or Polluted Water," presented to eighth graders.

Name of teacher
Age of students—14 or 15 years
Area of health education—Community Health Problems
Unit Title—Purified or Polluted Water
Objectives of the Unit
1. To be aware of the extent of water pollution
2. To avoid polluted water
3. To take action in solving the community's water pollution problem
4. To familiarize others with the necessity of purified water
Lessons of the Unit
1. Water pollution
2. Diseases resulting from polluted water
3. Purification of community water supplies

## PURIFICATION OF COMMUNITY WATER SUPPLIES

| Content | Methods | Materials of Instruction |
|---|---|---|
| *Review*<br>1. Diseases resulting from polluted water<br>  a. Typhoid fever<br>  b. Amebic dysentery<br>  c. Bacillary dysentery<br>  d. Diarrhea<br>  e. Hookworm disease | Question and answer<br>Class discussion | Poster illustrating five diseases |
| 2. Characteristics of diseases resulting from polluted water<br>  a. Causative agent<br>  b. Signs<br>  c. Transmission<br>  d. Effects<br>  e. Treatment<br>  f. Immunization, if available | Student committee reviews characteristics | Poster illustrating characteristics of each disease |
| *New Content*<br>1. Methods of water purification for a community<br>  a. Aeration<br>  b. Sedimentation<br>  c. Filtration<br>  d. Coagulation<br>  e. Disinfection | Student committee explains exhibit<br><br>Experiments to illustrate sedimentation and filtration | Exhibit to show how a water purification plant operates<br>Laboratory equipment |
| 2. Sanitary analysis of a sample of water<br>  a. Physical tests<br>  b. Chemical examination<br>  c. Microscopic examination<br>  d. Bacteriological examina- | Invited speaker: Sanitary Engineer employed by the city health department<br><br>Experiments done to show these analyses | Microscope<br>Slides<br><br>Laboratory materials to do experiments |
| 3. Vocabulary list:<br>sedimentation<br>filtration<br>aeration<br>coagulation<br>disinfection<br>bacteriological<br>microscopic | | |
| *Conclusion*<br>1. Summary of the unit<br>  a. Water pollution<br>    1) Types of pollution<br>    2) Sources of pollution<br>    3) Extent of pollution | Student panel | |
|   b. Consumption of water in the United States<br>    1) 325 billion gallons consumed each day<br>    2) 160 billion gallons consumed by industry each day<br>    a) Number of gallons needed to produce a pound of high-grade paper | Student panel | Chalkboard |

## PURIFICATION OF COMMUNITY WATER SUPPLIES

| Content | Methods | Materials of Instruction |
|---|---|---|
| b) Number of gallons needed to produce 30,000 pounds of aluminum<br>3) 141 billion gallons consumed by agriculture each day<br>c. Diseases resulting from polluted water<br>d. Methods of water purification for a community<br>e. Orientation procedures for field trip to the community's water purification plant<br>　1) Checklist of methods of purification<br>　2) Checklist of sanitary analyses of water supplies | Question and answer<br><br>Class discussion<br><br>Field trip | Model of water purification plant<br><br><br>Checklist made by students |

*Evaluation*

1. Are the students, as a result of the unit, participating in community action to solve the water' pollution problem?
2. Did the students discuss the importance of water purification methods in other courses in the school?
3. Are the students aware of the sources of polluted water in the community?
4. Have the students discussed the importance of water purification with their parents, friends, and brothers and sisters?

*Teacher References*

1. American Public Health Association: *Control of Communicable Diseases in Man.* 11th ed. New York: The Association, 1970.
2. Anderson, C. L.: *Community Health.* St. Louis: The C. V. Mosby Company, 1969.
3. Smolensky, J., and Haar, F. B.: *Community Health.* 3rd ed. Philadelphia: W. B. Saunders Company, 1972.

The fifth of these lessons is the second of a four-lesson unit, "Venereal Diseases" taught to 15-, 16-, and 17-year-old students.
Area of health education—Prevention of Diseases
Unit Title—Venereal Diseases
Objectives of the Unit
1. To be aware that promiscuous sexual relations are the means of spreading venereal diseases
2. To recognize the signs of syphilis, gonorrhea, and other venereal diseases
3. To seek medical care if the signs of venereal disease appear
4. To assist in the eradication of venereal diseases
Lessons of the Unit
1. The VD picture today!
2. Syphilis
3. Gonorrhea
4. Other venereal diseases

## SYPHILIS

| Content | Methods | Materials of Instruction |
|---|---|---|
| *Review*<br>1. Venereal diseases<br>　a. Syphilis<br>　b. Gonorrhea | Panel of four students | Poster with names of venereal diseases |

## SYPHILIS

| Content | Methods | Materials of Instruction |
|---|---|---|
| c. Granuloma inguinale<br>d. Lymphogranuloma venereum<br>e. Chancroid<br>2. Incidence of syphilis and gonorrhea<br>   a. Teenagers<br>   b. Adults<br>   c. Geographical areas of the United States | | *VD FACT Sheet,* Washington, D.C.: Gov't Printing Office (annually). Spot map |
| *New Content*<br>1. Syphilis<br>   a. Causative agent<br>   b. Transmission<br>   c. Four stages<br>     1) Primary<br>     2) Secondary<br>     3) Latent<br>     4) Late | Class discussion | Pamphlets from American Medical Association, United States Public Health Service, and local and state health departments |
|    d. Characteristics of primary stage<br>   e. Characteristics of secondary stage<br>   f. Characteristics of latent stage | Slides made from photographs from Center for Disease Control, Atlanta, Georgia | "Lack of Reporting Masks VD Climb," *Medical News,* Jan. 6, 1969. |
|    g. Characteristics of late stage<br>   h. Blood tests<br>   i. Treatment<br>   j. Congenital syphilis<br>2. Finding syphilis<br>   a. Contact tracing<br>   b. Premarital examinations<br>   c. Examination of food handlers<br>3. Vocabulary list:<br>   chancre<br>   latent<br>   congenital<br>   *Treponema pallidum*<br>   antibiotics | Filmstrip, "Venereal Disease: A Present Danger," Guidance Associates, 1968. | Filmstrip |
| *Conclusion*<br>1. Mass blood testing for syphilis | Debate<br>(Topic assigned to eight class members at previous lesson) | |
| 2. Summation of facts on syphilis | Programmed instruction | Schwartz, *Student's Manual on Venereal Diseases, Facts About Syphilis and Gonorrhea,* Parts I, II, III. Amer. Assoc. for Health, Physical Education and Recreation, 1965. |

*Evaluation*

1. Do the students recognize the signs of syphilis?

2. Are students able to disprove misconceptions about syphilis?

3. Do the students accept the immediate

need for medical treatment of syphilis?

4. What student opinions were expressed in the debate on mass blood testing for syphilis?
5. What suggestions did the students give for community action in eradicating syphilis?

*Student References*

1. Haag, J. H.: Venereal diseases. In *Focusing on Health (High School)*. Austin, Tex.: The Steck-Vaughn Company, 1972.
2. Morton, R. S.: *Venereal Diseases*. Baltimore: Penquin Books, 1966.
3. Schneider, R.: *The Venereal Diseases*. Boston: Allyn and Bacon, Inc., 1968.
4. Webster, B.: *What You Should Know About VD*. New York: Scholastic Book Services, 1967.

*Teacher References*

1. American Association for Health, Physical Education and Recreation: *Venereal Disease Resource Unit—Senior High School*. Washington, D.C.: The Association, 1967.
2. American Public Health Association: *Control of Communicable Diseases in Man*. 11th ed. New York: The Association, 1970.
3. Bureau of Disease Prevention and En-

vironmental Control, National Communicable Disease Center: *Syphilis: A Synopis*. 1968.
4. Top, F.: *Communicable and Infectious Diseases*. 6th ed. St. Louis: The C. V. Mosby Company, 1968.

The sixth of these lessons is the first of a four-lesson unit, "Pregnancy and the Birth of the Baby" presented to high school seniors.

Name of teacher
Age of students—17 or 18 years
Area of health education—Family Life and Sex Education
Unit Title—Pregnancy and the Birth of the Baby
Objectives of the Unit
1. To realize that the quality of prenatal care not only influences the health of the pregnant woman but also the health of the unborn child
2. To understand the changes that occur to the unborn child during the nine months of pregnancy
3. To become familiar with the reasons for multiple births
4. To disprove the fallacies concerning pregnancy and birth of a baby.
Lessons of the Unit
1. Pregnancy through the fourth month
2. Pregnancy from fifth month until birth
3. Labor and birth of the baby
4. Multiple births

## PREGNANCY THROUGH THE FOURTH MONTH

| Content | Methods | Materials of Instruction |
|---|---|---|
| *Introduction* | | |
| 1. Importance of having children and establishing a home | Role playing by group of students | |
| 2. After a reasonable adjustment to the marriage, first pregnancy | | |
| *New Content* | | |
| 1. Full-term human pregnancy lasts about 266 days | | |
| a. Zygote | Slides | Slides of human zygote |
| b. Embryo—first eight weeks of pregnancy | Slides | |
| c. Fetus—from the third month until birth | Slides | |
| 2. Early signs of pregnancy | Invited speaker: obstetrician | |
| 3. Prenatal care | | |

## PREGNANCY THROUGH THE FOURTH MONTH

| Content | Methods | Materials of Instruction |
|---|---|---|
| 4. Danger signs of pregnancy<br>  a. Toxemia<br>  b. Vaginal bleeding<br>  c. Amniotic fluid escapes<br>  d. Pains or contractions before labor<br>  e. Chills and fever<br>  f. Adverse effects from unprescribed medication | | Poster with danger signs of pregnancy |
| 5. Smoking and pregnancy | | |
| 6. First month of pregnancy | Conceptual approach, 3M Co., Sub-Concept: "Explaining Conception, Prenatal Stages of Development and the Birth Process," #4462, Level 4, 1967 | |
| 7. Second month of pregnancy<br>  a. Broad mouth<br>  b. Eyes shift<br>  c. Eyelids<br>  d. Brain<br>  e. Limb buds<br>  f. Muscles<br>  g. No sex emerged | | Transparencies |
| 8. Third month of pregnancy<br>  a. Tooth buds<br>  b. Vocal cords<br>  c. Digestive system<br>  d. Liver<br>  e. Kidneys<br>  f. Facial bones and muscles | Conceptual approach | Maternity Center Association, New York, N.Y.; teaching aids<br><br>Sex Information and Education Council of the United States: teaching aids |
| 9. Fourth month of pregnancy<br>  a. "Quickening"<br>  b. Head<br>  c. Finger- and toeprints<br>  d. Skin | Conceptual approach | |
| 10. Growth from first through fourth month<br>  a. Length<br>  b. Weight | | |
| 11. Vocabulary<br>  zygote<br>  embryo<br>  fetus<br>  toxemia<br>  amniotic<br>  placenta<br>  umbilical | | |
| *Conclusion*<br>1. Disprove fallacies about pregnancy | Class discussion | |
| 2. Assignment: During the development of the unborn baby, at what month<br>  a. Is the enamel and dentin formed?<br>  b. Does a paste-like substance cover the fetus? | | Chalkboard |

## PREGNANCY THROUGH THE FOURTH MONTH

| Content | Methods | Materials of Instruction |
|---|---|---|
| c. Are the eyeballs completely formed?<br>d. Are the tastebuds present?<br>e. Are the finishing touches made to the brain and central nervous system?<br>f. Is there sensitivity to light touch on the palm?<br>g. Does the fat form under the skin?<br>h. Is the pigmentation of the skin slight? | | |

*Evaluation*

1. Do the young adults accept the importance of high-quality health care for the pregnant woman?
2. Do the young adults understand the changes occurring to the unborn child from conception through the fourth month of pregnancy?
3. Are the young adults aware of the responsibilities of the mother and father during pregnancy?
4. Did the young adults disprove any fallacies concerning pregnancy?
5. What changes have occurred in the young adults' attitudes about pregnancy?

*Student References*

1. Blue Cross Association: *The Modern Baby.* Chicago: The Association, 1967.
2. Haag, J. H.: Pregnancy and birth of the baby. In *Focusing on Health (High School).* Austin, Texas: The Steck-Vaughn Company, 1972.
3. Hofstein, S.: *The Human Story: Facts on Birth, Growth, and Reproduction.* Glenview, Ill.: Scott, Foresman & Company, 1967.
4. Levine, M. I., and Selgman, J. H.: *A Baby Is Born.* rev. ed. New York: Golden Press, 1966.

*Teacher References*

1. American School Health Association, Committee on Health Guidance in Sex Education: *Growth Patterns and Sex Education, Kindergarten through Grade Twelve.* Kent, Ohio: The Association, 1967.
2. Burt, J., and Brower, L. A.: *Education for Sexuality: Concepts and Programs for Teaching.* Philadelphia: W. B. Saunders Company, 1970.
3. Kilander, H.: *Sex Education in the Schools.* New York: The Macmillan Company, 1970.
4. Schulz, E., and Williams, S.: *Family Life and Sex Education: Curriculum and Instruction.* New York: Harcourt, Brace, and World, Inc., 1969.

### References for Further Study

Cornacchia, H., Staton, W., and Irwin, L.: *Health in Elementary Schools.* 3rd ed. St. Louis: The C. V. Mosby Company, 1970.

Kilander, H.: *School Health Education.* 2nd ed. New York: The Macmillan Company, 1968.

Mayshark, C., and Irwin, L.: *Health Education in Secondary Schools.* 2nd ed. St. Louis: The C. V. Mosby Company, 1968.

Smolensky, J., and Bonvechio, L. R.: *Principles of School Health.* Boston: D. C. Heath and Company, 1966.

Willgoose, C.: *Health Teaching in Secondary Schools.* Philadelphia: W. B. Saunders, 1972.

# Chapter 16

# *METHODS AND MATERIALS OF INSTRUCTION*

## AN INCIDENT

The curriculum director of a school system has asked elementary school and health education teachers to use the conceptual approach, critical incident technique, demonstrations, experiments, and other methods rather than showing films as the usual method of instruction. Also, the curriculum director has requested that the school health educator display and explain some of the materials used in health education. The curriculum director has indicated that health education could be more effective if a variety of methods and materials were included in each lesson plan.

Each lesson of the previous chapter included mention of possible methods and materials of instruction. In order to clarify the content, methods and materials of instruction must be skillfully used by the teacher and students. At no time should the methods and materials overshadow the content. The methods and materials of instruction are supplementary devices to enhance the pupil's learning.

## METHODS OF INSTRUCTION

The methods are "how" the lesson is done. Many instructional methods can change an uninteresting lecture into meaningful pupil learning experiences. Some of these methods are described.

### Conceptual Approach

Educational literature for the past sixty years or more has included studies about concepts. Within the past decade, the identification, nature, and use of concepts have gained attention. Particularly the use of concepts in organizing knowledge has gained prominence. For curriculum planning, Woodruff has defined a *concept* as "some amount of meaning more or less organized in an individual mind as a result of sensory perception of external objects or events and the cognitive interpretation of the perceived data."[1] The School Health Education Study states, "identifying representative concepts of a field of knowledge serves as a basis for the selection of subject matter content and teaching procedures that will give meaning to the concepts."[2] In addition, the concept may reflect how the individual accounts for his responses to a situation. Sometimes the concept is a mental image, a symbolic response, or an overwhelming belief.

The School Health Education Study stresses three facets of a concept of health —physical, mental, and social—which focus upon the individual, family, and community. Three key concepts serve to unify the health education curriculum. These three concepts are

1. Growing and Developing: The dynamics of the growing and developing individual—like all other persons, like some others, and like no other person.
2. Decision Making: Decisions an individual makes in taking or not taking action or in choosing between alternatives.

[1]Asabel Woodruff: The use of concepts in teaching and learning. *J. Teacher Education* 15 (March, 1964) :81-97.
[2]School Health Education Study: *Health Education: A Conceptual Approach to Curriculum Design.* Minnesota: 3M Education Press, 1968. p. 6.

3. Interacting: An individual's interactions with his environment including the social, physical, economic, psychological, and cultural forces.

In the second level of the concept hierarchy are ten subordinate concepts related to the three key concepts. *Two* concepts are related to Growing and Developing:

1. Growth and development influences and is influenced by the structure and functioning of the individual.
2. Growing and developing follows a predictable sequence, yet is unique for each individual.[3]

*Four* concepts are related to Decision Making:

1. Personal health practices are affected by a complexity of forces, often conflicting.
2. Utilization of health information, products, and services is guided by values and perceptions.
3. Use of substances that modify mood and behavior arises from a variety of motivations.
4. Food selection and eating patterns are determined by physical, social, mental, economic, and cultural factors.[3]

*Four* concepts are related to Interacting:

1. Protection and promotion of health is an individual, community, and international responsibility.
2. The potential for hazards and accidents exists, whatever the environment.
3. There are reciprocal relationships involving man, disease, and environment.
4. The family serves to perpetuate man and to fulfill certain health needs.[3]

From these ten concepts emerge subconcepts which apply to physical, mental, and social health. The establishment of long-range goals completes the conceptual approach. Goals serve as guides for determining the desired outcomes for each of the ten concepts from kindergarten through grade twelve. The goals are divided into cognitive, affective, and action domains.[4] The conceptual approach is an identification of major concepts and supporting ideas so that there can be an organization of knowledge and a structure for meaning-

ful relationships. In Chapter 15, the conceptual approach was used as a method of instruction in the lesson ' "Sniffing" and "Pot"'; in the lesson "Case against Tobacco"; and the lesson "Pregnancy through the Fourth Month."

## Critical Incident Technique

Mayshark and Foster have given a thorough review of the critical incident technique as a method of instruction. The critical incident technique requires six steps. In the *first* step, a thumbnail sketch of an incident is read. This sketch should take three to five minutes to read. In the *second* step, each class member will ask one question pertinent to the ultimate solution. Since the thumbnail sketch of the incident does not present sufficient information to reach a conclusion, the class members will be seeking further information. Two or three minutes are allowed for the class members to write out their questions. Discussion of major issues is the *third* step. This step can begin with the question of what needs to be decided immediately. The class members need to decide what action should be immediate and what should be done in the future. Since the incidents involve a time element, solutions require immediate action as well as planning for the future. In step *four*, a class member summarizes the discussion of the class. This discussion should lead the class members to decide the course of action. One student could be appointed at the beginning of the incident to serve as an observer-reporter of the discussion in order to give an analysis of the discussion, mentioning its successes and failures and its conclusions. In step *five*, students record their decisions as to what action they would take to solve the problem described in the incident. Usually, ten minutes is necessary. The *sixth* step involves a group decision. For the first time, the teacher involves himself as an impartial discussion leader. The teacher points out facts that were omitted in earlier discussion. He guides the class in revision of individual and class decisions. The teacher tells the class of the actual decision, if known. In summary, Mayshark and Foster have indicated the advantages of the critical incident technique: (1) it requires no advance preparation by teacher or pupils; (2) it im-

[3]*Ibid.*, pp. 21-23.
[4]*Ibid.*, pp. 25-28.

proves the decision-making skills of the teacher; (3) it permits greater class participation; and (4) it builds the teacher's confidence to make wise and spontaneous decisions.[5]

## Educational Television

Reaching millions of viewers, the programs on educational television are selected with the assumption that the viewers have diversified interests and abilities. There are two types of educational television, "instructional or in-school" and "adult programming." "Instructional" television consists of lessons and units of subject-matter fields for elementary school, secondary school, and college students. "Adult programming" includes programs for the general public.

Educational television is transmitted by either closed- or open-circuit systems. Closed-circuit television operates over cables like the telephone. It does not require television channels because it does not send the picture and sound through the air. Open-circuit television requires federal allocation of an assigned television frequency. It has wider geographical coverage than closed-circuit television has. The majority of educational television programs for elementary and secondary schools are broadcast on open-circuit systems. Closed-circuit systems may be used on college campuses.

Videotape is a system of high-quality recording of the sound and picture of a television lesson on magnetic tape. These tapes are permanent records of the lessons taught and can be duplicated and used by different television stations. In contrast, "live" telecasts send their picture and sound simultaneously over two or more educational television stations.

The television teacher must not only be a "master" teacher in knowledge of subject matter and in teaching ability but also be able to adjust to the demands of television and work with the persons who operate television facilities. Even though the television teacher determines what he says and the method of instruction, techni-

cal personnel advise the television teacher how he can best present the subject matter and best use the methods of instruction. These technical personnel include television producers, directors, cameramen, lighting experts, studio artists, and other technicians.

Effective teaching on television demands precise planning of the lesson. Each part of a lesson must have a definite time allotment, as the television teacher cannot linger for several minutes to clarify a point. The teacher cannot end the lesson five minutes ahead of time, nor can the teacher wander from the subject matter outlined in the classroom teacher's study guide. The teacher's personality and enthusiasm are vital to the success of television teaching for a dull lesson devoid of subject matter can be simply ended with a flick of the television dial.

## Demonstrations

In the lesson "Tooth Brushing after Eating," in Chapter 15, a demonstration of tooth brushing is necessary.

Following the teacher's demonstration, the pupils practice tooth-brushing procedures in the classroom and brush their teeth after the midmorning snack and noonday meal. As a teaching method, the *techniques of demonstration can be outlined to include* the following:

1. Teacher should be fully acquainted with each phase of the demonstration.
   a. Verbal explanations accompany each phase.
   b. Skills are used in each phase.
   c. Demonstration is practiced by teacher before presenting it.
2. All equipment and supplies to be used in demonstration should be within arm's reach of the teacher.
3. Teacher explains "why" the demonstration is being made.
4. Teacher takes each phase of demonstration slowly, carefully, and emphasizes the "how" of each phase.
5. Teacher finishes the demonstration by emphasizing the highlights of the demonstration and the importance of each phase.
6. Teacher repeats the complete demonstration (#3 through #5).

[5]Cyrus Mayshark and Roy Foster: *Methods in Health Education, A Workbook using the Critical Incident Technique.* St. Louis: The C. V. Mosby Company, 1966, pp. 5-7.

7. Students follow the teacher as the teacher demonstrates a third time.
8. Students not having a chance to follow the teacher, as stated in #7, follow teacher demonstration the fourth time.
9. Students practice skills without teacher demonstration. Teacher moves around the classroom checking each student's attempts and corrects and approves these attempts.
10. Pitfalls of teacher demonstration:
    a. The teacher may not be fully acquainted with the verbal explanations and skills necessary for the demonstration.
    b. Supplies and equipment may be insufficient and not accessible.
    c. The class may be poorly organized for student practice sessions.
    d. Classroom space may be inadequate for pupil practice.
    e. The teacher may not check on students' practice attempts.
    f. Students' practice attempts may not be included in the evaluation of the students' skills at the close of the unit.

When can the *demonstration* be used? The following are a few of the many ways in which demonstrations can be used as an instructional method in health education:

American Red Cross First Aid
    Bandaging, treatment for shock, control of bleeding, fractures, artificial respiration, treatment of wounds, care of internal poisoning, treatment of simple emergencies, transportation, etc.
Facial skin care
Shampooing of the hair
Care of the hands and nails
Preparation of a vegetable salad as a part of a unit in meal planning
Bicycle safety skills
    Riding, hand signals, care of bicycle parts, parking bicycle, etc.
Weighing and measuring height
Fire drills and disaster self-preservation procedures
Safety in handling a gun
Using a snake-bite kit
Lifting objects, such as a table or chair, from floor
Handling a knife, ax, hammer, saw
Using a fire extinguisher

## Experiments

One of the most effective experiments is the "Clinitest," a test for sugar in the urine, in a unit on diabetes. The kit containing an eye dropper, test tube, and reagent tablets can be obtained from any pharmacist.

In addition, two containers of tap water and a specimen of urine are needed. Procedures of the experiment:

1. Collect urine in a clean container.
2. With dropper in an upright position, place 5 drops of urine in the test tube.
3. Rinse dropper.
4. Add 10 drops of water to urine.
5. Drop 1 reagent tablet in test tube.
6. Do not shake test tube during reaction nor for 15 seconds.
7. After 15 seconds, shake tube gently.
8. Compare with color chart.
9. Color chart:

| Blue | 0% | Negative |
|---|---|---|
| Dark green | $\frac{1}{4}\%$ | Trace |
| Green | $\frac{1}{2}\%$ | One plus |
| Brown-green | $\frac{3}{4}\%$ | Two plus |
| Brown | 1% | Three plus |
| Orange | 2% | Four plus |

10. Should color rapidly "pass through" green, tan, and orange to dark greenish-brown, record as over 2% sugar.
11. Conclusion: Amount of sugar in urine specimen is determined by the color of the solution in the test tube.[6]

Another highly successful experiment is one dealing with animal feeding and effects of different diets on rats. Three diets are used: (1) diet of enriched whole-wheat bread and water; (2) diet of whole pasteurized milk and water; and (3) diet of enriched whole-wheat bread, whole pasteurized milk, and water. Teacher should be familiar with the following information before attempting an animal-feeding experiment.

1. Where to obtain rats
2. Materials used in experiment
3. Materials used in building cages

[6]Instructions accompanying Clinitest kit and reagent tablets. Ames Company, Elkhart, Ind.

4. How to build cages
5. Planning experiment with students
   a. Purpose
   b. Number of rats and condition of each rat at the first day of the experiment
   c. Diet of each rat
   d. Conditions of rat to be observed daily
   e. Handling and weighing rats
   f. Recording daily weight of rats
   g. Daily cleaning of cages
   h. Precautionary measures
6. Conclusions drawn from experiments

Many health education lessons can utilize experiments. Experiments showing the effects of sedimentation, filtration, and sanitary analysis of water are used in the lesson "Purification of Community Water Supplies" in Chapter 15. Other possible experiments are testing the reaction time and hand-eye coordination of an abstainer of alcoholic beverages and of a problem drinker, preparing homemade butter, making a homemade fire extinguisher, showing the amount of carbohydrates in food, indicating tar and nicotine from different brands of cigarettes, and hatching a chick from a fertilized hen egg.

## Field Trips

Community facilities can be visited on field trips. Some of these relevant to health education are the water-purification plant, sewage-treatment plant, bakeries, dairies, restaurants, food-processing plants, voluntary health agencies, police department, self-service grocery stores, and solid-waste disposal plants. The teacher should be familiar with seven steps necessary to a successful field trip. *First*, the teacher should visit the establishment several weeks before the class field trip. At that visit, the purpose of the field trip should be explained, and arrangements should be made to secure a guide. At the time of the teacher's visit, the trip can be arranged for the hour best suited to the establishment's work schedule. *Second*, the school principal must approve and give permission for the field trip. He should be informed that the field trip may take more time than originally allotted. *Third*, safety precautions should be taken by the teacher before the trip. He must also provide for bus

transportation and chaperons. *Fourth*, a check list should be made by students before they go and after the teacher has explained each phase of the establishment's work. The student check list will serve to pinpoint the important highlights of the trip. *Fifth*, students should prepare questions to ask the guide during the trip. *Sixth*, discussion should be held in the classroom after the trip to discuss the highlights. *Seventh*, a letter of appreciation should be sent to the manager of the establishment and the guide by the students. If the field trip is to be meaningful, each student should contribute to the class discussion to make sure that the purpose of the trip is clearly understood.

## Dramatizations

Skits, plays, pageants, monologues, marionette and puppet shows, charades, and pantomimes are some of the possible forms of dramatization. Dramatizations can be used in many health education areas of instruction—mental health, nutrition, family life and sex education, care of the human body, safety education, and consumer health. For example, a skit can portray the acceptance of a classmate with a chronic health condition. A play can emphasize the importance of a well-balanced breakfast. Pageants can reveal measures to prevent fires in the home, school, and community. Monologues might be used to evaluate advertising of a charlatan. Marionette and puppet shows have been used widely in primary grades. Charades and pantomimes lend themselves to health education at the middle or junior high school level.

## Invited Speakers

Community workers can be invited to class as speakers to supplement the content of the health education lesson. Before presenting the speaker to pupils, the teacher should visit his headquarters. A member of the staff of many community organizations is usually designated to speak in schools. Some nonofficial health and safety agencies have speakers for different topics and age groups. City police and fire departments have staff members who work with teachers on safety problems. During the visit, the teacher can inform the speaker of the purpose of the speech, the age level of the students, their in terests in the topic, the content of the health education unit, and the best time for the speaker's visit. If audiovisual aids borrowed from the speaker's headquarters have been used, the speaker should know this to avoid duplication. Pupils should be familiar with the speaker's topic and should have questions to ask the speaker after his speech. Class discussion can follow the question period. A summation of the pertinent parts of the speech can be made by a student chairman or by the teacher. A letter of appreciation should be sent following the speaker's visit.

## Problem Solving

Problem solving can be used in lessons within units of these areas of health education: "American Red Cross First Aid," "Consumer Health," "Nutrition," "Safety Education," "Community Health Problems," and "Family Life and Sex Education." There are eight steps to problem solving:

1. Recognizing a problem
2. Defining the problem
3. Selecting procedures for its solution
4. Collecting data
5. Analyzing and interpreting data
6. Preparing conclusions
7. Applying conclusions to a plan of action or solution of the problem
8. Evaluating the results.

Problem solving is one of the most practical methods for changing student health practices. The scientific approach is used to solve personal and community health problems. Students collect data, analyze and interpret data, and differentiate between misconceptions, half-truths, and valid facts.

## Programmed Instruction

These self-instruction devices with information to be learned and arranged in sequence are available so that the student is led through a series of steps of learning. The student may answer a question, solve a problem, or respond in some other way. When the student gives the correct answer, he is so informed and proceeds to the next stage in programmed instruction. The student moves at his own pace. Programmed instruction was listed in the lesson on "Syphilis." There are arguments for and against programmed instruction. Some areas of health education might lend themselves to programmed instruction. However, class discussions, panels, debates, and other methods requiring a verbal exchange between students or the students and teacher are lost by using programmed instruction.

## Other Methods of Instruction

*Student reports* can be the result of individual or committee research as in the lesson "Purification of Community Water Supplies." Student reports can supplement the content of a health education lesson; for example, one lesson of a cancer unit for high school students might include oral reports on cancer research. A committee of students might report on the World Health Organization during a unit on international health problems. Oral reports should utilize such references as *Today's Health* and publications of official and nonofficial health agencies.

Many teachers prefer *group discussion* during health education lessons. The group discussion can result from a student report or can be stimulated by questions asked by the teacher. There are many ways in which the teacher can create effective group discussion. She may, for example, keep the main topic under discussion before the group, encourage the participation of all students, use frequent summaries as the discussion progresses, and answer a pupil question with another question.

In the previous chapter, *question and answer, exhibits, panels, surveys,* and *role-playing* were mentioned as possible methods of instruction in ' "Sniffing" and "Pot," ' "Case Against Tobacco," "Purification of Community Water Supplies," "Syphilis," and "Pregnancy Through the Fourth Month." The *question-and-answer* method can be employed by the pupils as well as by the teacher. *Exhibits* can be made by students to clarify the explanation by the teacher or students. A *panel* can use student reports as the basis for the discussion among panel members. A *survey* by students can collect information about adults' and students' health practices. *Role-playing* is unrehearsed acting out of a situation by two or more students. Role-playing helps students to understand how their classmates feel in a given situation and can bring about changes in their attitudes.

Successful role-playing depends upon (1) the situation's being clearly defined to the students who are to act it out so that each knows what is expected of him; (2) observers who need to discuss in advance what they should detect in the role-playing; (3) the teacher's selection of those students for role-playing so that no one will be in a role which causes embarrassment or emotional conflict; and (4) discussion and evaluation following the completion of the role-playing.

Other health education methods of instruction are *debates, buzz sessions, published and teacher-made health education measuring devices* (Chapter 22), *creative experiences, storytelling, classroom games, brainstorming,* and *independent study. Classroom games* may include the many varieties of pencil-and-paper games, quiz programs, and variations of spelling "bees." The class may be divided into small groups in *buzz sessions*. Each group discusses a problem or formulates questions around a problem. Each group selects a leader who summarizes the group's discussion and presents the discussion to a group. *Creative activities* may be writing a play, preparing a telecast, or writing articles for a school newspaper. These activities should be performed by students with only minimum teacher guidance. *Brainstorming* is an attempt to solve a problem by all students in a class, or a type of problem solving. Any solution offered by a student, regardless of how extreme, is accepted. There is free association of ideas in brainstorming. *Films, filmstrips,* and *slides* will be discussed in the next section of this chapter, even though they can be classified as methods of instruction.

The *question box* can be used for written questions from students not wishing to be identified. Used during a unit from family life and sex education, the question box can indicate to the teacher health problems students wish to have discussed. It was used in the lesson "Case Against Tobacco."

A method of instruction that has tremendous possibilities is the *case study*. Actual situations in public schools can be used for case studies. Group discussion, panel, and role-playing can be used, but at least two hours is needed for discussion and analysis. Hamburg and Hamburg advocate using the case study as a method in health education. Solutions to each case study are omitted so that many possible ways to handle the case can be discussed by the class.[7]

## MATERIALS USED IN HEALTH EDUCATION

Health education materials of instruction are unlimited. The materials are objects, not subject matter. Only materials used most frequently will be mentioned in this section.

*Community resources* can be used to clarify explanations of health education topics. During instruction on community health problems, the water purification plant, food-processing and frozen-food locker plants, bakeries, restaurants, the local health department, and the sewage-treatment plant are resources that can provide sites for field trips and speakers. Supermarkets, dairies, school and hotel kitchens, and drive-in eating establishments are community resources that can be used for instruction in nutrition. Teachers should not overlook police departments, fire stations, and community health agencies as potential sources.

Lunchrooms, as *school facilities*, are teaching laboratories, as are fire and disaster drills, which utilize many parts of school buildings. First-grade children should learn how to operate drinking fountains, use hand washing facilities outside the lunchrooms, and handle the toilet room facilities. School grounds, playing fields, auditoriums, library, gymnasium, laboratories, and shops, as well as classrooms, corridors, and stairs, are utilized in safety education.

Black-and-white or color sound *films* have influenced the content and methods of health education. The number of health education films is countless. Validity of the health information, techniques employed to convey it to the audience, scope of the information covered, relevance of the information to the health needs and interests of a particular age level and community, possibilities of use with more than one unit of health education, and innumerable other criteria should be used in evaluation of

[7]Morris Hamburg and Marian V. Hamburg: *Health and Social Problems in the School*. Philadelphia: Lea & Febiger, 1968, pp. 1-242.

films. Before previewing any film, a selection of several films appropriate to the health education content should be made. On a film-preview evaluation sheet, the teacher should indicate the following information:

Title and source of film
Color or black and white
Topic covered on film
Time length
Defects of film
Terminology in film—valid, up-to-date, correlation with health education content, and specific facts
Techniques employed to convey health information
Scope of health information
Motivating qualities of film
Is the sound clear and distinct?
Is word usage appropriate for the grade level of intended use?
Are the pictures appropriate to the health education topic?
Possibilities for use of the film

The teacher should preview the films a second time before final selection of a film is made. The teacher then orders the film and gives the time, date, and location of the school and classroom where the film is to be shown.

The students should have a complete orientation to the topic covered before the film is shown. During the orientation, specific health information should be emphasized so that students are aware of what they should learn from the film. Some teachers summarize the film with an outline or a list of highlights on the chalkboard. Regardless of the technique employed, the orientation should be thorough and fully descriptive.

The teacher might also use an evaluation sheet to show the students' reactions. Could the students hear and see the film from all parts of the classroom? What highlights of the film, pertinent to the health education content, did the students overlook after the second showing? Did the students gain any specific health information from the film? Did the students like the film?

A second showing of the same film is valuable at every grade level, because students gain more specific information from two viewings than from one. Following the second showing, students can answer pre-pared lists of questions or can complete check lists. Some teachers prefer group discussion to using prepared questions or check lists. Students should have an opportunity to reveal whether they did or did not gain specific health information, whether they agreed or disagreed with the point of view expressed in the film, and whether they wish to raise questions concerning the film's information.

In addition to films, *filmstrips* and *slides* are extremely useful materials in health education. They can be teacher- or pupil-prepared, as well as commercially made. Teacher-prepared slides depicting students' posture can be an excellent way to show deviations in lateral and anterior-posterior posture. Facial features of students should be blacked out, and the students should have suitable attire.

In schools that cannot purchase human anatomy and physiology charts for health education, teacher-prepared slides of drawings from human anatomical and physiological texts can be substituted for the charts. The same drawings might be used with an opaque projector, which enlarges the drawing on the chalkboard, where it can be traced. The filmstrip can be a record of a field trip to the water purification plant, or show a series of self-preservation procedures to be followed during a disaster drill.

*Other Materials of Instruction*

Radio
Television
Recordings
Transcriptions
Dioramas
Models
Specimens
Microscope slides
Petri plates with nutrient fluid
Microscopes
Materials used in laboratory experiments
Puppets
Marionettes
Dramatization materials (scripts, costumes, props)
Cartoons
Flash cards

Charts
Maps (spot, geographical)
Graphs (area, bar, pictorial)
Flannelgraphs and feltboards
Posters
Flat or still pictures (photographs, magazine pictures)
Manikins
Newspaper clippings
Nostrums
X-ray viewer and x-rays
Platform scales
Visual and hearing screening instruments and records
Health Records

Diagrams
Labels from drugs
Pesticides
Food additives
Transparencies and transparency projector
Facsimiles of dangerous drugs, narcotics, and hallucinogens
Programmed instruction materials
Dental health materials (full-mouth x-rays, mouth mirrors, probes, etc.)
Advertisements
Samples of health insurance policies
Reaction-time testing devices
Nutrition education materials (food samples, exhibits, laboratory equipment analyzing foods, labels from food products, etc.)
Chest x-rays and tuberculin testing materials
Check lists and questionnaires
Rating scales and surveys
Pupil diaries
Interest-inventory scales

Shadow boxes
American Red Cross first-aid equipment
Testimonials
Prescription drugs
Over-the-counter drugs
Cosmetics
Pamphlets, bulletins, and other printed materials from quacks
Filmstrip projector
Film projector
Objects used by narcotic addicts; e.g., "cooker"
Syringes
Bicycles, guns, swim fins
Small power-driven automobiles
Salk and Sabin vaccines, insulin, and other vaccines with syringe, alcohol, and cotton
Classroom games
Bulletin boards
Chalkboards
Scrapbooks
Published and teacher-made health knowledge, attitudes, and practices measuring devices
Question boxes
Homemade movies

*Printed health education materials* include a wide variety of bulletins, pamphlets, statistical tables, periodicals, such as *Today's Health,* textbooks, single mimeographed or printed pages, research reports, and medical dictionaries. The effectiveness of pamphlets needs continuous teacher evaluation. Some of the questions raised about the effectiveness of pamphlets:

1. Has a qualified person or agency been the author of the pamphlet?
2. Is the subject matter or content of recent date?
3. Is the subject matter or content specific and detailed?
4. Is the type large enough to read?
5. Are references given?

Not listed above among the materials of instruction are the *health museums* found in various sections of the nation. In these museums, elementary and secondary teachers can gain a wealth of ideas for teaching methods and materials. The "try-it-yourself" exhibits, three-dimensional models, automat serving the "meal of your choice," and quiz games are a few of the many devices used by health museums. Popular with persons of all ages, these museums have contributed greatly to the health education of the nation.

## References for Further Study

Anderson, C. L.: *School Health Practice*. 5th ed. St. Louis: The C. V. Mosby Company, 1972.

Cornacchia, H., Staton, W. M., and Irwin, L. W.: *Health in Elementary Schools*. 3rd ed. St. Louis: The C. V. Mosby Company, 1970.

Fodor, J. T., and Dalis, G. T.: *Health Instruction: Theory and Application*. Philadelphia: Lea & Febiger, 1966.

Grout, R. E.: *Health Teaching in Schools*. 5th ed. Philadelphia: W. B. Saunders Company, 1968.

Haag, J. H., and DeVault, M. V.: *Physiology*. (Demonstrations for pupils) Austin, Texas: The Steck-Vaughn Company, 1960.

Kilander, H.: *School Health Education*. 2nd ed. New York: The Macmillan Company, 1968.

Mayshark, C., and Irwin, L. W.: *Health Education in Secondary Schools*. 2nd ed. St. Louis: The C. V. Mosby Company, 1968.

Oberteuffer, D., Harrelson, O., and Pollack, M.: *School Health Education*. 5th ed. New York: Harper & Row, 1972.

Smolensky, J., and Bonvechio, L. R.: *Principles of School Health*. Boston: D. C. Health and Co., 1966.

Turner, C. E., Randall, H. B., and Smith, S. L.: *School Health and Health Education*. 6th ed. St. Louis: The C. V. Mosby Company, 1970.

Willgoose, C. E.: *Health Education in the Elementary School*. 3rd ed. Philadelphia: W. B. Saunders Company, 1969.

# Chapter 17

# COMMUNITY RESOURCES

## AN INCIDENT

A beginning teacher has obtained many types of printed health education materials from various voluntary community health agencies. The school health educator has compiled sources of health education materials from commercial and semicommercial groups. The members of the school health council have invited representatives of professional groups to attend the council's meetings. However, principals complain that some teachers are not familiar with community resources for health education.

Two terms, "official" and "nonofficial," applied to community health agencies, have appeared in public health publications. *Official health agencies* are those financed by taxation and authorized by state or federal legislative action to fulfill specific functions. *Nonofficial health agencies* receive their funds from private gifts, sale of advertised products, voluntarily subscribed memberships, and privately financed community projects.

## OFFICIAL AGENCIES

Two official agencies will be discussed: public health and public education. Both of these agencies have federal, state, and local divisions with separate responsibilities.

### Public Health—Federal

The federal agency is the United States Public Health Service under the direction of the Secretary of Health, Education and Welfare. Established in 1798, the Service has undergone many changes in its funding, organization, functions, and name. In 1912, it was named the United States Public Health Service, and in 1953 it became a part of the newly established Department of Health, Education and Welfare. The Service has three agencies: the Food and Drug Administration, Health Services and Mental Health Administration, and the National Institutes of Health.

There are ten National Institutes of Health. They are the National Cancer Institute, the National Eye Institute, the National Heart and Lung Institute, the National Institute of Allergy and Infectious Diseases, the National Institute of Arthritis and Metabolic Diseases, the National Institute of Child Health and Human Development, the National Institute of Dental Research, the National Institute of Environmental Health Sciences, the National Institute of General Medical Sciences, and the National Institute of Neurological Diseases and Stroke. These Institutes "conduct, foster, and support research and research training . . . collaborate with other institutions and organizations engaged in similar research . . . collection and disseminate information on research findings."

There are three major functions of the United States Public Health Service. First, the Service identifies health hazards in man's environment and in the products and services which he uses in order to develop, promulgate, and assure compliance with standards for control of such hazards. Second, it supports the development of, and helps to improve the organization and delivery of, comprehensive and coordinated physical and mental health services for all Americans, and it provides direct health care services to some federal beneficiary groups. Third, the service conducts and supports research in the medical and related sciences, promoting the dissemination of knowledge of these sciences and furthering the development of health education and training to insure an adequate supply of qualified health manpower.

The Food and Drug Administration protects the public health of the Nation by insuring

> that foods are safe, pure, and wholesome; drugs are safe and effective; . . . products are honestly and informatively labeled and packaged; dangerous household products carry adequate warnings for safe use and are properly labeled; counterfeiting of drugs is stopped; and interstate travelers are afforded adequate levels of sanitation and control of health hazards.[1]

Seventeen district offices and ten regional offices serve the United States. There are four Bureaus: Bureau of Foods, Bureau of Product Safety; Bureau of Drugs; and Bureau of Veterinary Medicine.

## Public Health—State

At the state level, there are numerous health services dispersed by separate departments of state governments. Each state, however, has one particular agency charged with the overall health program of the state. This agency is usually called the State Department of Health.

The functions of state health departments differ greatly from the functions of local health departments. A state health department furnishes consultant and advisory services to local communities, while local health departments provide direct health services to their communities.

A state health department may administer financial assistance to local health departments. State legal requirements are enforced by a state health department, such as regulations concerning the control of communicable diseases. It often fosters research projects in local health departments, and some of the state personnel may work with local health departments on research projects and special assignments.

There are four basic functions of a state health department. The first is health surveillance, planning, and program development. The state health department assists

in developing comprehensive health programs and in financing these programs with state and federal funds. The second function is the promotion of local health care. The state health department assists local health departments in meeting minimum criteria so that the people receive adequate health care. The third function is the establishment and enforcement of standards. The state health department certifies services and facilities participating in federal medical care programs. The fourth function is the provision of health services. The state health department focuses its attention on personal health services, environmental conditions, research, professional education, public health education, and administration.

Many divisions and bureaus may be found in state health departments. Some of these divisions and bureaus include those responsible for records and statistics; public health education; communicable diseases; and environmental health services such as milk and dairy products, food and drugs, occupational health, sanitary engineering, air pollution, vector control, radiation control, and wastewater technology. Other divisions and bureaus may supervise health facilities construction; local health services; laboratories; public health nursing; and preventive medical services such as problems of chronic diseases, dental health, and veterinary public health. In addition, there may be special health services such as crippled children's services, cancer and heart disease control, maternal and child health care, and tuberculosis control services; and medical care administration such as licensing of hospitals, home health services, and nursing and convalescent homes.

## Public Health—County

County health departments may serve one county, several counties, small cities, or a county and city. County health departments may offer the same services as local health departments, but their services extend over larger areas. General hospitals may be operated by county health departments so that residents may receive medical care close to their homes.

Some of the usual services fall into nine categories: (1) promotion of child health; (2) communicable disease control; (3) en-

[1]Office of the Federal Register. *United States Government Organization Manual—1971/72*, pp. 331-337.

vironmental health promotion; (4) promotion of maternal and child health; (5) keeping of vital statistics; (6) mental health promotion; (7) health education; (8) promotion of adult health; and (9) laboratory service. Public health nurses promote *child health* through assistance to parents in understanding the health problems of their children, securing medical services for their children, and providing home nursing. Some of the activities in *communicable disease control* are supplying immunizations, providing for quarantine and isolation of persons with communicable diseases, control of carriers of diseases, and case reporting. *Environmental health promotion* is accomplished by sanitarians who inspect water supplies, food and milk, sewage and waste disposal, insect and rodent infestations, along with other services. *Promotion of maternal and child health* is accomplished by public health nurses whose services are aimed at the health of expectant mothers and infants. *Vital statistics* reveal public health problems by application of statistical methods to the birth rate, death rate, infant mortality rate, maternal mortality rate, morbidity rate, and fatality rate. *Mental health services* provide the resident of the county with assistance in solving serious emotional problems. *Health education* is directed to all ages and aims to affect the people's health attitudes, health practices, and health knowledge constructively. *Promotion of adult health* emphasizes the health problems of the over-forty age group and elderly citizens. *Laboratory service* includes examination of water and food, contaminated food, and specimens used in medical diagnosis of disease.

A county health department can be organized when there are 50,000 residents in a county. Often small city and county health departments are consolidated to meet the needs of the residents more efficiently.

## Public Health—Local

The most common function of a local health department is providing nursing service. The public health nurse visits the homes of those citizens who need her services, works in clinics of the health department and hospitals, discovers hidden cases of disease and defects which need medical care, and educates her patients concerning their responsibilities in community health.

Local health departments may operate clinics for supervision of maternity patients and young children; dental health; immunization against communicable diseases; diagnosis and treatment of venereal diseases and tuberculosis; mental health; and diagnosis and treatment of cancer, diabetes, and heart disease. The local health department continuously checks radiation hazards and air pollution and is responsible for purified drinking water, adequate sewage treatment, proper disposal of solid wastes, sanitary food handling, supervision of milk production and distribution, and inspection of meat. It may provide diagnostic laboratory services, public health education, and nutrition services. The local health department is concerned with family planning. It collects and analyzes all data relative to vital statistics. The control of rats, insects, and rabid animals is another function of the local health department. It inspects nursing homes, privately operated hospitals, and other establishments that can affect the health of citizens, whether it is a beauty shop or a community-owned swimming pool.

The effectiveness of a local health department depends upon the amount of local financing available and the willingness of the local citizens to cooperate. Adequate funds from taxation allotted to a health department provide the needed facilities and equipment and enable the employment of personnel prepared to cope with the health problems of the community.

## Public Education

The federal education agency is the United States Office of Education under the direction of the Secretary of Health, Education and Welfare. Created in 1867, it has undergone changes in its functions and name. The Office of Education collects

statistics and facts as shall show the condition and progress of education, to diffuse such information as shall aid the people of the United States in the establishment and maintenance of efficient school systems, and otherwise to promote the cause of education.[2]

---

[2]*Ibid.*, p. 338.

There are a Bureau of Elementary and Secondary Education; Bureau of Adult, Vocational and Technical Education; Bureau of Education for the Handicapped; and Bureau of Higher Education. In addition, there are an Institute of International Studies, National Center for Educational Research and Development, Experimental Schools Staff, National Center for Educational Statistics, National Center for Educational Communication, Bureau of Educational Personnel Development, and Bureau of Libraries and Educational Technology.

The state agencies responsible for education have many official titles, such as State Department of Education, Department of Public Instruction, or Education Agency. Because Americans have vested the authority over public schools in the local school systems, the state education office has limited powers. However, it is usually responsible for the school census, teacher certification, accreditation of schools and school systems, lunch programs, bus regulations, vocational rehabilitation, veterans' education, financing through bonds and investments, trade and industrial education, establishment of specifications for new and remodeled school plants, curricular and instructional patterns, adoption of textbooks, approval of instructional materials, and other functions.

A board of education is the official governing group of the local elementary and secondary schools. The superintendent is responsible for the functioning of the school system. He has general and specific responsibilities within the school health program (Chapter 18).

## NONOFFICIAL AGENCIES

The nonofficial agencies are extensive and varied, and they provide a wide range of health services.

### Professional Groups

#### American Association for Health, Physical Education and Recreation

Among the many professional groups is the American Association for Health, Physical Education and Recreation, a National Affiliate of the National Education Association. The School Health Division of the association offers consultant services in health education, serves as a liaison agent between the National Education Association and the American Medical Association, cooperates with other nonofficial agencies and publishes many types of health education materials. The *School Health Review* and *The Research Quarterly* contain information about school health education.

### The American School Health Association

The American School Health Association was first organized in 1927 as the American School Physicians Association. Membership is drawn from physicians, nurses, dentists, health educators, nutritionists, school administrators, dental hygienists, public health educators, and other professional personnel interested in school health programs. Its purpose is to promote school health services, healthful school living, and health education. It publishes *The Journal of School Health*.

### The American Public Health Association

The American Public Health Association was organized in 1872 by a group of public health authorities who recognized the need for a national organization concerned with every phase of public health. This association is the largest and best-known organization of the public health professions. Its School Health Section, organized in 1942, has jointly held meetings with the Maternal and Child Health, Food and Nutrition, and Public Health Education Sections. *The American Journal of Public Health* is its official publication.

### The American Medical Association

Since 1921, the American Medical Association has published a popular health magazine. In 1950, the title was changed to *Today's Health*. The Department of Health Education of the association has sponsored, every odd-numbered year, a National Conference on Physicians and Schools to promote the total school health program. As a result of these conferences, data have been published on medical examinations, emergency care, control of communicable diseases, and physical and mental health guidance. It is through the efforts of the department that the Joint Committee on Health Problems in Education has worked with the National Education Association since 1911.

*The American Dental Association*

The American Dental Association has aided dental health through research and education and by increasing the scope of dental care. The Council on Dental Therapeutics of the association has been evaluating products used in the treatment and prevention of dental diseases since 1930. The first edition of *Accepted Dental Remedies*, which listed and evaluated dental products, appeared in 1934. Most educational materials on dental health are produced by the association. This service has been available to teachers since 1934. Because of the demand for educational materials, the association established a Bureau of Health Education in 1954.

*The American Nurses' Association*
and the *National League for Nursing*

The public health nurse working with the school health program and the school nurse are members of the American Nurses' Association and/or the National League for Nursing. In 1896, the American Nurses' Association was organized; its present name adopted in 1911. ANA members are professional registered nurses representing every occupational field of nursing. Following 10 years of preparation and planning, the National League for Nursing was formed in 1952. Professional and practical nurses and nursing aides, persons in allied professions, persons interested in good nursing, nursing services, and agencies and institutions with educational programs in nursing are members of the NLN.

*Other Professional Associations*

Other professional groups contributing to elementary and secondary school health programs are:

American Academy of Pediatrics
American Dental Hygienists' Association
American Dietetic Association
American Home Economics Association
American Optometric Association
American Pharmaceutical Association
American Physical Therapy Association
American Society of Heating, Refrigerating
  and Air-Conditioning Engineers
Child Study Association of America, Inc.
Illuminating Engineering Society
National Health Council
National Safety Council
Society of Public Health Educators

**Voluntary Community Health Agencies**

Voluntary community health agencies consist of many diversified groups. The purposes of the agencies tend to vary with the needs for particular services in different communities, and not all communities have local chapters or units of each agency. The agencies are so numerous that it is impossible to list all of them here. Only a few of the most prominent will be mentioned.

*The American Cancer Society*

The American Cancer Society had its origin in the American Society for the Control of Cancer founded by a small group of physicians and laymen in 1913. In 1944, the present name of the society was adopted. The public education goal is to save lives by teaching the importance of early cancer detection and of prevention where applicable. The society's education programs emphasize ways for persons to protect themselves against cancer: (1) adopt preventive habits; avoid cigarette smoking, overexposure to sunlight, and other possible factors causing cancer; (2) have an annual medical examination; (3) learn the warning signals of cancer and go to a physician if one should occur. The society's professional education goal is to communicate information concerning cancer to the medical and allied professions, to stimulate interest in the overall problem, and to assist members of these professions in acquiring the skills necessary for the detection, diagnosis, and treatment of cancer. The society's goal for research is to treat those persons who have cancer and to save others through prevention. The long-range goal of cancer research is the total control of cancer. In July 1969, the society initiated a program to speed basic research findings to the cancer patient through its Clinical Investigation Program. The society's service program has as its goals the provision of earlier and improved treatment of cancer in order to save lives and the continuing evaluation of the end results.

*The American Diabetes Association*

The American Diabetes Association was organized in 1940 by physicians and other scientists concerned with diabetes mellitus and related problems. The association has four goals: first, to create a better understanding of diabetes mellitus among patients and their families; second, to facilitate a free exchange of knowledge and the care of the patient among physicians and other scientists; third, to disseminate accurate information about the importance of early recognition and medical supervision of diabetes to the general public; and fourth, to promote research by universities, hospitals, clinics, and individual scientists.

*The American Heart Association*

In 1924, the American Heart Association was founded by a group of physicians to combat heart disease through scientific and educational activities. In 1948, the association was reorganized as a national voluntary health agency. The program of the association is divided into research, community action, and education. The aim of research is to find the basic causes of cardiovascular disorders and to develop ways of treating and preventing them. The community phase of the program is to encourage early diagnosis and treatment of cardiovascular disorders and to help cardiac patients regain their economic independence. The education phase of the program is (1) to inform physicians about new developments in the care for cardiovascular patients and (2) to give people the facts which will help them protect their hearts.

*The American National Red Cross*

The interval between 1882 and 1914 is considered the formative period of the American National Red Cross. During 1908 and 1909, the First Aid Service was organized to fill the need for a nationwide program of instruction in emergency care of the injured. The Red Cross Public Health Nursing Service originated in 1912. The Life Saving and Water Safety Service was established in 1914. The nutrition program was expanded in courses of Home Hygiene and Care of the Sick during 1939. Safety Services fused together first aid, water safety, and accident prevention in 1947. Services available in local chapters include: (1) services to members of the armed services and their families; (2) services to veterans and their families; (3) disaster services; (4) blood program; (5) nursing programs; (6) safety programs: first aid, small craft safety, water safety; and (7) international rela-

tions. Youth programs are organized for elementary school students through Junior Red Cross; for secondary school students through High School Red Cross; for colleges and universities through College Red Cross.

*The American Social Health Association*

The American Social Health Association was founded in 1912; it then had as its major objectives the control of venereal disease and combatting of prostitution. In 1961, the association added as an objective the eradication of drug abuse. The association has been a leading force in supporting state laws and local ordinances against prostitution. In 1962, the association made a nationwide survey of private physicians to determine the size of the venereal disease problem. The association was the first national voluntary agency to establish a major program of public education on drug abuse, defined as both misuse of drugs and narcotic addiction. Indiscriminate use of barbiturates and amphetamines is considered as much of a problem as narcotic addiction. The association's sex education program has been broadened to include family life education which has been introduced into the curricula of elementary and secondary schools.

*The National Association of Hearing and Speech Agencies*

Formerly the American Hearing Society, the National Association of Hearing and Speech Agencies was established in 1966. The association promotes high standards of professional service and of community organization in identification, diagnosis and assessment, treatment, rehabilitation, education, and research in the various areas of communication disorders. This purpose is carried out by assisting local communities and agencies to establish, maintain, and improve hearing, speech, and language services. Also, the purpose is promoted by conducting the planning, programs, and activities necessary to provide the leadership required for solving the collective problems which occur at the local, state, national, and international levels. NAHSA's programs fall into administrative services, communication, education and training, field services, and special projects.

## The National Association for Mental Health

As a result of a 1909 classic autobiography, *A Mind That Found Itself* by Clifford Beers, the National Committee for Mental Hygiene was founded. In 1950, the National Association for Mental Health was organized. There are four basic programs. The first program emphasizes improved care and treatment for mental hospital patients. Its aim is to see that the mental hospital provides the best available treatment aimed at the patient's earliest possible return to the community. The second program emphasizes aftercare and rehabilitation services. Its aim is to see that persons recovering from mental illness are provided with these services in each community. These services should restore the patient to the fullest physical, mental, social, vocational, and economic usefulness of which he is capable. The third program emphasizes the treatment, education, and special services for the mentally ill child. Its aim is to see that the child is provided with the diagnosis, treatment, education, and rehabilitation that he needs. The fourth program emphasizes community mental health services. Its aim is to see that the mentally ill have a sequence of comprehensive, coordinated, and professionally directed services for diagnosis, treatment and rehabilitation, close to home and suited to the person's needs.

## The National Foundation—March of Dimes

In 1958, the National Foundation for Infantile Paralysis, because it had expanded its program to other fields, changed its name to the National Foundation. When it was founded, in 1937, it realized that an attack on poliomyelitis would succeed if the attack was waged vigorously. Thus, in the intervening years, the NFIP supported investigators who worked in the field of virology as well as those concentrating on polio. With the success of the Salk and Sabin vaccines for polio, the National Foundation focused its attention on a fight against birth defects in 1958. The National Foundation defines "birth defect" as "a structural or metabolic disorder present at birth, whether genetically determined or a result of environmental influence during embryonic or fetal life." Four approaches in the fight against birth defects are used. First, research seeks the causes and cures;

faster, more accurate diagnostic methods; and more effective treatment techniques. Second, patient services include a nationwide network of Birth Defects Centers dedicated to raising the standards of medical care for affected children. Third, professional health education helps to teach and educate many types of health personnel required in the care of children with birth defects. Fourth, public health education provides information to American families to help them help themselves in the prevention of birth defects.

## The National Easter Seal Society for Crippled Children and Adults

The present day Easter Seal movement began in 1919. Each year more than 250,000 crippled children and adults are served by the Easter Seal Society. Rehabilitation and treatment centers; clinics; camps; sheltered workshops; home employment; physical, occupational, and speech therapy programs are operated by state and local affiliates. The national staff includes consultants in care and treatment organization, public education, and research. In 1953, the society established the Easter Seal Research Foundation. The society has an Easter Seal Library, a major source of information about the handicapped and rehabilitation progress. In addition, the society operates the most comprehensive personnel service in the rehabilitation field.

## The National Society for the Prevention of Blindness, Inc.

Founded in 1908, the National Society for the *Prevention* of Blindness works closely with professionals and professional organizations concerned with the preservation of sight and serves as a clearing house on all aspects of eye diseases and disorders and eye health and safety. Some of its major functions are vision screening of children, glaucoma program through education and screening, professional education, promotion of understanding of dyslexia, eye safety campaign, and public education. The vision screening of children has as its prime target the discovery of amblyopia in preschool children. The eye safety campaign aims to reduce eye injuries in industry and schools, from fireworks, and from hazardous toys, as well as encouraging the use of safety lenses in all eyeglasses and sunglasses, and issuing safety glasses to armed forces personnel who wear prescription glasses. Pamphlets, a film library, professional journals, and exhibits are some of its promotional materials for public education.

## The National Tuberculosis and Respiratory Disease Association

In 1892, the Pennsylvania Society for the Prevention of Tuberculosis was founded in order to eradicate tuberculosis. The National Tuberculosis Association was established in 1904, following the pattern of the Pennsylvania Society. Between 1905 and 1912, the National Tuberculosis Association stimulated the organization of state and local associations. In 1907, Emily Bissell held the first American sale of Christmas Seals in Delaware.

In 1967, the National Tuberculosis Association became the National Tuberculosis and Respiratory Disease Association. The NTRDA promotes "programs directed toward the eradication of tuberculosis, the control of respiratory diseases, the elimination of cigarette smoking, the conservation of air, and improvement of community health and welfare."[3] Through education efforts and promotion of legislation, the association calls for special efforts for the benefit of TB-RD patients and their families in deprived areas. In addition, the association's specialists work with comprehensive health planning, regional medical programs, and other federal activities.

Professional education and research have been given a new priority in the NTRDA's program upon the urging of physicians. The number of persons involved in the health care of a respiratory disease patient, the vast amount of unknown information about respiratory disease, and the increase of knowledge about respiratory disease among physicians, nurses, and therapists necessitated the priority of professional education and research.

## Planned Parenthood—World Population

Margaret Sanger opened the first birth control clinic in the United States in 1916.

As a result of her pioneering efforts, the Planned Parenthood Federation of America, Inc., was established in 1961. Planned Parenthood—World Population helps national family planning organizations in more than 100 countries. There are five principal goals·

1. To help make information and effective means of family planning, including contraception and voluntary abortion and sterilization, available and fully accessible to all
2. To educate all American parents to the fact that it serves their own family well-being and the common good to limit family size
3. To stimulate relevant biomedical, socio-economic and demographic research
4. To combat the world population crisis by helping to bring about a population of stable size in an optimum environment in the United States
5. To support the efforts of others to achieve these goals in the United States and throughout the world.[4]

Planned Parenthood—World Population is a charter member of the International Planned Parenthood Federation. This worldwide organization provides technical consultants to the United Nations in its programs concerned with population and family planning.

Among other agencies providing health services are these:

Alcoholics Anonymous
American Foundation for the Blind
American Institute of Family Relations
American Parkinson Disease Association
Arthritis Foundation
Association for Family Living
Epilepsy Foundation of America
Leukemia Society of America, Inc.
Maternity Center Association
Muscular Dystrophy Associations of America, Inc.
Myasthenia Gravis Foundation, Inc.
National Council on Alcoholism
National Cystic Fibrosis Research Foundation
National Hemophilia Foundation
National Kidney Foundation
National Multiple Sclerosis Society
Sex Information and Education Council of the United States (SIECUS)
United Cerebral Palsy Associations, Inc.

[3]Jules Saltman: NTRDA's New Directions for the Seventies. VTRDA Bulletin 56 (May, 1970):5-9.

[4]Planned Parenthood—World Population: The future is now. New York: The Association, 1970.

## Youth Groups

The third group of nonofficial agencies differs in its organization, programs, and purposes, and in the manner in which its functions are related to school and community life. Some of the agencies are found entirely within schools; others act as independent community organizations. Among the youth groups are 4-H Clubs, Future Farmers of America, Future Homemakers of America, Boy Scouts of America, Girl Scouts of America, Boys' Clubs of America, Camp Fire Girls, American Junior Red Cross, Young Women's Christian Association, and Young Men's Christian Association.

## Civic, Social, Service, Child Welfare, and Other Community Agencies

The fourth group of nonofficial agencies includes community service organizations, social clubs, fraternal organizations, recreation agencies, religious associations, labor unions, patriotic organizations, the Salvation Army, United Fund, National Congress of Parents and Teachers, and child welfare associations. These civic, social, service, child welfare, and other community agencies contribute to projects in their local communities or to state or national projects benefiting the health of children and youth. Some of their projects are:

1. Assistance to child-care centers and day nurseries
2. Camps for children with chronic health problems
3. Clinical services for children with eye, ear, nose, and throat problems
4. Dental care and treatment
5. Purchase of mechanical aids for the handicapped
6. Provision of speech teachers
7. Care and treatment of crippled children
8. Organization of school safety patrols
9. Employment of American Red Cross first-aid or water-safety instructors
10. Assistance to school lunch activities
11. Provision of summer and year-round youth recreation
12. Assistance of cancer, glaucoma, diabetes, and cardiac detection clinics

## Foundations

Many foundations have been established to aid in the promotion of the health of this nation. These foundations assist in the preparation of physicians, public health personnel, nurses, school health educators, dentists, nutritionists, and research scientists in the health professions. They provide information on community and personal health problems. They finance research on the cause, prevention, and treatment of diseases. They assist in solving problems of hospital administration and allied health fields.

## Commercial and Semicommercial Groups

This sixth group of nonofficial agencies may be sustaining and associate members of community voluntary health agencies. Single *commercial* organizations may supply to public school personnel health teaching aids, consultant services, and funds for in-service health education. *Semicommercial* groups are composed of many commercial organizations of the same type. The semicommercial groups supply reliable health information and teaching aids as one of their many services. Appendix B contains commercial and semicommercial groups.

## SCHOOL PERSONNEL'S USE OF OFFICIAL AND NONOFFICIAL AGENCIES

The functions of official and nonofficial agencies are broad in scope, and school personnel should be aware of the extent of their activities. If the health agency has a local headquarters, school personnel should visit the agency. The local health agency may be able to furnish printed materials, such as posters, bulletins, pamphlets, graphs, charts, research abstracts, and textbooks for reference use by teachers. In addition, the local agency may be able to provide films, filmstrips, slides, models, exhibits, and other audiovisual aids. The health agency may also provide speakers for certain lessons in health education in the intermediate elementary and secondary school. A field trip to the local health agency may be planned for the class in health education. Consultants from health agencies may assist teachers in preparing health education units, in planning demonstrations and research studies in health education, and in enriching the health education curriculum. Such consultants may serve on the school health council, participate in the school health program, and promote school-community health projects.

In summary, the official and nonofficial agencies can provide school personnel with (1) printed health materials; (2) audiovisual teaching aids for health education; (3) special speakers; (4) locations for field trips; (5) consultants on health education, especially curriculum, demonstrations, and research studies; (6) members of the school health council; (7) participants in the school health program; and (8) resource people for school-community health projects.

## IMPLICATIONS FOR HEALTH EDUCATION

Repeated studies have revealed that young adults are not familiar with the health agencies that promote and protect the health of all Americans. These young adults are not aware of how taxes are used to support the official health agencies and how donations support the activities of voluntary community health agencies. Nor are the services of professional health groups or the commercial groups known to young adults. These agencies protect the consumer, provide funds for research, help to educate the public, and contribute to solving national health problems. In the area of "Community Health Problems," there could be units on the United States Public Health Service, state health department, and nonofficial health agencies. In the area of "Consumer Health," there could be units on the Food and Drug Administration and commercial groups.

## References for Further Study

Beyrer, M. K., Nolte, A. E., and Solleder, M. K.: *A Directory of Selected References and Resources for Health Instruction.* 2nd ed. Minneapolis: Burgess Publishing Company, 1969.

Biddle, W., and Loureide, J.: *Encouraging Community Development.* New York: Holt, Rinehart and Winston, Inc., 1968.

Conant, R. W.: *The Politics of Community Health, National Commission on Health Services.* Washington, D.C.: Public Affairs Press, 1968.

Fry, H. G.: *Education and Manpower for Community Health.* Pittsburgh: The University of Pittsburgh Press, 1967.

Hanlon, J. J.: *Principles of Public Health Administration.* 5th ed. St. Louis: The C. V. Mosby Company, 1969.

Herman, H., and McKay, M. E.: *Community Health Services.* Washington, D.C.: International City Managers' Association, 1968.

Katz, A., and Felton, J., eds.: *Health and the Community.* New York: The Free Press of Glencoe, 1965.

Lecht, L.: *Manpower Needs for National Goals in the 1970s.* New York: Frederick A. Praeger, Inc., 1969.

National Commission on Community Health Services: *Action Planning for Community Health Services.* Washington, D.C.: Public Affairs Press, 1967.

National Institutes of Health: *The Advancement of Knowledge for the Nation's Health.* 1967.

Porterfield, J.: *Community Health: Its Needs and Resources.* New York: Basic Books, Inc., 1966.

Sanders, I. T.: *The Community.* 2nd ed. New York: The Ronald Press, 1966.

Warren, R. L.: *Perspectives on the American Community.* Chicago: Rand McNally and Company, 1966.

# Part IV

*ORGANIZATION AND ADMINISTRATION
OF THE SCHOOL HEALTH PROGRAM*

# Chapter 18

# *RESPONSIBILITIES OF THE SUPERINTENDENT OF SCHOOLS*

## AN INCIDENT

A medium-sized school system wishes to develop a school health program. Problems have arisen with the organization and administration of the school health program. A well-organized and successfully functioning health department is found within the community. The local medical officer, who administers the health department, has proposed that the school health program be completely under his control. The superintendent of schools and board of education have rejected this proposal because they feel that the health needs of elementary and secondary school students can best be served by placing the administration of the school health program with the school superintendent.

Each board of education should determine the extent of health problems among elementary and secondary school students and school personnel and the relation of these problems to the health problems of the entire community. In order to discover these problems, the medical officer of the community, the school superintendent, and the health coordinator have to examine many types of information from numerous sources. In addition, the following questions will be asked: Shall a school health program consist of school health services, healthful school living, and health education? Who supplies funds for the total program? Do the local public schools or the local health department have facilities for the total program? With whom do state education departments work? Who has the equipment and supplies for the total program? Who employs the teachers and the

supervisor of health education? Do the local public schools or the local health department provide regularly scheduled health education, for students of the ages 6 through 18, meeting requirements of state education departments?

Byrd[1] and Mayshark and Shaw[2] have suggested different concepts for the organization and administration of the school health program. Byrd indicates that if the school administrator accepts that the fundamental purpose of the school is to educate the pupil, then, the school health program must be primarily educational. Also, an effective and well-functioning school health program is dependent upon community cooperation.

Mayshark and Shaw have given reasons for joint administration of the school health program by the board of education and the board of health. First, dual administration combines the specialities of educational method and preventive medicine to serve the student most effectively. Second, joint administration fosters cooperation between teachers and public health personnel. Third, the local health department and public schools share the responsibility for healthful school living. Fourth, public health personnel have better rapport with teachers when the public health personnel are seen as members of the school staff. Fifth, curriculum revision requires the experience and advice of public health personnel as well as teachers. Although joint administration may be ideal, most school

[1]Oliver E. Byrd: *School Health Administration*. Philadelphia: W. B. Saunders Company, 1964, pp. 3-9.
[2]Cyrus Mayshark and Donald D. Shaw: *Administration of School Health Programs*. St. Louis: The C. V. Mosby Company, 1967, pp. 81-99.

health programs, however, are controlled by local boards of education.

## BOARD OF EDUCATION

The legal control of the total school health program is placed with the local board of education, which delegates the responsibility for the program to the superintendent of schools. Funds for the three parts of the school health program are designated in the board of education budget. These funds may provide the facilities, equipment, and supplies of the program as well as the salaries of school health services personnel. School health programs can be developed within school systems of all sizes. In each instance, the local board of education relies on the school superintendent for his knowledge, interest, and leadership in developing the total school health program.

## SUPERINTENDENT OF SCHOOLS

It is possible that a school system may have no professionally prepared teacher of health education and no administrative or supervisory personnel familiar with the total school health program. Also, it is possible that the school nurse employed by the board of education may have little understanding of her functions in school health services. Thus the development of the total school health program depends on the school superintendent. Some of his general functions in organizing and administering the school health program will be mentioned.

### Total Administrative Control

The superintendent of schools must have total administrative control over school health services, healthful school living, and health education. Even in school systems with full-time school physicians, the superintendent of schools has total administrative control of the school health program. The Joint Committee on Health Problems in Education of the NEA and the AMA and the American Association of School Administrators have emphasized this vital role of the school superintendent.[3]

[3]American Association of School Administrators: *Health in Schools.* (Twentieth Yearbook) Washington, D.C.: National Education Association, 1951.

In school systems with a full-time school physician, the superintendent of schools maintains total administrative control over the physician's functions. At no time may the physician assume the functions of the school superintendent in the school health program.

Regardless of the number of nurses employed by the local board of education, the school superintendent has total administrative control over all functions of school nurses. If there is a director or supervisor of school nurses, she is responsible to the school superintendent for all of nursing activities in school health services.

Dental hygienists, speech therapists, part-time dental specialists, psychiatrists, or other health services personnel must be aware that the superintendent of schools has total administrative control of the school health program. No member of the health professions can assume that he has been delegated the responsibilities of the superintendent of schools by the local board of education.

### Approval of Policies and Procedures

The superintendent of schools must approve all policies and procedures affecting the total school health program. Even if the school superintendent delegates certain responsibilities for the school health program to the health coordinator or supervisor of health education, every policy and procedure of the total program should be known to the superintendent. The complexity and scope of the total health program necessitate the superintendent's approval. These policies and procedures can affect every phase of school health services, healthful school living, and health education. Procedures for exclusion of a pupil with communicable diseases, readmission of a pupil following recovery from communicable diseases, required immunizations, and emergency care should be in written form and approved by the local board of education and the superintendent of schools.

### Supervision of Health Education

One of the recommendations for improved health education in the elementary and secondary schools from the School Health Education Study was to provide better supervision of health education.[4] With the increasing demands for health education in elementary and secondary schools, the wise superintendent will employ professionally prepared teachers of health education with supervisory credentials. In-service health education can be effectively conducted only by teachers whose major preparation has been school health education and whose teaching experiences have been in the same field. Because many elementary and secondary school health education textbooks are *not* adequate for proper instruction in health education, elementary and secondary school teachers need assistance in providing students with sound health education. Misconceptions and out-of-date information about health and poor planning of health education courses have created curriculum problems needing the assistance of professionally prepared teachers of health education.

The supervisor of health education may find that teachers do not attempt to discover the pupil's health needs and interests as a basis for determining the health education content. The supervisor may find that teachers show little variation in teaching methods and in the use of materials of instruction. The subject matter may be out of date and meaningless, and there may be no evaluation of health education. Many elementary teachers and secondary teachers assigned to teach health education have accepted the topics in textbooks without realizing that the topics may be duplicated, are outdated, and have little influence on the pupil's health practices, attitudes, interests, and knowledge. The functions of the supervisor of health education will be discussed more fully in Chapter 19.

## Funds

In order to have the best financial management of the school health program, the superintendent of schools might consider program budgeting, performance budgeting, and program evaluation and review technique (PERT). Some of these budget-

[4]School Health Education Study: *Summary Report of a Nationwide Study of Health Instruction in the Public Schools.* Washington, D.C.: The Study, 1964, pp. 40-45.

ing and accounting systems will be mentioned in Chapter 20. Current expenses of the school health program and financial demands of emergency situations need to be included. Travel expenses of school nurses, other health services personnel, and the supervisor of health education must be considered. There should be funds to buy vision and hearing screening devices, nurses' and American Red Cross first-aid supplies, and printed forms for records of the pupil's health status. School lunch activities will also have a budget to show outlay of expenses and different sources of funds. Costs of all instructional materials needed in elementary and secondary school health education must be budgeted.

## Facilities

Many types of facilities are needed for school health services, healthful school living, and health education. A health service unit may be found within a modern school building. In secondary schools, there should be health teaching laboratories for teacher demonstrations, pupil practice sessions, experiments, and student projects. School lunchrooms must have specific facilities in order to provide a Type A lunch or a nutritious noonday meal. A safe and healthful school environment is dependent on the school's facilities. Further information regarding facilities will be included in Chapter 20.

## Equipment and Supplies

The school health program requires not only facilities but also equipment and supplies. The budget of the local board of education must include funds to purchase equipment and supplies needed in school health services, healthful school living, and health education. A wise superintendent of schools may delegate to the supervisor of health education the responsibility of compiling the budget information with details about equipment and supplies needed in the health program. Inventories and requisitions of equipment and supplies must include health education as well as school health services. Specific equipment and supplies needed within the school health program will be discussed in Chapter 20.

## Legal Regulations

The public school health program is affected by many types of legal regulations. First, there are statewide regulations established by state boards of education and adopted by state legislatures. Second, there are the regulations of the local boards of education. Third, there exist statewide requirements established by state boards of health and adopted by state legislatures. Fourth, local health departments may enact regulations affecting the health of all public school pupils and personnel employed by local boards of education. Fifth, there are federal laws, such as Public Law 396—National School Lunch Act.

Legal regulations affecting the public school health program may be mandatory or permissive. An example of a mandatory regulation established by state boards of *health* is the requirement for certain immunizations as a prerequisite for attendance at school. New York has a public health law requiring immunization for smallpox, polio, and measles of all school children. Despite objections to this law, numerous court decisions have upheld the constitutionality of this public health law.[5] An example of a mandatory statewide regulation found in *education* statutes is the Pennsylvania statute which authorizes school authorities to exclude a pupil not vaccinated against smallpox. Permissive statutory provisions for examinations of school children are found in New Jersey. Legislation in New Jersey imposes the duty upon boards of education to determine the existence of "physical defects." However, each local board of education may determine which examinations shall be used.[6] Most educators prefer permissive legislation.

Statewide or local regulations that affect the public school health program vary from state to state and from community to community, but these legal regulations most often involve the following:

1. Administration of the school health program

2. Funds for the program
3. Construction of school buildings
4. Heating and ventilation, lighting, water supply, sewage disposal, plumbing, garbage and waste disposal, etc.
5. Safety regulations against fire and accident hazards
6. Medical examinations and diagnostic procedures and laboratory tests of all school employees
7. Certification requirements of secondary school teachers of health education and supervisors of health education
8. Health education preparation of elementary and secondary teachers as a prerequisite for provisional teacher certification
9. Immunizations of school children
10. Exclusion of pupils with communicable diseases from elementary and secondary schools
11. Readmission of pupils recovered from communicable diseases to the elementary and secondary schools
12. Tuberculosis screening of school children
13. Medical examinations of pupils
14. Medical treatment of pupils
15. Health records of pupils and school employees
16. Parents' being notified of child's chronic health condition
17. Health requirements of food workers in the school lunchroom
18. Sanitation of food preparation and serving and of school lunchroom facilities and equipment
19. Health education in elementary and secondary schools including:
    a. Alcohol, narcotics, and tobacco
    b. Physiology and hygiene
    c. Fire prevention and safety education
    d. Nutrition, etc.
20. Professional preparation, standards for employment, and functions of registered nurses, physicians, dentists, dental hygienists, and other health services personnel employed by local boards of education
21. School health councils
22. School bus transportation
23. Sick leave
24. Retirement plans of school employees
25. Educational television

Many of the regulations affecting the public school health program are widely accepted. Forty-nine of the 50 states have statutes requiring instruction about the use of alcohol and narcotics. With the increase of drug abuse among public school pupils, many state legislatures have recently passed additional requirements pertaining

[5]Dean F. Miller: Recent litigations relating to school health services. *J. School Health 40* (December, 1970):526.
[6]Nathan Hershey: Compulsory personal health measure legislation. *Public Health Report 84* (April, 1969):341.

to teaching about drug abuse. These requirements are not only general in their demands for basic information about drug use and abuse to be taught but also specific in requirements about time allotment, grade level, preparation of curriculum materials, and in-service education.

Student activists who deviate from the norm in dress, grooming, and hair style have been involved in court decisions. Considered as personal symbols of protest, these actions have not always been upheld by the courts. Thus, local boards of education have developed dress codes since, in most cases, the local board of education has the right to be the arbiter of student conduct.[7]

## Elementary and Secondary School Health Education

In their willingness to cooperate with local groups and in the absence of well-planned health education, school superintendents have scheduled lectures or mandatory units on drug abuse, smoking, alcoholism, venereal diseases, and sex education. These sporadic efforts are ineffective. The School Health Division, American Association for Health, Physical Education and Recreation has recommended there be a *"unified approach to health teaching— that is, a planned, sequential curriculum in health education throughout the school years."* Also, it has recommended that curriculum development in health education be undertaken to identify the content, learning activities, and evaluation of health education and that, in addition, those assigned to teach health education be specifically prepared in health education.[8]

At the 97th Annual Meeting of the American Public Health Association, the Governing Council passed a resolution supporting family life and sex education in school systems. In addition, the resolution pointed out the need for sound preparation of teachers in family life and sex education.[9]

Among the 1970 resolutions of the Governing Council of the American School Health Association was one urging the development of curriculum guides for comprehensive health education in the schools. The resolution indicated that curriculum guides can make significant contributions to the quality of health education.[10]

Too often, unfortunately, curriculum guides in health education ignore the *real* health problems of elementary and secondary school students, isolate health education from the total school health program, and stress noncontroversial topics. The attitudes of the committee preparing curriculum guides seem to be that "anything is better than nothing." The guides may be a hodge-podge of topics with little consideration for the *real* health problems of students. References in these poor curriculum guides often have no publishers, no dates of publication, and no edition; sources of printed materials are not given; depth of content is a rarity; controversial units or areas are ignored. One might ask where there is a secondary school curriculum guide in health education which has an in-depth outline of the subject matter of suicide, contraception, abortion, quackery, fluoridation of water supplies, water and air pollution, and health insurance?

## Noonday School Meals

The superintendent of schools should be aware of the values of sound dietary habits among pupils and school personnel. Many of these dietary habits are promoted by the noonday school meals. With the enactment of the National School Lunch Act and supplemental legislation, elementary and secondary schools may receive assistance from the federal government through state education departments. The assistance may be funds and surplus foods, such as milk and milk products, fruits and vegetables, meat, flour, and cereal grains. The noonday school meal, breakfast, and supplementary feeding provide many advantages to the pupil who has undergone recent surgery, has had prolonged illness, and has nutritional deficiencies. Further advantages of school nutrition were discussed in Chapter 10.

[7]Floyd G. Delon: The law and student activism in the public schools. *Educational Horizons—The Official Publication of Pi Lambda Theta 49* (Winter, 1970-71):45.
[8]A unified approach to health teaching—AAHPER position statement. *J. School Health 41* (April, 1971):171.
[9]Resolutions—Sex education in school systems. *Amer. J. Public Health and the Nation's Health 60* (January, 1970):186.

[10]1970 resolutions adopted by the Governing Council, the American School Health Association. *J. School Health 41* (January, 1971):22-23.

## Public Relations

The school health program should be accepted by the superintendent as an integral part of the school system's public relations. A diversity of school and community contacts exists within the school health program. The supervisor of health education and school nurses may desire uniform procedures when working with official and nonofficial health agencies.

Medical and dental examinations by family physicians and dentists necessitate pupil absence from school for appointments. How well do the public relations procedures handle these absences? Home visits by the school nurse may uncover the need for community assistance to a family. What are the methods of informing community agencies of a problem, and to what extent may the public schools work with these agencies?

Controversial issues can occur in school health services and health education. Teacher observations of possible pupil health difficulties create many questions among parents. Notices sent to parents giving the results of vision and hearing screening and tuberculin testing can create parental anxiety. Emergency care procedures and exclusion of a pupil with a communicable disease need to be understood and accepted by parents. Possible controversy caused by certain areas or units in health education needs to be ameliorated by the school system's public relations. It is possible that parents can misinterpret the need for instruction about family life and sex education, drug use and abuse, alcoholism, mental illness, suicide, venereal diseases, immunizations, quackery, fluoridation of water supplies, and other health education areas and units. The acceptance of health education in elementary and secondary schools by the community depends on the school superintendent's public relations policies and procedures.

There is need for specific public relations procedures appropriate to the entire school health program, for all school personnel, and for the entire year. It is possible that these public relations will be flexible, broad in scope, and penetrate into every part of the total school health program.

## Liaison Agent

Most superintendents of schools are aware that they or a professionally prepared teacher or supervisor of health education must serve as a liaison agent between the school and the community. In the school health program, the liaison agent has to interpret the problems and gain the cooperation of the professional health services personnel in the community and the school instructional staffs. School health concepts are held by family physicians and dentists, professional personnel in local health departments, workers in nonofficial health agencies, and citizens with no children in the public schools. Suggestions may be given by family physicians. These suggestions may need interpretation, however, for without interpretation they may go unheeded. Modern health education in elementary and secondary schools needs considerable explanation because of the outdated concepts of health education as "physiology and hygiene" still held by some persons in the community.

## In-Service Health Education

Because our teacher education institutions have generally not permitted sufficient time for the preparation of elementary and secondary school teachers for their functions in the school health program, continuous in-service health education must be provided. The in-service health education will serve to make each teacher aware of the program of school health services, healthful school living, and health education. Particularly, health education will demand a great deal of in-service education. Supervisors of health education spend the greater part of their time providing elementary and secondary school teachers with the subject matter of health education. Much of the in-service education by the supervisor is carried out in a series of direct contacts with the individual teacher. In addition, workshops held during the school year can focus attention on the overall curriculum planning of health education, grades K through 12. Since the subject matter of health education is changing from day to day, the individual teacher depends on the professionally prepared supervisor of health education to keep him informed.

In-service health education is usually requested by school nurses to assist them in providing school health services. Workshops, institutes, and seminars can be organized to offer the school nurse up-to-date information on many health problems of children and youth. It is of vital importance that the school nurse be well informed about the latest techniques of tuberculin testing, recognition of the emotionally disturbed child, types of children in special education, assistance from community official and nonofficial health agencies, and specific community health problems. Supervisors of health education should encourage school nurses to attend workshops in health education planned for teachers.

## Cooperation with the Local Health Department

The superintendent of schools should cooperate with the local medical officer and public health personnel in measures devised to control disease. There should be procedures for the exclusion of the pupil with a communicable disease and for the readmission of the pupil following recovery. Cases of impetigo, ringworm, measles, influenza, mumps, chicken pox, whooping cough, and other diseases should be reported to the local health department. Cooperation with the local health department can be secured when the school takes measures for controlling disease by proper disposal of solid wastes and sewage; by use of purified drinking water; and by other sanitation procedures. Adequate tuberculin testing, immunizations for entrance into local public schools, and cooperative procedures among school and public health nurses can foster excellent relations with the local health department.

## School Health Council

A resolution adopted by the Joint Committee on Health Problems in Education of the NEA and the AMA in 1971 recommended that "component parts of a health program in a school system be coordinated by an advisory school health council consisting of representatives of the administration, instructional staff, students, parents,

employees, and the health disciplines."[11] The school superintendent should be an active member or appoint an administrative official to represent him on the school health council. The supervisor of health education may be delegated this responsibility by the school superintendent. School health councils assist in solving school health problems that affect pupils and school personnel. If there is no professionally prepared teacher or supervisor of health education, the school superintendent should participate actively in the council's actions. Because the health council draws its membership from both the school and the community, community health problems can be brought to the attention of the school superintendent. In addition, the superintendent can discover community personnel interested in school health. Chapter 21 will present more information concerning school health councils.

## Evaluation of the Program

The superintendent of schools must evaluate the school health program for effectiveness and growth. School health services, healthful school living, and health education should be evaluated. Many questions can be asked about the total school health program.

Evaluation will determine the effectiveness of leadership in the total program. Does the leadership attempt to coordinate school health services with health education? Does the superintendent clarify the purposes of the total school health program? Does the leadership promote teamwork among school and community personnel?

The need for in-service health education and professionally prepared teachers and supervisors of health education will be disclosed through evaluation of the school health program. Does health education contribute to the pupil's health attitudes, practices, interests, and knowledge? Is there a planned health education curriculum based on the pupils' health needs and interests

[11]Resolutions adopted by the Joint Committee on Health Problems in Education of the National Education Association and the American Medical Association, Washington, D.C., February 13-16, 1971. *School Health Review* 2 (April, 1971):26.

for grades 1 through 12? Is the subject matter of health education current and valid? What controversial health education units are taught? Are there planned facilities for health education in the secondary schools?

In 1965, an investigation of selected Indiana public high schools was conducted for the purpose of evaluating the health programs in these schools. High schools from eight areas of the state and with three different classifications of student enrollment were selected. Seventeen high schools with fewer than 200 students, seventeen with enrollments between 200 and 499 students, and eighteen with enrollments of 500 or more students were included. A survey instrument of four parts: (1) administration of the school health program; (2) healthful school living; (3) health education; and (4) school health services was used. Some of the findings of the evaluation:

1. In all 52 high schools, the administration of the school health program ranged from 5 to 44.6% of possible achievement, indicating a need for improvement in the administration of the school health program.
2. Health councils were practically non-existent.
3. Of the parts of the school health program, health education ranked lowest in achievement. There was little evidence of curriculum planning. The quality of the health education curriculum was judged to be poor.
4. Physical educators taught 90% of the health education classes.
5. Schools with small enrollments had inadequate equipment, facilities, and materials of instruction for health education.
6. In school health services, procedures for emergency care were inadequate. Communicable disease control, follow-through by the school nurse, and screening examinations ranked first,

second, and third. Tuberculin tests were given in all schools.
7. In healthful school living, the environmental factors, school nutrition, and school day needed vast improvement. Disaster drills were lacking.

Principals of the 52 high schools indicated that they understood the concept of the school health program. However, these principals achieved only 28.2% of their functions in the administration of the school health program.[12]

## References for Further Study

American Association for Health, Physical Education and Recreation: *Approaches to Problems of Public School Administration in Health, Physical Education and Recreation.* Washington, D.C.: The Association, 1969.

Bolmeier, E.: *The School in the Legal Structure.* Cincinnati: The W. H. Anderson Company, 1968.

Bucher, C.: *Administration of Health and Physical Education Programs.* St. Louis: The C. V. Mosby Company, 1971.

———: *Administration of School and College Health and Physical Education Programs.* 4th ed. St. Louis: The C. V. Mosby Company, 1967.

Gauerke, W.: *What Education Should Know About School Laws.* Englewood Cliffs, N.J.: Prentice-Hall, Inc., 1968.

Hanlon, J., and McHose, E.: *Design for Health: School and Community.* 2nd ed. Philadelphia: Lea & Febiger, 1971.

Hanlon, J.: *Principles of Public Health Administration.* 5th ed. St. Louis: The C. V. Mosby Company, 1969.

Johnson, G.: *Education Law.* East Lansing: Michigan State University Press, 1969.

Jones, J.: *School Public Relations.* New York: Center for Applied Research in Education, 1966.

Leibee, H.: *Tort Liability for Injuries to Pupils.* Ann Arbor, Mich.: Campus Publishers, 1966.

Nolte, M.: *Guide to School Law.* West Nyack, N.Y.: Parker Publishing Company, 1969.

Seaton, D., Stack, H., and Loft, B.: *Administration and Supervision of Safety Education.* New York: Macmillan Company, 1968.

*Yearbook of School Law, 1970.* Danville, Ill.: The Interstate Printers and Publishers, 1971.

[12]Donald J. Ludwig: Evaluation of school health programs in selected Indiana public high schools. Presented before the Research Council, American School Health Association, Chicago, October 17, 1965.

# Chapter 19

# SCHOOL AND COMMUNITY PERSONNEL IN THE HEALTH PROGRAM

## AN INCIDENT

A state board of education has recommended that each school superintendent develop a total school health program: school health services, healthful school living, and health education. A health coordinator is to work with the school superintendent in developing the school health program. A consultant or supervisor of health education is to provide the in-service health education for elementary school classroom teachers and for those assigned to teach health education in the secondary schools. Two semesters of regularly scheduled health education are to be taught in the junior or middle school and two semesters of regularly scheduled health education in the senior high school. At least 200 minutes a week of health education are to be provided, through direct instruction, in the elementary schools. These recommendations are the result of studies of the health problems of elementary and secondary school students.

Teamwork is necessary among school and community personnel to develop the total school health program. Each person should understand his own functions and their importance. Many family physicians and dentists will be involved in the program. Parents are team members, and pupils and school personnel share in the development of the program. Many community workers contribute to the health program in schools. When a health coordinator is employed, he brings together the functions of school and community personnel to develop the health program. Where there is no health coordinator, the school superintendent has the task of de-

veloping teamwork. Without teamwork, the school health program degenerates to a few unrelated, fragmentary actions of spasmodic concern to schools and communities.

## HEALTH EDUCATION PERSONNEL

Various health education personnel may participate in the development of school health program. These may be the school health educator or teacher of health education in the secondary schools, consultant or supervisor of health education, health coordinator, community health educator, and public health educator.

### School Health Educator or Teacher of Health Education

The main function of a school health educator is to teach the regularly scheduled health education courses in secondary school. In addition, he assists the health coordinator to develop the school health program in the secondary school where he teaches. In small school systems, it is possible that the school health educator may also perform some of the functions of the health coordinator if there is no health coordinator.

As early as 1896, the preparation of a teacher of health education was recognized as necessary for the secondary schools. At that time, school hygienists were being prepared in Europe, but teachers of health education were nonexistent in the United States.[1] Professional societies, voluntary health agencies, and national conferences

[1]Richard K. Means: *A History of Health Education in the United States.* Philadelphia: Lea & Febiger, 1962, pp. 61-62.

recommended the need for teachers of health education. By 1924, four states had certification requirements for health education teachers in the secondary schools.[2] However, not until 1931 and 1937, was the preparation of teachers of health education dealt with extensively at the two National Conferences on College Hygiene.[3] Within the period of 1937 to 1947, health education as a single subject-matter field became an essential part of the school curriculum. Abernathy[4] has summarized the numerous conferences and committee actions taken to promote the preparation of teachers of health education from 1947 to 1967. In 1949, only five states certified teachers of secondary school health education, but by 1970, 22 states had certification requirements. The school health program as a course of study was either required or suggested for potential health educators in eight states.[5]

The preparation of the school health educator falls into four groups. The first group provides a broad preparation in the natural and behavioral sciences, in addition to other academic requirements. Anatomy, physiology, microbiology, and chemistry are among the natural sciences and sociology, psychology, and anthropology are among the behavioral sciences most often studied. The second group includes the *specialized curriculum* in *health education:*

1. School health program
2. Nutrition
3. Safety education
4. Community health
5. Disease prevention and chronic health conditions
6. Family life and sex education
7. Drug abuse, narcotic addiction, smoking, and misuse of alcoholic beverages
8. Health education curriculum and evaluation

The third group consists of the professional education courses of study: growth and development, adolescent psychology, secondary school organization, methods and materials in health education, and student teaching in health education.[6] The fourth group is preparation for a second teaching field commonly taught in the secondary schools, of at least 24 semester hours. Biology may be the second teaching field.

At the National Professional Preparation Conference in 1962, a statement was given regarding the goals of the specialized curriculum in health education. Each professionally prepared teacher should:

Prepare the student to understand and know how to determine and utilize health needs and interests of children and youth in the curriculum development.

Enable the student to understand the total school health program and the responsibilities of various school and community personnel involved, as well as to develop the necessary skills to perform his responsibilities.

Give the student a thorough comprehension of the content areas included in the scope of health instruction and ways of organizing the content for teaching and learning experiences.

Provide for the development of skills in the use of a variety of teaching methods and materials that motivate the learner to translate knowledge into desirable health behavior.

Provide the student with a knowledge of the community resources that contribute to health and knowledge of how to use these resources. . . .

Develop an understanding of the teacher's role in maintaining and promoting pupil health and safety, including the development of skill in pupil health appraisal procedures.[7]

During the freshman and sophomore years of the preservice preparation, the program director with the assistance of other faculty members should regularly observe, compile data about, and confer

[2]U.S. Office of Education: *Requirements by State Departments of Education for Teachers and Supervisors of Physical Education and Health Education in Elementary and Secondary Schools.* Circular #35. Washington, D.C.: U.S. Office of Education, 1924, pp. 1-16.

[3]Means, *op. cit.*, p. 277.

[4]Ruth Abernathy: Teacher preparation in health education, yesterday, today, and tomorrow. *School Health Review 1* (February, 1970):26-35.

[5]Jessie Helen Haag: Comparisons on the preparation of health education teachers in the United States: 1949-1970. *Inter. J. Health Education 13* (#4):163-168.

[6]Recommended standards and guidelines, teacher preparation in health education. *J. Health, Physical Education and Recreation 40* (February, 1969):31-38.

[7]American Association for Health, Physical Education and Recreation: *National Conference for the Professional Preparation in Health Education, Physical Education and Recreation Education.* Washington, D.C. The Association, 1962, p. 42.

with the future school health educator. Program directors of the undergraduate preparation of the school health educator should have the same preparation as the undergraduate and have experiences teaching regularly scheduled health education in the secondary schools. Some of the personal qualities of the school health educator are "self-direction, the ability to communicate, sound personal health, self-renewal with a commitment to continued education, the ability to stimulate others to progressive learning and excellence, and self-actualization."[8]

The school health educator must be able to interpret, explain, and clarify the vast amount of information related to the health problems of secondary school youth and their communities. He must be a scholar who is sensitive to a changing society. His enthusiasm and interest in health education are shown by his thoroughness of preparation and creativity in teaching. He cannot permit himself to get bogged down in the technology of educational methods and materials, thus forgetting the humanness of each student.

## Consultant or Supervisor of Health Education

One of the problems of health education cited by school administrators in the School Health Education Study was the lack of consultative and supervisory services.[9] Among the recommendations of the School Health Education Study was

A person with specialized preparation in health education and who possesses other desirable attributes should be designated to assume responsibility in each school system for the overall coordination of the health instruction program and to provide supervisory assistance. . . .

In-service opportunities [should be made] available to teachers for strengthening and expanding their professional competencies in health education.[10]

These tasks require that the consultant or supervisor of health education has the equivalent of the undergraduate preparation of the school health educator or teacher of health education. In addition, the consultant or supervisor must complete graduate studies in school health education beyond the bachelor's degree. Areas of the graduate program in the specialized school health education core include research and research techniques in school health education and health-related fields; supervision of health education; curriculum problems in health education; in-depth subject-matter concentration: consumer health, mental health, international health, public health, drug abuse, and nutrition; and internship as a consultant or supervisor of health education. Most likely the consultant or supervisor will have to complete certain other graduate requirements for a supervisory certificate. In addition, upper division or graduate courses should be taken in sociology, psychology, anthropology, microbiology, anatomy, physiology, and other health-related sciences. The program director for the graduate studies should possess an earned doctorate with graduate preparation similar to that required of the consultant or supervisor of health education. The program director should have had experiences as a consultant or supervisor of health education or as a teacher of regularly scheduled health education in secondary schools.

The *main* function of the consultant or supervisor of health education is to strengthen and improve the health education curriculum, K through 12. The consultant or supervisor of health education works with all elementary school classroom teachers, junior or middle school teachers assigned to teach health education, and those assigned to teach health education courses in the senior high schools, such as physical education teachers. Usually, the consultant or supervisor focuses his services on those teachers with little or no preparation and understanding of health education. Even though in-service health education may be given to groups of teachers, often it is directed individually to one teacher needing and requesting help in teaching health education. Some of the *specific* functions of the consultant or supervisor of health education are

[8]Recommended standards & guidelines, teacher preparation in health education: *op. cit.*, p. 37.

[9]School Health Education Study: *Summary Report of a Nationwide Study of Health Instruction in the Public Schools, 1961-1963.* Washington, D.C.: The Study, 1964, p. 12.

[10]*Ibid.*, pp. 14-15.

1. assisting teachers in their discovery of health problems of students
2. assisting teachers in their discovery of community health problems and the means to eradicate the problems
3. assisting teachers in obtaining valid health information from official and non-official health agencies
4. developing curriculum guides, K through 12, in health education with teachers and students cooperating
5. demonstrating new methods of health instruction; e.g., critical incidence technique
6. assisting teachers in the evaluation of materials of health instruction; e.g., film-strips on drug abuse
7. assisting teachers in developing teacher resource units and lesson plans in health education
8. being continuously informed about the in-depth content of the thirteen areas of health education so that teachers can have a dependable source of information
9. assisting teachers in the construction of teacher-made health knowledge tests and measuring devices for health attitudes, practices, and interests
10. assisting teachers and librarians in developing and evaluating library materials in health education useful to both students and teachers
11. assisting principals in scheduling health education
12. securing necessary teaching facilities for health education with adequate equipment in each classroom or laboratory
13. assisting principals in assigning teachers who are enthusiastic and eager to learn about health education to junior or middle schools and high schools
14. conducting research projects to improve the content, methods, and materials of health education, K through 12
15. evaluating the health education curriculum, K through 12, with the assistance of students, teachers, principals, and parents
16. developing procedures for teaching controversial areas or units in health education

The consultant or supervisor of health education can prevent the pitfalls of the controversial areas or units by developing procedures as given in Chapter 13. Careful orientation must be given to the school superintendent and principals, parents, and instructional personnel so they understand the content and the purposes of these areas and units. Not only the content but also the methods and materials of instruction and parental responsibilities must be included in the orientation procedures.

## Health Coordinator

The *main* function of the health coordinator is to develop a total school health program. He must bring together the parts of the program within a school building and within a school system. The report of the School Health Education Study stated "better articulation of school health services with the health instruction program is needed . . . [and] some type of organizational framework that will assure continuity in dealing with school health problems should be considered."[11]

These tasks require that the health coordinator have undergraduate and graduate preparation in school health education. The graduate program should include research and research techniques in school health education and health-related fields; organization and administration of the school health program; curriculum problems in health education; problems in the school health program: health counseling, legal liability, and public relations; school-community health programs; school and community health councils; and internship as a health coordinator. Most likely the health coordinator will also have to complete certain graduate requirements in educational administration. In addition, upper division or graduate courses should be taken in sociology, psychology, business administration, and journalism. The program director for the graduate studies should possess an earned doctorate with graduate preparation similar to that required of the health coordinator. The program director should have had experiences as a health coordinator or as a teacher of regularly scheduled health education in secondary schools.

The *specific* functions of the health coordinator are that he

1. works with the superintendent of schools in the organization and administration of the school health program
2. serves as a liaison agent between the school personnel and the professional health services and public health personnel

[11]*Ibid.*

3. coordinates school health services with healthful school living and health education
4. establishes and guides school health councils
5. works with health services personnel employed by the board of education in developing school health services
6. works with school principals in maintaining a healthful and safe school environment, adequate school nutrition, and promotion of the health of school personnel
7. assists in the development of public relations necessary for the school health program
8. coordinates the services of community workers in the school health program
9. reports to the superintendent of schools the strengths and weaknesses of the total school health program in specific school buildings and in all schools of that school system
10. evaluates the total school health program on a day-to-day basis

Among the 1971 Resolutions of the Joint Committee on Health Problems in Education of the NEA and AMA was one dealing with accountability in school health. It stated:

WHEREAS, Teachers are being asked to account for their instructional efforts in terms of preconceived goals, specific pupil performances, and other behavioral changes, therefore be it RESOLVED, that the total school health program be directed to give more attention to student behavioral change through such evaluations as parent, teacher, peer interviews and case studies, and review of school records.[12]

This resolution might be fulfilled if a health coordinator was employed by the board of education.

## Community Health Educator

A community health educator may be employed by a voluntary health agency, a local or state health department, a commercial or semicommercial agency, a professional society, or a college. The School Health Education Study[13] listed

### Degree Offered

| Bachelor's | Master's | Doctoral |
|---|---|---|
| 21a | 14a | 3a |
| 8b | 6b | 3b |

a Institutions offering specialization in community health education
b Institutions in process of development of community health education programs

To compare the number of institutions preparing the community health educator to the number preparing the school health educator:[14]

### Degree Offered

| Bachelor's | Master's | Doctoral |
|---|---|---|
| 21c | 14c | 3c |
| 87d | 73d | 30d |

c Institutions—community health education
d Institutions—school health education

At least 104 institutions offered some undergraduate and graduate preparation in school health education in 1970. At the same time, 35 institutions were in the process of developing programs for preparation in school health education.[15]

Since the preparation of the community health educator varies from one institution to another, the best way to obtain information about preparation is to write directly to the institution. A listing of the institutions, their addresses, degree programs, and persons in charge of the program was given by the School Health Education Study.

## Public Health Educator

Public health educators are employed by local and state health departments, the United States Public Health Service, and institutions preparing public health personnel. The School Health Education Study listed 11 institutions accredited to prepare public health educators of the 18 institutions accredited in public health by the American Public Health Association.[16]

[12]Resolutions adopted by the Joint Committee on Health Problems in Education of the National Education Association and the American Medical Association, Washington, D.C., February 13-16, 1971. *School Health Review 2* (April, 1971):26.

[13]School Health Education Study: *Institutions Offering Programs of Specialization in Health Education for Schools, Colleges, Communities at the Undergraduate and Graduate Levels and Schools of Public Health.* Washington, D.C.: The Study, 1970, pp. 46-49, 56-58.
[14]*Ibid.*, pp. 15-20.
[15]*Ibid.*, pp. 50-55.
[16]*Ibid.*, pp. 59-60.

The specialized preparation of the public health educator usually takes place at the graduate level. Some of the applicable graduate studies are introduction to public health, problems in health education, public health problems, principles of epidemiology, school health education, principles of environmental health, community organization in health education, specialized field work in public health education, and related fields in health education.

## ELEMENTARY SCHOOL CLASSROOM TEACHER

The teacher most likely to influence the health practices, attitudes, and interests of pupils is the elementary school classroom teacher; too often, however, he may not be aware of the health problems of children and how he can determine what those problems are through the school health program. Often in the preservice preparation, the elementary teacher has had no opportunity to learn of the different types of health appraisal, ways to prevent and control diseases, recognition of chronic health conditions, procedures for emergency care, follow-through by the school nurse, and changes occurring during mixed dentition. In addition, the teacher does not know that health education should be based upon a discovery of the health problems of the child. The methods of discovering these problems from school health services and healthful school living are unknown to many teachers. Among school personnel who have seen how little teachers recognize the health problems of elementary school children is the school nurse.

Irma Fricke, Director of School Nursing, Evanston Public Schools, wrote an editorial, in the *Journal of School Health*, about the preparation of teachers:

> Classroom teachers too often [come] with little or no knowledge whatsoever of health services or health education. Few know how to make the best use of health services and fewer still are prepared to teach health in a vital, dynamic, and meaningful manner. . . .
>
> . . . [The] relationship between health and everyday living too often does not "come through."[17]

There is a tendency to assume that the health course for college freshman is sufficient preparation for the elementary school classroom teacher, but in this course there is disregard for the health problems of children and how these problems are found in the school health program. Recently, a course dealing specifically with drug abuse has been required of elementary teachers in many states. This course cannot, however, with its special emphasis, take the place of the course concerned with the health problems of children and health education.

In 1924, the Joint Committee on Health Problems in Education of the NEA and the AMA stressed the need for a course where the health program is considered as a whole and synthesis occurs.[18] Many elementary school classroom teachers are not aware of the numerous signs of possible visual difficulties, hearing difficulties, nutritional deficiencies, dental health problems, posture conditions, skin infections, diseases and defects of vision and hearing, chronic health conditions, and diseases ranging from colds to whooping cough occurring to children and how to relate this information to health education. The relation of school nutrition to nutritional deficiencies of children, the relation of school furniture to posture conditions of children, or the relation of fire and disaster drills to accident prevention are not recognized. How school health services and healthful school living are related to health education is ignored. The health problems of elementary school children are pushed aside for further learning of anatomy, physiology, and physical education in "health."

In 1970, the Ohio Department of Education in cooperation with the State Planning Committee for Health Education in Ohio assigned high priority to the following topics in the preparation of elementary teachers:

1. Need for School Health Programs
2. Teacher's Role in the Health of Children
3. Determining the Health Needs of Pupils and What To Teach
4. Nature and Scope of School Health

[17]Irma Fricke: An editorial: inadequate teacher preparation for health education. *J. School Health* 41 (February, 1971):74.

[18]Joint Committee on Health Problems in Education of the National Education Association and the American Medical Association: *Health Education.* New York: The Committee, 1924, p. 76.

5. Teacher's Responsibilities for School Health Services
6. Role of the Teacher in the School Health Environment Program
7. Making Health Instruction Effective
8. Selecting and Using Health Materials and Resources.[19]

They also indicated that, among the many challenges facing education, one of the most urgent is that of improving health education: "Better-prepared teachers are needed now."[20]

## PHYSICAL EDUCATION TEACHER

Physical education is education through physical activities. The objectives, course content, methods and materials of instruction, and the activities themselves differ considerably from those of health education. Physical education has a very definite place in the curriculum of elementary and secondary schools; however, combining two very different types of program under the term "health and physical education" has not benefited either physical education or health education. Both subject-matter fields have suffered from the use of this term. Too often, to meet the demands of administrators unaware of the values of health education and physical education, time allotted to physical education has been relinquished to health education to meet local and state requirements.

The School Health Education Study reported that over 65% of the health education courses in grades 7, 8, and 9 and 90% of the health education courses in grades 10, 11, and 12 were taught by a teacher with a specialization in physical education.[21] Dees' study of health education in selected Texas secondary schools in 1966 disclosed that those assigned to teach health education were physical educators who were actually teaching anatomy and physiology. Also, these teachers were not complying with the Texas Education Agency's minimum requirements for time

and content of health education, effective in 1962, and they were generally not aware of the students' health problems.[22]

Who prepares teachers of physical education to teach health education? Mayshark and Kirk revealed that physical educators are predominant among instructors of personal health, the freshman college health course in junior and community colleges.[23] Torrance reported that 91% of the college teachers of health education in those teacher education institutions with the largest number of graduates in Texas were physical educators. Also, there was a clear lack of professional interest and participation in research in health education.[24] Since physical educators, in the majority of instances, prepare those who will teach health education in secondary schools, there is a question of the qualifications of these physical educators to teach health education in the secondary schools. In 1970, 24 states certified a person to teach health and physical education in the secondary schools. Of these, 11 states required a mean of 10.09 semester hours in health education. Among the health education courses or topics required or suggested were the school health program, first aid, personal health, and safety education.[25] Because physical educators have accepted the fact that they often will be assigned to teach health education, many prospective physical education teachers, at the preservice level, select health education as a second teaching field. Or, at the graduate level, the physical educator sometimes chooses the major field of health education.

Some of the functions of the physical education teacher in the total school health program include:

1. observation of signs indicating possible defects, diseases, or injuries among pupils

---

The Ohio Department of Education in Cooperation with the State Planning Committee for Health Education in Ohio: *A Guide for Preparing Elementary Teachers in Health Education.* Columbus: The Department, 1970, p. 5.

*Ibid.*, p. 7.

School Health Education Study: *Summary Report of a Nationwide Study of Health Instruction in the Public Schools, 1961-1963, op. cit.*, p. 10.

[22]Myron H. Dees: Status of health education in selected Texas secondary schools in 1966. Unpublished doctoral dissertation. The University of Texas at Austin, 1968, p. 154.

[23]Cyrus Mayshark and Robert H. Kirk: Status of the personal health course in junior colleges. *School Health Review 2* (April, 1971):19.

[24]Shelby F. Torrance: Undergraduate health education in approved teacher education programs in selected Texas colleges and universities, 1969-1970. Unpublished doctoral dissertation. The University of Texas at Austin, 1971, pp. 90-91.

[25]Haag, *op. cit.*, pp. 166-167.

2. utilization of a health grade classification by a physician to indicate the type of physical education for each student
3. exclusion of pupils with communicable diseases and readmission of pupils recovered from communicable diseases
4. completion of emergency care procedures
5. provision of adapted physical education or physical education for the handicapped
6. prevention of dental and eye injuries in physical education activities
7. promotion of sanitation and accident prevention procedures in the physical education facilities
8. provision of posture screening
9. promotion of desirable pupil health and safety practices in all daily physical education activities
10. recognition of fatigue among pupils and adjustment of daily physical education activities to pupil health needs

Foremost, the physical education teacher should recognize his role as a team member participating in the school health program. As a team member, he needs to accept the functions of the school health educator, health coordinator, elementary school classroom teacher, school or family physician, school or public health nurse, and other school and community personnel in the school health program.

## SPECIAL EDUCATION TEACHER

The teacher working with children who are physically handicapped or those children significantly below or above the average mentality is the special education teacher. The child may be hard of hearing or deaf. The child may have orthopedic defects. Different types of speech defects and disorders may be found among pupils. The child may partially see or be blind. The child may be mentally retarded. Some children may be mentally gifted. Teachers of special education work with children having cerebral palsy, muscular dystrophy, birth defects, and other handicapping health conditions. Throughout this text, mention is made of the special education teacher as a member of the school health team. Some of the *specialized* undergraduate preparation for the teacher of special education includes a survey of the types of exceptional children, language problems of exceptional children, visual problems of exceptional children, special instructional

media, and education of children with retarded mental development. In addition, education of children with crippling and other special health problems, therapeutic procedures for the cerebral palsied, education of children with visual and hearing disabilities, and education of the deaf are required or suggested.

## SCHOOL PHYSICIAN

In 1965, Wagner and others reported upon the school physician's functions in the Los Angeles City Unified School District. The functions were divided into three general types. First, individualized health examinations included routine medical examinations, special referral examinations, and athletic examinations. Second, in-school contacts were the physician-nurse contacts, physician-principal contacts, physician-teacher contacts, and physician-parent contacts. Third, the community contacts involved the members of medical profession and nonmedical community agencies.[26]

The American Academy of Pediatrics' Committee on School Health[27] indicated the duties and responsibilities of the school physician in (1) administration; (2) health services; (3) special education; and (4) psychological services. Some 16 duties and responsibilities were listed under health services. *The Forty-fifth Annual Report of the Department of Health Services, Denver Public Schools, 1969-1970,* listed five full-time and nine part-time physicians who gave 8365 routine pupil medical examinations, who gave 1169 immunizations to pupils, and who did 2718 pre-employment and annual health evaluations on adults. Other functions reported were carrying out of a citywide mass rubella vaccination program; psychiatric consultative services; medical examinations of new pupils and special pupil referrals; medical appraisal of pupils with problems interfering with learning; medical appraisals of pupils in special education; medical reports on "battered" children; and assistance with health

[26]Marsden G. Wagner, Carl S. Shultz, and Marian Heller: A study of school physician behavior. *Am. J. Public Health 58* (March, 1968):517.
[27]*Report of the Committee on School Health of American Academy of Pediatrics.* Evanston, Ill.: Academy, 1966, pp. 4-6.

disability, and retirement leaves for adult personnel.[28]

School physicians might also:

1. participate in the planning of school health services
2. give medical examinations to pupils who have no family physician and to athletes
3. classify students for physical education activities
4. work with school nurses, the health coordinator, and the school superintendent on exclusion and readmission procedures and emergency care procedures
5. work with school nurses, the health coordinator, and special education personnel on vision and hearing screening procedures
6. assist in the special education activities
7. work with school nurses, the health coordinator, and the school superintendent to devise forms for health records and other types of records used in school health services
8. administer tuberculin testing and immunizations
9. develop screening of heart conditions and diseases
10. encourage and conduct screening procedures of nutritional status and orthopedic cases
11. work with school counselors and the health coordinator to discover and assist the emotionally disturbed child
12. be available to school personnel to help with their own health problems
13. work with teachers of health education and the health coordinator in strengthening the total school health program
14. assist with the supervision of sanitary conditions in the school building

The American Academy of Pediatrics suggests that school physicians must possess special skills and knowledge if they are to function effectively in school health programs. School physicians must have special competence in providing medical care for the health problems of children and youth. Also, school physicians must be knowledgeable concerning the total school health program, particularly the organization of school health services; and the contributions of educators, nurses, and other school and community personnel to the school health program.[29]

## SCHOOL NURSE

In 1966, the American Nurses' Association published *Functions and Qualifications for School Nurses*. This publication placed the functions of the school nurse into five categories, including how to plan, implement, and evaluate the functions. In addition, the qualifications for a school nurse in a staff position and in supervisory, consultative, or administrative positions were given. For the school nurse in a staff position, there was recommended a basic program of study in school health, among other programs.[30]

In the Denver Public Schools, Division of Health Services, there were 78 full-time school nurses and 10 part-time school nurses employed in 1969-1970. Some of the services of these nurses included routine vision screening, participation in pupil discussion groups to modify behavior, classroom inspections for scalp ringworm and other diseases, screening for hearing and physical growth, assistance to teachers in sex education, tuberculosis education and skin-testing procedures, follow-through with counseling, and assistance in first-aid care of injuries.[31]

The National Council of School Nurses, American Association for Health, Physical Education and Recreation has made seven recommendations endorsed by AAHPER Board of Directors. These recommendations were that

1. local boards of education employ school nurses
2. minimum professional preparation for a school nurse should include being a registered professional nurse and having a baccalaureate degree including preparation in school health
3. state departments of education adopt certification requirements based upon standards of professional associations

[29]*Report of the Committee on School Health of the American Academy of Pediatrics, op. cit.*, p. 3.
[30]American Nurses' Association: *Functions and Qualifications for School Nurses*. New York: The Association, 1966.
[31]*Forty-fifth Annual Report of the Department of Health Services, Denver Public Schools, Colorado, 1969-1970, op. cit.*

[28]*Forty-fifth Annual Report of the Department of Health Services, Denver Public Schools, Colorado, 1969-1970*. Denver: Division of Health Services, Denver Public Schools, 1970, 1-48.

4. continuing education and graduate study should be pursued and nurses should belong to and participate in the activities of professional associations
5. written policies and procedures for school nurses should be developed by local school districts
6. supervision of school nurses should be provided by local school districts
7. supervision of auxiliary personnel in school health services should be the responsibility of school nurses

Along with these recommendations is the statement that "school health services are best administered by the local board of education to provide the most effective integration of health services with the instruction program."[32]

The School Nursing Committee of the American School Health Association prepared guidelines for school nursing in 1967. These guidelines were divided into eleven sections, among which were sections dealing with the responsibilities of the nurse in the school health program, the school nurse as educator, the school nurse as counselor, educational preparation for school nurses, factors influencing the pupil load of the school nurse, supervision in school nursing, and evaluative criteria for school nursing.[33] These guidelines have been extremely helpful to school superintendents.

In addition to the functions mentioned, the school nurse may also

1. participate in the in-service health services education of school personnel
2. work with special education teachers on vision and hearing screening
3. assist in the control of communicable diseases
4. work with school and family physicians in developing efficient health services
5. develop records for school nursing activities
6. work with physicians, the superintendent of schools, and the health coordinator on exclusion and readmission procedures and on emergency care procedures
7. work with school and family physicians on immunizations and tuberculin testing

8. assist school counselors, the health coordinator, and teachers in discovering the emotionally disturbed child
9. work with the Parent-Teacher Association on the readiness-for-school medical examination
10. assist teachers of health education and the health coordinator in developing the total school health program

Boards of education not able to employ a school nurse usually seek assistance from local or county health departments. Public health nurses have often worked with public school teachers in performing some of the functions of the school nurse.

## FAMILY PHYSICIAN

Throughout the literature of school health education there is frequent reference to the family physician. The family physician is a medical doctor licensed to practice medicine in the state where he resides. It is important that school personnel do *not* accept persons who practice medicine without a license. When the student has no family physician, the school nurse or the health coordinator can ask the local health department or school health committee of the local medical society to submit a list of physicians from which the parents can select a family physician. If the family cannot afford the services of a family physician, the local health department should be notified. The family should be aware of the importance of the pupil's health status being known to a physician.

## DENTIST AND DENTAL HYGIENIST

The dentist is the doctor of dental surgery licensed to practice dentistry in the state where he resides. Among the dental specialists are the oral surgeon, orthodontist, pedodontist, periodontist, and public health dentist. Dental hygienists work under the supervision of licensed dentists. The hygienist cleans teeth, takes x-rays, and teaches patients how to take care of their teeth.

Hayden[34] has offered six advantages for having the dental examination and referral program in the school setting.

[32]AAHPER position statement, the school nurse in education. *School Health Review 2* (February, 1971):36.
[33]The School Nursing Committee, American School Health Association: The nurse in the school health program. *J. School Health 37* (February, 1967):2a.
[34]Charles H. Hayden: Preventive dental procedures adaptable to school health programs. *Amer. J. Public Health 59* (March, 1969):522.

1. Dental health education given by teachers will be reinforced by the dental examination and referral program
2. There is more opportunity to share dental experiences among children
3. Overall dental problems in schools can be assessed
4. Dental health problems will be brought to the attention of the school nurse who can include them in the follow-through
5. Dental health problems of children will be brought to the attention of school personnel so that community resources can be utilized to solve these problems
6. Fears or misconceptions about dental examinations can be overcome by teachers and dentists working together

In some states, the dental hygienist is the dental hygiene teacher. In the Port Chester, New York, school system the dental hygiene teacher makes annual dental inspections. During the inspection, the student is informed of his dental health status and is given individual instruction in tooth brushing. Parents are notified of the need for professional care by their family dentist. Teachers are informed of, the number of pupils needing professional dental care and are given lists of dental defects occurring among pupils. When informing parents of their child's apparent dental defects, the dental hygiene teacher assists parents in understanding the need for professional dental care. Particular attention is paid to physically and mentally handicapped children and their dental health problems.[35]

## OTHER PERSONNEL IN HEALTH SERVICES

Some large city school systems have certain medical specialists on a part-time or consultative basis. These specialists include ophthalmologists, otologists, pediatricians, and psychiatrists. Occasionally, an orthopedic surgeon and cardiologist are listed as consultants to school health services.

School systems having special education facilities may employ a registered physical therapist to work with pupils having orthopedic problems and cerebral palsy. Other personnel in special education may be speech and hearing therapists, audiometrists, and psychologists. Psychiatric social workers are employed by some school systems. Podiatrists, optometrists, and specialists in preventive medicine might also serve as consultants.

## LOCAL HEALTH DEPARTMENT

Rosner and others[36] have reported on the improved use of health professionals in the New York City schools; this report should be of interest to public health nurses and medical officers in local health departments. Public health assistants, according to this study, were effective in reducing the technical and clerical subprofessional activities of school nurses.

Public health nurses and the local medical officer can assist school personnel in developing *health services* in the elementary and secondary schools. In school systems not able to employ full-time school nurses, the public health nurses may assume some of the responsibilities of the school nurse, with the consent of the board of education and the board of health. These responsibilities may include the follow-through, control of communicable diseases by exclusion and readmission procedures, immunizations, and tuberculin testing. The local medical officer may assume some of the responsibilities of the school physician, with consent of the board of education and the board of health. These responsibilities may include formulation of health records, establishment of exclusion and readmission procedures and of emergency care procedures, and care of the handicapped child.

Sanitary engineers, sanitarians, inspectors, public health nurses, and the local medical officer can work with school personnel in maintaining a *healthful and safe school environment.* Supervision of purified water supplies, adequate disposal of sewage and garbage, inspection of food and milk, control of insects and rats, sanitation in the school lunchroom, and accident and fire prevention may be among the many measures taken by public health personnel to promote a healthful and safe school environment. Careful inspections, suggestions to eradicate diseases, and assistance in

[35]Dental health service in the Port Chester School System. *J. School Health 38* (October, 1968):511.

[36]Lester J. Rosner, Olive E. Pitkin, and Lucille Rosenbluth: Improved use of health professionals in New York City Schools. *Amer. J. Public Health 60* (February, 1970):328.

solving environmental health problems are given by public health personnel.

The public health educator can assist the school health educator by sharing information related to community health problems, arranging field trips to the health department, and scheduling public health personnel to provide demonstrations in *health education* courses. The public health educator, local medical officer, public health nurses, or other public health personnel should select a representative of the local health department to serve as a member of the school health council.

## NONOFFICIAL HEALTH AGENCIES

In Chapter 17, there are suggestions for the school personnel's use of nonofficial health agencies. These agencies include professional groups, voluntary health agencies, civic and service community agencies, foundations, and commercial and semicommercial groups found within the local community. Too often, school personnel are not aware of the local medical and dental societies, units or chapters of national voluntary health agencies, and community welfare and civic groups. These nonofficial

health agencies should be represented on school health councils.

## References for Further Study

Anderson, C. L.: *School Health Practice.* 5th ed. St. Louis: The C. V. Mosby Company, 1972.

Byrd, O. E.: *School Health Administration.* Philadelphia: W. B. Saunders Company, 1964.

Freeman, R.: *Community Health Nursing Practice.* Philadelphia: W. B. Saunders Company, 1970.

Joint Committee on Health Problems in Education of the National Education Association and the American Medical Association: *Healthful School Environment* (1969); and *School Health Services* (1964). Washington, D.C.: National Education Association.

Kilander, H. F.: *School Health Education.* 2nd ed. New York: The Macmillan Company, 1968.

Mayshark, C., and Shaw, D. D.: *Administration of School Health Programs.* St. Louis: The C. V. Mosby Company, 1967.

Oberteuffer, D., Harrelson, O., and Pollock, M.: *School Health Education.* 5th ed. New York: Harper & Row, 1972.

School Health Division, American Association for Health, Physical Education and Recreation: *Appraisal Guide for Professional Preparation in Health Education.* Washington, D.C.: The Association, 1967.

Turner, C. E., Randall, H. B., and Smith, S. L.: *School Health and Health Education.* 6th ed. St. Louis: The C. V. Mosby Company, 1970.

Willgoose, C. E.: *Health Education in the Elementary School.* 3rd ed. Philadelphia: W. B. Saunders Company, 1969.

Young, W. O., and Striffler, D. F.: *The Dentist, His Practice and His Community.* 2nd ed. Philadelphia: W. B. Saunders Company, 1969.

# Chapter 20

# FUNDS, FACILITIES, EQUIPMENT, AND SUPPLIES

## AN INCIDENT

To develop a school health program, the school superintendent has asked the health coordinator and the consultant or supervisor of health education to indicate what funds, facilities, equipment, and supplies are needed. The health coordinator has agreed to do this for school health services. To develop a curriculum in health education from kindergarten through 12th grade, the consultant or supervisor of health education will designate the funds, facilities, equipment, and supplies needed. School nurses, teachers in the elementary schools, teachers assigned health education in the junior or middle schools, and school health educators have been called upon to assist in this task.

Probably no other phase of a school system's organizational and administrational structure is as grossly neglected as the school health program. In a large city school system, school health services may be adequately developed while health education is totally ignored in the curriculum. In a small school system, there may be very little evidence of school health service and only small concern about health education. Funds, facilities, equipment, and supplies for the school health program are assigned with *no relation to the health problems of pupils*, if they are assigned at all.

## FUNDS

School administrators should be able to justify the allocation of, account for the expenditure of, and manage the use of *funds* for the school health program. Some administrators use the *line item budget*, a listing on a line-by-line basis. Often those items at the end of the line item budget are decreased or eliminated, which may happen in the school health program. Other administrators use an *object budget* which groups items of cost into classifications; e.g., instructional salaries. The object budget can permit increases or reductions as programs change, which may account for some school systems with staffs of school nurses while no teachers of health education are employed. The teachers of health education would be placed under "instructional salaries" while school nurses would be classified under "school health services." The *program budget* seeks to bring all costs associated with one program together as one expenditure. This type of budget, when used in local health departments, may not give equal consideration to health education since most funds are spent for patient care. The *performance budget* places its emphasis upon the result or end product to be obtained. Work-measurement procedures are established so that each task performed can be matched against the funds assigned. *Alternative budgeting* takes into consideration when an item on the budget can be best done, how it can be best done, and by whom it can be best performed. However, all parts of the school health program, in each school building and reaching each pupil, would have to be considered.[1]

One would believe that the school health programs are adequately financed with all

[1]Cyrus Mayshark and Donald D. Shaw: *Administration of School Health Programs*. St. Louis: The C. V. Mosby Company, 1967, pp. 338-350.

the federal, state, and local funds reaching schools. However, seldom is the total school health program adequately funded.

Funds for the total school health program may be distributed among several divisions of the budget of the local board of education. The health coordinator may be listed under "administrative salaries" and the consultant or supervisor of health education under "supervisory salaries." Salaries of teachers of health education are usually listed under "instructional salaries." It is possible that "school health services" may be a separate item on the budget. School nutrition may be listed as "food services" or "school lunch." Supplies and equipment for maintaining a sanitary school environment may be placed under the item "maintenance."

Within *school health services* funds must be secured to pay the salaries and transportation expenses of school nurses and buy all equipment and supplies used in school health services. Part-time physicians, dentists, dental hygienists, or other health services personnel employed by the local board of education must be paid from funds allocated to school health services. In addition, funds must cover the construction, equipping, and maintenance of health service units within school buildings.

The efficient operation of school lunchrooms depends, in addition to cash sales, on funds allocated to *school nutrition.* These funds pay the salaries of the school lunch director and managers, cooks, helpers, attendants, cashiers, and other food workers. Utility bills must be paid. In addition, funds are needed to purchase equipment for the dining, kitchen, dishwashing and storage areas. Food must be purchased, and supplies are needed to dispense the prepared food as well as to prepare the food.

In Chapter 10, the National School Lunch Act and its amendments were described. However, school administrators and teachers have found that children needing the school lunch do not always receive it. The National School Lunch Act requires that each state provide $3 of matching funds for every federal dollar the state receives. In some states, the matching funds are the moneys that school children pay for lunch, while in other states, no state matching funds are provided. Or,

the states divert the federal funds for school lunches into other aspects of the school lunch instead of feeding needy children. The National School Lunch Act indicates that school systems accepting federal funds must serve a lunch without cost or at a reduced cost to those children unable to pay, but those children unable to pay must be determined by local school authorities. The standards by which children are judged eligible for free lunches vary widely. In some school systems, children on welfare are eligible but not those from families with marginal incomes. Sometimes, one child within a family qualifies while a brother will not. Too often, the availability of free lunch for needy children is not known to teachers, parents, and the community. The idea that a hot lunch must be served has denied many needy children of a nutritious meal because school administrators claim they cannot finance the facilities and equipment for serving a hot lunch. It is estimated that nine of every ten schools that do not serve federally funded school lunches are elementary schools, in which the damage by hunger and malnutrition is the greatest. Every teacher and principal needs to evaluate the school lunch program in their building carefully to see if needy children and those children from marginal-income families are receiving the free lunches.

Salaries of the teacher of health education and the elementary school classroom teacher are paid from funds allocated to instructional salaries. In addition, *health education* requires funds for instructional supplies. The School Health Education Study[2] revealed a shortage of instructional materials and failure to provide these materials for health education; in addition, it showed the lack of financial support to health education. Some of the necessary instructional materials are textbooks, supplemental reference materials, audiovisual aids, filing cabinets and demonstration table, materials for teaching first aid, and items for experiments and demonstrations. Funds are needed to purchase standardized

[2]School Health Education Study: *Summary Report of a Nationwide Study of Health Instruction in the Public Schools, 1961-1963.* Washington, D.C.: The Study, pp. 40-44.

health education tests, library materials, exhibits, and forms for pupil records. There should also be some money available to assist the teacher of health education in the preparation of classroom materials.

The multiplicity of custodial supplies and maintenance equipment needed to maintain a sanitary *school environment* should be of utmost importance on the board of education budget. Sanitary conditions in the toilet rooms, classrooms, lunchroom, and physical education facilities reduce the incidence of disease. Under the budget item of "maintenance," salaries of custodians and maids should be placed. Many secondary schools have a laundry which provides clean towels for physical education activities, home economics classes, health service unit, and lunchroom. Each time a student has a physical education class or participates in after-school physical education activities, he receives a clean towel. Some secondary schools use the laundry to provide clean gym clothing or athletic uniforms. However, though a sanitary school environment is the main responsibility of the custodial staff, it is not their responsibility alone; teachers and pupils also have specific daily responsibilities in maintaining sanitary surroundings.

## FACILITIES

Three types of *facilities* in the school health program will be considered: the health service unit, food-service areas, and the health education classroom. School facilities used in health services are called the "health service unit," "health room," or "health suite." For simplification, the term "health service unit" will be used.

The amount of space needed for the *health service unit* will depend on the enrollment in the school building the unit serves, the kinds of services to be rendered within the unit, and the ages of the pupils using the unit. Some of the services may include emergency care of the ill or injured pupil, medical examinations, dental examinations, screening procedures for vision and hearing, tuberculin testing, nutrition and posture screening, exclusion and readmission procedures, and health counseling. In addition, the unit may be used by the school health educator for demonstrations during health teaching. Community health agencies may schedule well-child

conferences, preschool health activities, and adult education meetings in the health service unit. School disaster procedures will designate the health service unit as the central first-aid station.

The health service unit should be located on the first or ground floor near a main entrance to the building. The unit should be close to the principal's office. In secondary schools, the health classroom should have direct access to the unit. The unit should be acoustically treated. The colors of the walls, ceiling, trim, and floor should create a warm and cheerful atmosphere. Flooring should be nonabsorbent, easily cleaned, and light in color. Wall construction used to divide the health service unit into separate rooms needs careful consideration.

The number of square feet recommended varies from 470 to 500 square feet for the health service unit in elementary schools and from 560 to 870 square feet for the health service unit in secondary schools. Some of the activities in the health service unit, in addition to the services mentioned above, are conferences between health services personnel and teachers, parents, and students; and maintenance of records.

Schools having enrollments of 300 or more pupils or ten classrooms should have a waiting room. It should be separated from other rooms of the unit by a wall to the ceiling and should be accessible to a corridor and evaluating room.

Every school with 180 or more pupils and six or more classrooms should have an evaluating room in the health service unit. This room should also serve for vision screening and, therefore, should have an uninterrupted length of at least 20 feet. It should be connected with resting rooms, waiting rooms, and offices. In small schools, the evaluating room may be a resting room. The types of activities that take place in the evaluating room will determine the size of the room.

All schools should have separate resting rooms for each sex within the health service unit. High schools having an enrollment of 300 or more students need separate resting rooms. In schools not having full-time health service personnel, the resting rooms should be located near the principal's office or the health classroom. Resting rooms may be used by pupils needing rest during

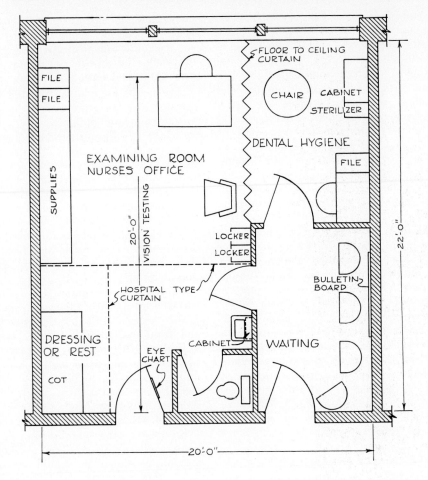

Figure 18. Suggested health suite for up to 300 pupils.

Figures 18, 19 and 20 adapted from the Division of School Buildings and grounds, State Education Department, The University of the State of New York.

the school day, pupils injured and receiving emergency care, and pupils with illnesses other than communicable diseases.

Toilet rooms should be accessible to resting rooms. In schools with 300 or more pupils, toilet rooms should be provided for each sex. These toilet rooms should be well ventilated. Washbasins might be operated by waist, knee, or foot.

Opening off each resting room should be storage space with linens, pillows, blankets, and other supplies. Movable storage cabinets are preferred.

In addition to resting rooms, there should be a small isolation room for pupils with communicable diseases. The room should be connected with the evaluating room.

When the dental services of the school are performed in the health service unit,

the evaluating room is extended so that a floor area of approximately 100 square feet is provided for these services.

The need for office space within the health service unit will depend on the amount of time health service personnel spend within a school. When provided, this office should be connected with the evaluating room and waiting room. The office space may be used as a counseling room where the physician, nurse, teacher, and parent can discuss the child's health.

The *food service* areas should be above ground, have an accessible loading area, be located away from playing fields and student traffic, and be isolated from classrooms. The receiving area should have a loading platform so that food can be taken into the inside receiving space. The storage

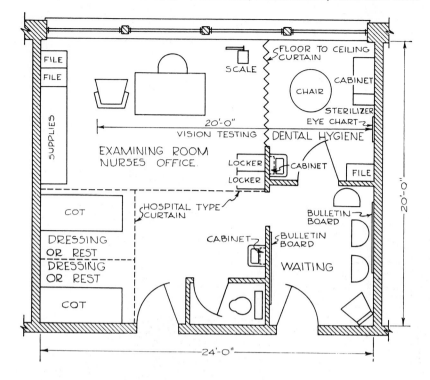

Figure 19. Suggested health suite for 300 to 800 pupils.

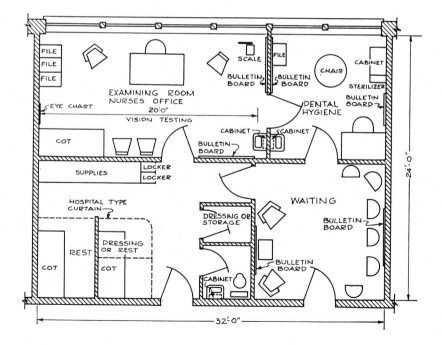

Figure 20. Suggested health suite for more than 800 pupils.

area should be close to the receiving area and kitchen. The serving area consists of the kitchen and the area for dispensing of food. Milk service and hot and cold food sections are in the serving area. A lavatory with hot and cold running water and mixer faucets, soap, and individual towels must be near the serving area. The dining area is where the students eat. Some schools have the noonday meals delivered from the kitchen to the individual classrooms on portable food carts. Other schools prepare "bag" lunches which are delivered to the classrooms. In these schools, a dining area is not necessary. The dishwashing area is best located near an exit and should be out of the way of cross traffic. The soiled dish area must have sufficient length to provide space for scraping dishes and for dish racks. The clean dish area must allow for the air drying of dishes.

The *health education classroom* in the secondary school should be designed for the type of instruction that takes place there. Unfortunately, the School Health Education Study[3] reported that in the secondary schools of the study, "any classroom available" was reported as the most common facility for health education by 50 to 80% of the respondents. The adequate health education classroom is described as follows: It has adjustable and movable desk-chair furniture for no more than 35 pupils and the teacher's desk and chair. Windows have opaque shades so that films and other projected materials can be viewed in a darkened room. The classroom has work tables, a demonstration table for the teacher, filing cabinets, a poster cabinet, a vertical file, open-shelved bookcases, storage cabinets, and a sink. The room is acoustically treated and air conditioned. Bulletin boards are found on the inner corridor wall, and chalkboards are placed on the front wall. There are electrical outlets on each wall. Sufficient storage space should be provided for bandages, splints, life-size manikin, microscopes, experimental equipment, and teacher- and pupil-made materials. A locked filing cabinet is necessary to store teacher-made and standardized tests, insulin and facsimiles of drugs and narcotics, course and unit outlines, and other materials.

[3]*Ibid.*, p. 30.

## EQUIPMENT AND SUPPLIES

The *equipment* needed within the *health service* unit will depend on the size of the unit, the services to be performed, and enrollment of the school. Cots with mattresses and bed linen will be needed in the resting rooms. A desk, chairs, a typewriter, filing cabinets, a telephone, and wastebaskets should be available. Electric outlets of proper size and type are necessary. Platform scales, vision and hearing screening devices, and a full-length mirror are necessary for certain types of screening procedures. A sterilizer and an instrument table, a foot-operated disposal can, cup and towel dispensers, and a first-aid supply cabinet will be of value to physicians and nurses. Hooks for hanging wraps and clothing as well as shelves for books should be accessible. Physicians, dentists, and dental hygienists may request additional equipment depending on the services rendered within the health service unit.

The *supplies* that should be found in school health services will include all necessary first-aid items, health and emergency care records, nurse's and other health service records, and materials for immunizations if completed in the health service unit. In some schools, records concerning teacher-parent conferences on the pupil's health are kept in the health service unit.

The *equipment* and *supplies* necessary to maintain a *healthful school environment* have multiple purposes. Some equipment and supplies are used to clean, disinfect, and remove odors; other equipment and supplies are necessary to repair, replace, and prolong the usefulness of the school environment. To ensure the efficient use of custodial equipment and supplies, some school systems require custodians to undergo in-service training.

The *equipment* and *supplies* for *school nutrition* depend on the amount of money available and on the expected scope of school lunch activities. Fixed equipment includes sinks, stoves, ovens, canopies, cabinets, dishwashers, refrigerators, counters, freezers, racks, steamers, choppers, and peelers. Hand equipment, such as bowls, cutlery, beaters, brushes, ladles, measures, openers, pots and pans, sieves, stools, trays, and thermometers, will also be required. In addition, there must be plates, silverware, and drinking glasses and cups. Necessary supplies include pest-control materials, garbage and waste-disposal cans, soap and detergents, disinfectants, and other items for sanitation purposes. Supplies necessary in the preparation of the noonday school meal will be condiments, baked goods, cereals, flour, dairy products, meats, fruits and vegetables, sugar, soup, preserves, and other food items.

Among the *equipment* and *supplies* necessary for *health education* are textbooks. The School Health Education Study[4] has recommended that the study of research findings on the accuracy and readability of health education textbooks will be helpful to teachers in evaluating textbooks. Benedict[5] analyzed health-related textbooks to determine their coverage of communicable diseases prevalent in Texas according to the morbidity reports of the Texas State Department of Health, 1935-1965. The 94 textbooks, including all those adopted for school use, were those dealing with elementary school health education, life science, physiology, biology, and secondary school health education. Some of the findings of this study were as follows:

1. Of the diseases listed in morbidity reports from 1935 to 1965, seldom was any one disease given sufficient coverage.
2. None of the textbooks was outstanding in the quality of its content about communicable diseases.
3. Gonorrhea and syphilis were not discussed in any textbook.
4. Information on communicable diseases only supplemented discussions of human anatomy and physiology.
5. Discussions of communicable diseases were

not grouped but were scattered throughout the textbooks.
6. Unnecessary repetition of the information about communicable diseases was found in the elementary school health education textbooks.
7. Discussions of basic concepts of communicable diseases (e.g., method of transmission of the causative agent) were omitted.
8. Of the 101 authors, the greatest number were physicians and public school administrators. Only three authors were professional health educators.

New editions and revisions of textbooks do not necessarily contain updated information. Equipment and supplies other than textbooks necessary for health education have been explained in Chapter 16, "Methods and Materials of Instruction." Published tests for health education classes will be mentioned in Chapter 22, "Evaluation of the School Health Program."

## References for Further Study

American Association of School Administrators: *Schools for America.* Washington, D.C.: National Education Association, 1967.

Anderson, C. L.: *School Health Practice.* 5th ed. St. Louis: The C. V. Mosby Company, 1972.

Byrd, O. E.: *School Health Administration.* Philadelphia: W. B. Saunders Company, 1964.

Hanlon, J. J., and McHose, E.: *Design for Health: School and Community.* 2nd ed. Philadelphia: Lea & Febiger, 1971.

Joint Committee on Health Problems in Education of the National Education Association and the American Medical Association. *Healthful School Environment* (1969); and *Suggested School Health Policies* (1966). Washington, D.C.: National Education Association.

Kilander, H. F.: *School Health Education.* 2nd ed. New York: The Macmillan Company, 1968.

Oberteuffer, D., Harrelson, O., and Pollock, M.: *School Health Education.* 5th ed. New York: Harper & Row, 1972.

Southern State Work-Conference: *School Food Service Policies and Standards.* 3rd ed. Tallahassee: Florida State Department of Education, 1967.

West, B. B., Wood, L., and Harger, V. F.: *Food Service in Institutions.* 4th ed. New York: John Wiley & Sons, 1966.

Willgoose, C. E.: *Health Education in the Elementary School.* 3rd ed. Philadelphia: W. B. Saunders Company, 1969.

---

[4] *Ibid.*, p. 31.
[5] Irvin J. Benedict: Analysis of health-related textbooks adopted in Texas, 1935-1965, in relation to their coverage of communicable diseases prevalent during the period. Unpublished doctoral dissertation. The University of Texas at Austin, 1968, pp. 212-245.

# Chapter 21

# SCHOOL HEALTH COUNCIL

## AN INCIDENT

A school superintendent in a small school system has asked principals in the elementary schools to organize a school health council. A superintendent in a medium-sized school system has requested the school health educator in one high school to establish a health council in that school. The board of education of a large school system has asked the health coordinator to organize a school health council representing elementary and secondary schools in the various areas of the school system.

A functional and effective school health program is dependent on community understanding and support. The school health council, with its participating members drawn from school personnel and students, parents, community physicians and dentists, representatives of local health agencies, and public health personnel can interpret the broad scope of the school health program to the community. Before attempting to explain the council, it is necessary to differentiate between the school health *committee* and the school health *council*. The committee may be one of many committees subordinate to a council, as different projects are assigned by the council to separate committees. The school health council may be concerned with an individual school, the entire system, or several school systems.

## PURPOSE OF THE COUNCIL

School health educators and coordinators are often asked why health councils are important. The council *assists in solving* school health problems. These problems

concern both pupils and school personnel, and many of the solutions will affect community life. The council has limitations in that it has no legal administrative authority and its members cannot assume the responsibilities of the school superintendent in the development of the school health program. The school health council as an advisory body is a definite part of the American public school traditions and functions. It operates within a local school or school system and is not under the jurisdiction of any state or federal agency.

## OPERATING PROCEDURES

Among the 1971 resolutions adopted by the Joint Committee on Health Problems in Education of the National Education Association and the American Medical Association was the resolution

> that the component parts of a health program in a school system be coordinated by an advisory school health council consisting of representatives of the administration, instructional staff, students, parents, employees, and the health disciplines.[1]

The school health council

1. discovers pertinent school health problems having direct relation to community health
2. compiles all data concerning school conditions that create these health problems
3. plans a course of action to solve the pertinent problems and to improve the health of all school personnel and students
4. suggests to the school superintendent the

[1]Resolutions adopted by the Joint Committee on Health Problems in Education of the National Education Association and the American Medical Association. *School Health Review* 2 (April, 1971):26.

course of action or, with the superintendent's approval, carries out the course of action

5. evaluates and revises plans of action so that other problems appearing in the future can be easily handled
6. makes recommendations for long-term planning that include both school and community health

In order to discover the pertinent school health problems, the council members can use the survey method. The student members might employ self-rating scales or questionnaires. The school faculty and community personnel might utilize check lists, conferences, anecdotal records, and interviews. The school health problems that appear with the greatest frequency become the problems the council attempts to solve. It may be necessary for the chairman of the council to designate committees to gather data on school conditions that create these problems. Investigation of various parts of the facilities, school activities, and curricular patterns may provide up-to-date and valid data. Often the chairman of the council will appoint a committee to appraise the effects of existing conditions on community health. When data on the conditions are compiled, the results of the compilation will focus attention on the most outstanding health problem. The members of the council pool their knowledge, interests, and efforts in planning a course of action to solve the pertinent problem. After several plans of action have been proposed, the members decide the course of action that is not only the most expedient and effective but also the most likely to gain school and community support.

The chosen course of action must have the superintendent's approval. Carrying out the program may be the duty of a particular committee of the council or may need the concentrated efforts of all members. However, the course of action, once put into effect, needs continuous evaluation and revision because many school personnel, students, and school facilities will be involved. With each course of action, the council should make recommendations for long-term planning so that problems that have been solved will not reappear. Such long-term planning will necessitate a broad probing into the entire school health program.

## MEMBERSHIP

The members of a school health council in a single *school building* are the principal, the school health educator/coordinator, a physician and a dentist interested in the school's health problems, a school nurse, three teachers, students representing various grade levels, the school counselor, the school lunch manager, a custodian, a representative from the Parent-Teacher Association, two members of voluntary community health agencies, and a member of the local health department.

If the school health council is to be concerned with several school buildings within a *school system*, the members include:

1. an administrative official of the school system
2. the school health educator or the health coordinator
3. a physician and a dentist interested in the school system's health problems or the physician and dentist cooperating in school health services
4. a supervisor of school nurses or a representative of the school nurses
5. teachers elected from different school buildings
6. students chosen from various school buildings and age levels
7. a counselor
8. a lunchroom director
9. the chief of the school system's custodial services
10. two representatives of the Parent-Teacher Association who may be chairmen of the health committees of their local associations
11. two members from different voluntary community health agencies
12. two personnel from the local health department

## ACTIONS

In order to function successfully, the school health council should have the school health educator or coordinator as leader because he has had experience with the functioning of a health council. As a part of his undergraduate preparation, the school health educator shared the problems of school and community health with numerous community workers. These might have been a public health nurse, a community sanitarian, a field representative of the local tuberculosis association, or a staff member of a community welfare agency. Having been a member of a school health council and having prepared for school health education, the school health educator or coordinator is the person best qualified to assume leadership in the council.

To function successfully, the council should:

1. rotate the chairmanship at the close of a school semester
2. have an agenda of each meeting drawn up by a steering committee
3. solve problems by action that can be completed within a school semester
4. have documentary evidence of all committees' work
5. encourage equal participation of all members
6. have faith that the problems to be solved will be solved
7. release reliable publicity frequently, stressing the work of the council's members
8. furnish an annual report easily understood by the whole community

As the leader of the council, the school health educator or coordinator should not accept its chairmanship. He obtains permission from the administrator for the survey methods employed by the council members in compiling data on pertinent school health problems. He informs the administrator and acquires the administrator's approval of the council's actions, revisions in plans of action, evaluation of actions, and long-term planning. He works with the steering committee in planning the agenda of meetings. He guides the council's attempts to solve pertinent school health problems and encourages the members to contribute unselfishly of their time, efforts, and knowledge. The educator or coordinator interprets policies and procedures of the school health program to council members. He is aware of community and school personnel who are interested in the school health program and who might replace other council members who become ill, move from town, or are too frequently absent from meetings. He serves as a liaison agent between the public school and the community personnel on the council. He publicizes the work of the council members through many media, strives to have continuous and reliable publicity, and assists in the publication of an annual report of the council's actions. He has information available for solving school health problems. He seeks new ways

for evaluating the effectiveness of the school health council.

## Actions in School Health Services

School health councils can assist the development of the total school health program in many ways. In *health services*, at the meetings of the council family physicians and dentists can acquaint school personnel with the incidence of remediable health difficulties among students. The number of dental health problems, inadequacy of immunizations, incidence of diseases and accidents, types of chronic health conditions, and emotional health problems among pupils can be disclosed. The incidence of emergency cases of illness or injury will be reported.

The representatives of voluntary community health agencies and public health personnel can inform the council members of interagency cooperation in the care of students with communicable disease or mental illness. These representatives can report the incidence of community health problems and can reveal public ignorance of particular community health problems. Problems facing the public health nurse during home visits will be disclosed. Interagency cooperation in providing medical and dental care to indigent pupils can be arranged.

Many of the problems pertaining to school health services may be solved through exchange of ideas by the professional health services personnel, public health workers, and the public school personnel at council meetings. A common problem in school health services is the provision of adequate routine medical examinations by family physicians so that data on the health status of each student can be gathered and used for classification in physical education. Reduction of the number of medical excuses prohibiting students from participating in physical education is another problem. Adequate school-community dental health programs also present a challenge. Assembling a panel of physicians to take care of emergency cases of illness or injury is another problem. Parent education in the importance of immunization must be considered. Better exchange of information about pupils between family physicians and school personnel may be needed. The provision of adequate vision and hearing screening for all students is another problem. There is need for parent education so that the excluded ill child is kept at home rather than allowed to play in the neighborhood. Parent education in the care of the child's deciduous and permanent teeth is often inadequate.

The health council can be active in promoting the physical and mental *health of the school personnel* by advocating that personnel have annual medical examinations and chest x-rays, group health insurance plans, and adequate sick leave. In addition, the council can alert school personnel to environmental factors which may cause injury to personnel.

### Actions in Healthful School Living

School health problems arising from the condition of the school *environment* can be corrected by action from the school health council. One of these conditions might be the existence of an unsafe playing area that serves as a collection spot for tin cans and bottles, provides no parking areas for bicycles, has unsupervised activities, and has no designated areas for young children.

A playground safety patrol might be organized by the school health council to establish rules and regulations for different activities and to designate play areas for children of different ages. The patrol might provide areas for parking bicycles or install bicycle racks. It could remove stones, bottles, and tin cans. It might provide supervision by patrol members for each play period and conduct a safety court for violators of playground rules.

Improvement of sanitary procedures in the environment might be a project of the council. Plans to improve existing conditions, such as the untidy appearance of toilet rooms, soiled dishes remaining on cafeteria tables, scraps of paper dropped in corridors and on auditorium floors, and disorderly corridor lockers, might be suggested. An investigation of the lunchroom sanitation procedures might be the means of reducing the incidence of streptococcal infections and food-borne diseases common to the school population. This inspection might result in the hiring of additional workers, improved solid-waste disposal methods, better sanitizing of dishes and glassware, and pupil assistance in removing soiled dishes from tables.

A check list of accident and fire hazards might indicate the need for safety procedures in the environment. A survey of the school building's lighting and furniture might be completed. The school health council might be the organization which plans fire and disaster procedures for the school building and conducts frequent school fire and disaster drills and fire prevention campaigns.

The health council can stimulate student interest in school *nutrition*. The lunch manager is a member of the council; she can therefore make many suggestions that will promote school nutrition. Because the council's membership is drawn from the community professional health services personnel, it is an excellent forum in which to discuss school and community nutritional problems, propose plans to solve them, and take action to eradicate them. A continuous program of in-service nutrition education might be suggested. Another possibile action is a program of "A Good Breakfast" sponsored by the health council.

### Actions in Health Education

Finally, the school health council can compile objective data used in discovering pupil health needs and interests as a basis for *health education*. For example, the council may conduct a survey of accidents occurring to secondary school students and the forms of self-medication applied to injuries. The results of the survey would be objective data for the teacher of health education to use in safety education and American Red Cross First Aid classes. A survey might be conducted to learn students' dietary likes and dislikes in order to pinpoint the need for nutrition education in health education classes. Another possibility for research is the accumulation of statistical evidence of common health problems reported by professional health services and public health personnel. The dentist, who is a member of the school health council, has considerable data on the dental health problems of school-age children. A check list, used by the student representatives of the council, can indicate health misconceptions of school personnel and students.

The council's actions in improving the school environmental conditions, promoting school nutrition, and establishing more meaningful school health services reveal information that is usable by the teachers of health education. The school health council is an invaluable ally to the school health educator because it accumulates data pertinent to health education, such as information revealing community and school problems. The council members will be aware of the necessity for direct health instruction in the elementary and secondary schools. Council members will ask, "What is being done about this problem in teaching?" In all probability, the council members will support regularly scheduled health education classes in the secondary schools and recommend increased emphasis on health education in the elementary schools.

## References for Further Study

Anderson, C. L.: *School Health Practice.* 5th ed. St. Louis: The C. V. Mosby Company, 1972.

Cornacchia, H., Staton, W. M., and Irwin, L. W.: *Health in Elementary Schools.* 3rd ed. St. Louis: The C. V. Mosby Company, 1970.

Hanlon, J. J., and McHose, E.: *Design for Health: School and Community.* 2nd ed. Philadelphia: Lea & Febiger, 1971.

Joint Committee on Health Problems in Education of the National Education Association and the American Medical Association: *Healthful School Environment.* Washington, D.C.: National Education Association, 1969.

Kilander, H. F.: *School Health Education.* 2nd ed. New York: The Macmillan Company, 1968.

Oberteuffer, D., Harrelson, O., and Pollock, M.: *School Health Education.* 5th ed. New York: Harper & Row, Publishers, 1972.

Smolensky, J., and Bonvechio, L. R.: *Principles of School Health.* Boston: D. C. Heath and Company, 1966.

Turner, C. E., Randall, H. B., and Smith, S. L.: *School Health and Health Education.* 6th ed. St. Louis: The C. V. Mosby Company, 1970.

Willgoose, C. E.: *Health Education in the Elementary School.* 3rd ed. Philadelphia: W. B. Saunders Company, 1969.

# Chapter 22

# *EVALUATION OF THE SCHOOL HEALTH PROGRAM*

## AN INCIDENT

The school superintendent has been asked by the board of education to evaluate the total school health program. Particular emphasis in the evaluation is to be placed upon health education. Also, the board of education needs justification for the use of local tax funds for the employment of school nurses, screening of pupils' vision and hearing in the elementary schools, school lunch when supplemented by state and federal funds, and the employment of a health coordinator.

Evaluation can reveal progress, existing conditions, needed improvements, and future developments of the school health program. Evaluation can include school health services, healthful school living, health education, and the total health program. It can be done on a day-to-day basis or at any time during a school day. School health services can be evaluated separately from health education or these two parts of the health program can be evaluated at the same time. Many types of evaluative materials can be used, including check lists, observations, questionnaires, surveys, records, tests, and reports. Objectivity, validity, and reliability should be stressed. Personal bias and self-interest are eliminated when objectivity is present. Validity is the extent to which an evaluative criterion measures what it intends to measure. The consistency of measurement is reliability. Who participates in the evaluation of the school health program? Pupils, parents, school personnel, community workers in health, and local citizens. The main purpose of evaluation is to determine the ef-

fects of the health program on the pupils' physical and mental health status, and on the pupils' health practices, attitudes, interests, and knowledge.

## SCHOOL HEALTH SERVICES

Every division of school health services can be evaluated by research techniques to appraise (1) the pupils' health status; (2) the activities of the school nurse; (3) the measures taken for prevention and control of diseases; (4) the status of pupils' dental health; (5) the amount and quality of care for those with chronic health conditions; (6) the effectiveness of emergency care; and (7) the health of school personnel.

### Appraisal of the Pupil's Health Status

Many sources of information can be used to determine the pupil's health status. The teachers' and nurse's *observations* can indicate possible pupil health problems. To improve the validity of observations, the teacher and nurse should be aware of the signs and the types of common pupil health problems (Chapters 2, 4, 5, 6, 7, 10). Skill and accuracy must be developed in recognizing the pertinent signs of each particular health problem, and observations must be recorded continuously throughout the school day. Accurate, up-to-date records should be kept of the pertinent signs of each pupil's health problems.

Readiness-for-school, routine, referral, and special *medical examinations* by family or school physicians can be forms of evaluation. The results of these examinations can identify students needing medical care, classify students for physical education, identify students with chronic health conditions, and disclose which students need modification of their school work. Medical examinations can be among the most effective techniques of appraisal of a pupil's health status.

Many *screening procedures*, used in the appraisal of the pupil's health status, were discussed in Chapter 2. These procedures can be evaluative criteria as they indicate, to some extent, the pupils' visual and hearing difficulties, heart diseases, posture conditions, and nutritional deficiencies.

## Activities of the School Nurse

The School Nursing Committee of the American School Health Association[1] has published "The Nurse in the School Health Program—Guidelines for School Nursing" which includes (1) an evaluation report and (2) a self-evaluation questionnaire for school nurses. Byrd[2] has adapted the Poe and Irwin study[3] into a check list which may be used to compare the work of school nurses with the standards of the study group. Also, Byrd has prepared a check list for the evaluation of the school nurse by the administrator.[4] A study by Rosner and others[5] disclosed methods of making better use of school nurses in New York City schools. The experimental school health team of this study (1) reduced the time spent by nurses in nonprofessional activities and (2) was effective in reducing technical and subprofessional activities of nurses. The publication of the American Nurses' Association[6] concerning school nurses might be used to establish evaluation criteria.

## Prevention and Control of Diseases

School personnel and parents should be informed about the importance of immunizations against specific diseases prev-

alent among elementary and secondary school pupils. Information about each pupil's immunizations should be included in the health history found in the health record. Study of all records can then indicate what preventive measures are necessary to combat diseases. The Center for Disease Control, United States Public Health Service, reported that, in 1970, 31 states had laws requiring immunization for a specific disease or diseases prior to school entry.[7]

Data about the incidence of diseases should be compiled so that school personnel can be familiar with the types of diseases commonly found among elementary and secondary school pupils. The repeated occurrence of "nuisance" diseases, such as head lice, is just as important as high incidence of the varieties of the common cold. Too often, teachers are unaware of the repeated incidence of particular diseases, such as streptococcal infections.

## Dental Health

Oral examinations and full mouth x-rays can indicate many types of pupil dental health problems. The dental hygienist's inspection can reveal group dental needs and the existence or nonexistence of professional dental care. In those school systems not having a full- or part-time dentist or dental hygienist, family dentists may compile the records about incidence of dental caries, periodontal diseases, and malocclusion among elementary and secondary school pupils.

## Chronic Health Conditions

Evaluative criteria can be applied to the special measures taken for many types of pupil chronic health conditions. School personnel should be aware of the incidence, severity of condition, private medical care, and educability of pupils with diabetes, epilepsy, cerebral palsy, cardiac conditions, defective vision, severe posture conditions, defective hearing, and muscular dystrophy. Rarely do evaluations of school health services include consideration of the amount and quality of care for those with chronic health conditions.

[1]School Nursing Committee of the American School Health Association: The nurse in the school health program—guidelines for school nursing. *J. School Health 37* (February, 1967):#2a.

[2]Oliver E. Byrd: *School Health Administration.* Philadelphia: W. B. Saunders Company, 1964, pp. 187-190.

[3]Nancy Poe and Leslie Irwin: Functions of a school nurse. *Research Quarterly 30* (December, 1959):452.

[4]Byrd, *op. cit.*, p. 193.

[5]Lester J. Rosner, Olive E. Pitkin, and Lucille Rosenbluth: Improved use of health professionals in New York City schools. *Amer. J. Public Health 60* (February, 1970):328.

[6]American Nurses' Association: *Functions and Qualifications of School Nurses.* New York: The Association, 1966.

[7]Center for Disease Control, United States Public Health Service: Immunization requirements prior to school entry, October 1970. *Morbidity and Mortality Weekly Report 19* (October 10, 1970):399.

## Emergency Care Procedures

Emergency care records of accidents and illnesses can provide information for evaluation of all procedures taken when a pupil is injured or ill. These records can also be used if school or community personnel claim that there was negligence during the care of the injured or ill child. In addition, these records can be used to identify accident hazards in the school environment, unsafe classroom equipment and activities, and needed safety education to prevent future injuries. Kilander[8] has prepared "A Checklist for the Emergency Care Program in Schools," which is helpful for evaluation.

## Health of the School Personnel

In school systems requiring school personnel to have an annual medical examination, a compilation can be made of all records of health problems of school personnel. This information can be used to identify common diseases, chronic health conditions, and injuries among school personnel. Pre-employment health appraisals required of teachers, clerical staffs, lunchroom workers, custodians, and other school personnel can also indicate specific health problems. There should be an attempt to discover emotional health disturbances, poor welfare practices, and on-the-job complaints of school personnel. The Joint Committee on Health Problems in Education of the NEA and the AMA's publication *Health of School Personnel*[9] might be used as a guide in the preparation of evaluative criteria.

## Evaluative Criteria in School Health Services

Wallace[10] has suggested that evaluative studies of personnel and funds in school health services can reveal the most efficient and effective use of personnel and funds. Comprehensive evaluative studies of

[8]H. Frederick Kilander: *School Health Education.* 2nd ed. New York: The Macmillan Company, 1968, pp. 510-514.
[9]Joint Committee on Health Problems in Education of the National Education Association and the American Medical Association: *Health of School Personnel.* Washington, D.C.: National Education Association, 1964.
[10]Helen Wallace: Evaluation of school health services. *J. School Health* 33 (April, 1963):171.

school health services are needed. The following sources are helpful for those who must determine evaluative criteria:

Neilson, Elizabeth: Analytical study of school health service practices in the United States. *J. School Health 30* (November, 1960):353.
Sellery, C. M., and Bobbitt, B. G.: Evaluation of health education and health services in the Los Angeles City Schools. Parts I and II. *J. School Health 30* (February and March, 1960):81 and 113.
Watters, R.: A scorecard for appraising the school health service program. In Mayshark, C., and Shaw, D. D.: *Administration of School Health Programs.* St. Louis: The C. V. Mosby Company, 1967, p. 246.
Young, M.: The Brookline school health study. *J. School Health 31* (February, 1961):47.

The evaluation of school health services can indicate the incidence and the effectiveness of medical care of known pupil diseases, emotional disturbances, chronic health conditions, injuries, operations, immunizations, visual and hearing difficulties, nutritional deficiencies, posture conditions, and so forth. The evaluation can reveal the many types of pupil dental health problems and the extent of treatment of these problems. The evaluation of the follow-through services by the school or public health nurse can show parental cooperation or neglect, teacher-nurse teamwork, and local physicians' efforts to reduce diseases among pupils. The effectiveness of teacher-nurse conferences, pupil referrals to medical and dental specialists, and home visits by nurses might be included in the evaluation of school health services. The modifications in the school schedule for the pupil with a specific health problem might be evaluated through school health services.

## HEALTHFUL SCHOOL LIVING

The three divisions of healthful school living—environmental factors, school nutrition, and the school day—can be evaluated. Personnel of the local health department, family physicians, and directors of nonofficial health agencies can assist in the evaluation of healthful school living.

## Environmental Factors

A check list may be used by personnel of the local health department in evaluation of the *water supply.* Some of the factors considered are the sources of the water supply, chemical and physical components of water, bacteriological quality, quantity of water required, location and characteristics of plumbing fixtures, and drinking fountains.

*Sewage disposal* can be checked after evaluation of the water supply. Adequate sewage disposal will not pollute drinking water supplies, will not pollute water for bathing and recreational activities, will not create odor or unsightly appearance, and will not be a breeding place for flies. With inadequate sewage treatment in many communities, sewage disposal in schools must be carefully inspected.

When *solid wastes* are improperly disposed of, they become the breeding place for flies and other insects, harbor rats, and encourage stray animals. Thus personnel of the local health department will check to see if solid wastes are disposed of as they should be. In this inspection, public health personnel will be sure that garbage cans have tight-fitting covers and are cleaned and disinfected daily. Also, public health personnel will inspect all methods of incineration.

*Heating, ventilation, and air conditioning* should also be evaluated. Air distribution can be measured per cubic foot per minute per person to determine if it is sufficient for the usual activity of each area of the school. The adequacy of heating and ventilating systems needs to be considered in any evaluation. Effectiveness of air conditioning, placement of the room-type units, and noise level of the air conditioning equipment are included in an evaluation. Nature of the school activities in specialized areas, such as the auditorium and the gymnasium, ages of the pupils, and construction of the building, should be included in any evaluation of heating, ventilation, and air conditioning.

*Noise and acoustical design* cannot be disregarded in an evaluation of the environmental factors. Noise can be measured within and outside the school building. Exposure to more than 95 decibels of noise is hazardous. Effectiveness of acoustical materials applied to ceilings, walls, and floors can be measured.

*Light and color* might be evaluated according to the criteria set by the Illuminating Engineering Society, the National Society for the Prevention of Blindness, and state departments of health. Both the quality of lighting and the level of illumination must be considered. Contrast, brightness, glare, reflection, and footcandles need to be understood by teachers as well as by persons evaluating light and color. Promotion of the individual pupil's eye health needs serious consideration.

Guides for the classroom teacher in checking the pupil's posture in relation to *school furniture* were given in Chapter 9. These simple procedures can prevent many of the common faults in sitting posture. Some of these faults result if the chair is too small, the chair seat is too deep from front to back, the chair seat is too high, the desk top is too low and flat, or the desk top is too high and far away from the pupil.

## School Nutrition

Many types of aids for evaluation of school nutrition have been published. Check lists have been developed to help in evaluating the quality of the school noonday meal, in measuring the quantity of food served, in comparing the meal served with the standards developed by federal and state agencies, and in determining food likes and dislikes of pupils. Surveys and questionnaires can be used to determine the efficiency and sanitation of food preparation and serving, of facilities in the kitchen and dining areas, and of procedures of lunchroom workers. Local and state health departments can develop evaluative criteria to assess the adequacy of sanitary measures of all school lunch activities. In addition, dietary studies can reveal nutritional deficiencies among elementary and secondary school pupils. The Food and Nutrition Service, United States Department of Agriculture, has prepared a series of questions used to evaluate the menus of the Type A lunch.[11] To evaluate the sanitation of school food-handling facilities, Anderson[12] has duplicated the inspection form developed by the Oregon State De-

[11]Food and Nutrition Service, United States Department of Agriculture: *A Menu Planning Guide for Type A School Lunches.* 1969, p. 17.
[12]C. L. Anderson: *School Health Practice.* 4th ed. St. Louis: The C. V. Mosby Company, 1968, pp. 362-363.

partment of Education and Oregon State Board of Health.

## School Day

Evaluation of the total health program in elementary and secondary schools must also include consideration of the school day and its relation to the pupil's total health. Some of the items to be scrutinized are time allotment, pupil grouping, daily program, teacher-pupil relations, teacher's organization of the school day, and methods of supervision.

## Evaluative Criteria in Healthful School Living

Helpful evaluative criteria can be found in the following:

Anderson, C. L.: Survey of healthful school living. *School Health Practice*. 4th ed. St. Louis: The C. V. Mosby Company, 1968, pp. 444-447.

Automotive Safety Foundation: *Guide To A School Pedestrian Safety Program*. Washington, D.C.: The Foundation, 1965, p. 31.

Byrd, Oliver E.: An administrative check list for evaluation of school lunchroom sanitation. *School Health Administration*. Philadelphia: W. B. Saunders Company, 1964, pp. 399-402.

Mayshark, C., and Shaw, D. D.: Checklist of the healthful school environment. *Administration of School Health Programs*. St. Louis: The C. V. Mosby Company, 1967, pp. 293-300.

National Commission on Safety Education, National Education Association: *School Safety Education Checklist: Administration, Instruction, Protection*. rev. Washington, D.C.: The Commission, 1967.

## HEALTH EDUCATION

What is evaluated in health education? The pupil's mental and physical health status and his health knowledge, attitudes, practices, and interests are evaluated. In a class of 30 pupils, can the teacher evaluate all these factors? Yes, when the teacher has the assistance of co-workers in the school and community in this evaluation. Yes, when the teacher is alert to changes in behavior, beliefs, interests, and appearance of pupils. Yes, when the teacher records the effects of the instruction on the pupil. Can this evaluation be done on the secondary level? Yes, when regularly

scheduled health education classes are held so that the teacher has the opportunity to do worthwhile evaluation, and when the content of these classes is based on the pupils' health needs and interests.

What is used in evaluation of the pupil's mental and physical health status, and the pupil's health attitudes, practices, interests, and knowledge? In order to answer this question, it is necessary to retrace the steps used to determine the health education content. In Chapter 13, methods used to discover pupil health needs and interests were discussed. This discovery of pupil health needs and interests resulted in a compilation of positive and negative findings for each pupil's mental and physical health status and his health knowledge, practices, attitudes, and interests. Negative findings appearing with the greatest frequency pointed to needs in the content of health education. Thus, an evaluation of health education will indicate whether the chosen content of health education did or did not change the pupil's mental and physical health status, and the pupil's health knowledge, attitudes, practices, and interests. When change was apparent, was the mental and physical health status of the pupil improved? Did this change foster desirable health attitudes, practices, and interests? How did this change affect the pupil's fund of health information?

If a teacher observes the signs of visual difficulties among his pupils, he recommends visual screening and encourages parents to take pupils to their family physicians. The teacher also includes "Eye Infections, Injuries, and Defects" (Chapter 14) in health education. What changes might occur in these pupils? In the evaluation of health education, it should be determined if the teaching influenced these pupils so that they asked parents to take them to their family physicians. Did the teaching reach parents through pupils' home conversations so that parents sought medical advice? Did the students' become aware of the need for proper lighting when reading? Were the students better informed about their eyes, care of their eyes, and the availability of medical specialists caring for the eyes? Did the students try to compensate for their visual difficulties? Did the students' attitudes toward the importance of vision change? To what extent did the students become interested in their own visual difficulties? Were there noticeable reductions in the students' visual difficulties after their visits to family physicians? What false beliefs and superstitions about the eyes were proved incorrect by the students? These are some of the questions that can be used to learn the results of health education.

## Some Sources of Information about Pupils Used to Evaluate Health Education

### Pupil Mental and Physical Health Status

1. Continuous and systematic teacher observation of pupil changes in appearance and behavior: visual difficulties, hearing difficulties, emotional health problems, communicable diseases, skin infections, nutritional deficiencies, posture conditions, dental health problems, and chronic health conditions
2. Results of follow-through given at teacher-nurse conference
3. Notification from family physician of completion of medical care
4. Results of immunizations and disease detection tests
5. Notification from family dentist of completion of dental care
6. Emergency care records
7. Results of second series of posture screening
8. Changes in pupil dietary habits at noonday school meal and supplementary feeding

### Pupil Health Practices

1. Continuous and systematic teacher observation
2. Follow-through
3. Immunization record
4. Emergency care record
5. Changes in incidence of pupil accidents and illnesses
6. Changes in pupil dietary habits at noonday school meal
7. Results of pupil demonstrations in American Red Cross First Aid
8. Results of pupil surveys
9. Results of pupil rating scales
10. Results of pupil check lists

11. Results of published measuring devices for health practices
    a. Colebank and Johns: *Health Behavior Inventory.*[13]
    b. Lawrence: *Getting Along: Grades 7, 8, 9.*[14]
    c. LeMaistre and Pollock: *Health: Behavior Inventory.*[15]
    d. Pollock: *Mood Altering Substances: A Behavior Inventory.*[16]
    e. Sallak: *Smoking Habits Questionnaire.*[17]
    f. Yellen: *Health Behavior Inventory: Elementary.*[18]

### Pupil Health Attitudes

1. Teacher-pupil conferences following first conference
2. Teacher-parent conferences following first conference
3. Follow-through
4. Health counseling
5. Screening procedures of vision, etc.
6. Changes in pupil conversations regarding his health
7. Sociodrama
8. Results of teacher-guided class discussions
9. Pupil questions directed to the teacher
10. Results of questionnaires
11. Results of attitude rating scales
12. Results of pupil panels and debates
13. Results of published measuring devices for health attitudes
    **Meise:** *A Scale for the Measurement of Attitudes toward Healthful Living.*[19]

---

[13]Albert D. Colebank and Edward B. Johns: *Health Behavior Inventory.* Monterey, Calif.: California Test Bureau, 1962.

[14]Trudys Lawrence: *Getting Along: Grades 7, 8, 9.* Temple City, Calif.: The Author, 6117 North Rosemead Boulevard, 1964.

[15]E. Harold LeMaistre and Marion B. Pollock: *Health Behavior Inventory: Senior High.* Monterey, Calif.: California Test Bureau, 1962.

[16]Marion B. Pollock: *Mood Altering Substances: A Behavior Inventory.* Los Angeles: Tinnon-Brown Publishing Company, 1968.

[17]V. J. Sallak. *Smoking Habits Questionnaire.* Buffalo: Buffalo and Erie County Tuberculosis Association, 766 Ellicott Street, Buffalo, N.Y., 1960.

[18]Sylvia Yellen: *Health Behavior Inventory: Elementary.* Monterey, Calif.: California Test Bureau, 1962.

[19]William C. Meise: *A Scale for Measurement of Attitudes toward Healthful Living.* Slippery Rock State College, Pa.: The Author, 1962.

*Pupil Health Interests*

1. Changes in pupil's choice of health reading materials
2. Changes in pupil written work in health education
3. Changes in pupil conversation
4. Results of pupil interest inventories
5. Pupil questions directed to the teacher
6. Changes in class discussion
7. Results of pupil experiments
8. Results of pupil-made surveys, check lists, questionnaires
9. Results of opinion polls

*Pupil Health Knowledge*

1. Changes in class discussion
2. Pupil questions directed to the teacher
3. Results of pupil panels and debates
4. Results of published measuring devices for health knowledge
   a. Crow and Ryan: *AAHPER Cooperative Health Education Tests: Junior High.*[20]
   b. Kilander: *Kilander Health Knowledge Test.* 6th ed.[21]
   c. _____ : *Information Test on the Biological Aspects of Human Reproduction.* 3rd ed.[22]
   d. _____ : *Information Test on Drugs and Drug Abuse.* 3rd ed.[23]
   e. _____ : *Information Test on Smoking and Health.*[24]
   f. _____ : *Nutrition Information Test.* 5th ed.[25]
   g. Klein: *Health Knowledge and Understanding Test for Fifth Grade Pupils.*[26]

h. McHugh: *A Venereal Disease Knowledge Inventory.*[27]
i. National Safety Council: *Bicycle Safety Information Test.*[28]
j. New York State Council on Health and Safety Education: *Health Knowledge Examination for the Secondary Level.*[29]
k. Schwartz: *Achievement Test on Syphilis and Gonorrhea.*[30]
l. _____ : *Teaching Test on Syphilis and Gonorrhea.*[31]
m. Speer and Smith: *Health Test.*[32]
n. Thompson: *Thompson Smoking and Tobacco Knowledge Test.*[33]
o. Veenker: *Health Knowledge Test for the Seventh Grade.*[34]

5. Results of teacher-made health education knowledge tests

**Teacher-Made Tests**

Teacher-made tests of health knowledge can be subjective or objective. Four common examples of the subjective type of knowledge tests follow: (1) A question is stated, "What are the seven warning signs of cancer?" (2) The teacher asks the pupil, "Explain the difference between benign and malignant cell growths or list the possible treatments used in the medical care of malignant cell growth." (3) A paragraph is given with specific information such as, "The American Cancer Society promotes research into suspected causes of cancer and into many radiation and surgical tech-

[20]Lester D. Crow and Loretta C. Ryan: *AAHPER Cooperative Health Education Tests: Junior High.* Princeton, N.J.: Educational Testing Service, 1972.
[21]H. Frederick Kilander: *Kilander Health Knowledge Test.* 6th ed. Staten Island, N.Y.: Glenn Leach, Wagner College, 1966.
[22]_____: *Information Test on the Biological Aspects of Human Reproduction.* 3rd ed. Staten Island, N.Y.: Glenn Leach, Wagner College, 1968.
[23]_____: *Information Test on Drugs and Drug Abuse.* 3rd ed. Staten Island, N.Y.: Glenn Leach, Wagner College, 1968.
[24]_____: *Information Test on Smoking and Health.* Staten Island, N.Y.: Glenn Leach, Wagner College, 1964.
[25]_____: *Nutrition Information Test.* 5th ed. Staten Island, N.Y.: Glenn Leach, Wagner College, 1968.
[26]Walter C. Klein: *A Health Knowledge and Understanding Test for Fifth Grade Pupils.* LaCrosse, Wis.: Northern Engr. and Mfg. Co., 1960.

[27]Gelolo McHugh: *A Venereal Disease Knowledge Inventory.* Durham, N.C.: Family Life Publications, Inc., 1966.
[28]National Safety Council: *Bicycle Safety Information Test.* Chicago: The Council, n.d.
[29]New York State Council on Health and Safety Education: *Health Knowledge Examination for the Secondary Level.* Cortland, N.Y.: John S. Sinacore, State University, 1962.
[30]William F. Schwartz: *Achievement Test on Syphilis and Gonorrhea.* Durham, N.C.: Family Life Publications, Inc., 1965.
[31]_____ : *Teaching Test on Syphilis and Gonorrhea.* Durham, N.C.: Family Life Publications, Inc., 1965.
[32]Robert K. Speer and Samuel Smith: *Health Test.* (Form A). Brookport, Ill.: Psychometric Affiliates, 1960.
[33]Clem W. Thompson: *Thompson Smoking and Tobacco Knowledge Test.* Mankato, Minn.: The Author, Mankato State College, 1963.
[34]C. Harold Veenker: *A Health Knowledge Test for the Seventh Grade.* Lafayette, Ind.: The Author, Purdue University, 1960.

niques used in treatment. What else does the American Cancer Society do?" (4) A paragraph of a designated length is to be written, for example, "Write a 50-word paragraph concerning the National Cancer Institute." Testing with subjective questions like these examples has advantages for the teacher. Students either know or do not know the answers and have no assistance as in recognition and recall objective test questions. The teacher can correct misspelled words. The students have an opportunity to organize their fund of information logically. Students reveal misinformation as well as false beliefs when they answer subjective test questions such as these. There are also disadvantages. Tests made up of subjective questions are time-consuming to grade; there is little chance to indicate the reliability and validity of the test item; and scores on these tests depend on the judgment of the grader.

The objective test can reveal the extent of the student's fund of information about specific and detailed items. It can cover a wide range of teaching content. Through item analysis, the objective test can indicate distinct weaknesses in test items as well as in the student's fund of information. Over the years, the test can be refined so that it has a reasonable degree of validity and reliability. The objective test is easier to grade, and scores do not rely on the whims of the grader; it is, however, much more difficult to construct.

Before attempting to devise an objective test, the teacher should review carefully the subject matter that was presented to students. From that subject matter alone, test items should be compiled, and items with no relation to the subject matter should be excluded. A careful check should be made so that there are significant items which test the complete range of the subject matter. Items generally accepted, controversial within a specific area of health education, too obvious, ambiguous, half-true, outdated, and misleading should be eliminated. The type of test form should be selected. Five possible test forms are these: recognition—(1) multiple choice and (2) matching; (3) recall-completion; (4) problem-to-be-solved; and (5) true-false.

The directions for the entire test should be placed in an introductory paragraph so that students will understand that there may be more than one part to the test. Each of the test forms might constitute a part of the test.

Before each part of the test, there should be a full set of directions which tell *how* to answer the items, with an example given. It is desirable to include the value of each test item with the directions, thus enabling the student to estimate his possible grade and to allot his time wisely when taking the test.

*Multiple Choice*

The teacher should be well informed about the construction of each test form. These suggestions will help him to devise multiple choice test form:

1. State the item briefly and give five choices listed alphabetically.
2. Have the student place his answer to the left of the item for ease in grading.
3. Word the choices concisely.
4. Make sure all choices are plausible.
5. Be sure one choice is *entirely* correct.
6. Avoid any set pattern of answers.
7. Watch sentence structure so that sentences are complete.
8. Score by counting correct answers.

PART I: Multiple Choice. In the bracket at the left of the question, place the letter of the best choice.
Example:
(a) The medical specialist who treats diseases of the eyes and performs eye surgery is an:
a. Ophthalmologist
b. Optician
c. Optometrist
d. Orthoptist
e. Otologist

( ) 1. When the eyeball is too long from front to back and the light rays converge in front of the retina, this visual defect is called:
a. Astigmatism
b. Hyperopia
c. Myopia
d. Presbyopia
e. Strabismus

*Matching Questions*

In devising matching questions, the

teacher may be helped by these suggestions:

1. Take the test items to be used in matching questions, and group into sets of five items each.
2. Select a topic in health education to be covered within each set, and relate each item to that topic.
3. Have the student place his choice in the bracket provided to the left of the first column for ease of grading.
4. Use single words in the left-hand column, if possible.
5. Give concisely, in incomplete sentences, the item to be matched in the right-hand column.
6. Alphabetize the items in the right-hand column.
7. Have each single word match only one statement of the right-hand column.
8. Scatter choices so that no pattern is established.
9. Draw a single line under each set of five items indicating that the topic within that set is complete.
10. Score by counting correct responses.

PART II: Matching Questions. In the bracket provided to the left of the single word, place the letter representing the best statement. *Do not use a letter more than once.*

Example:
(c) Heroin    a. Coca leaves
(b) Marijuana    b. "Pot"
(a) Cocaine    c. "Skin shots"
(d) Barbiturate    d. Sleeping powder
(e) Morphine    e. Used in small amounts to ease pain

( ) Tolerance (heroin)    a. Barbiturate trade name
( ) Hallucinogens    b. Diminished effort of same dosage of narcotic over a long period of time
( ) Seconal
( ) "Speed"    c. Gasoline, paint thinners
( ) Inhalants    d. Mescaline LSD, psilocybin
   e. Methamphetamine

*Completion*

Completion questions, a type of recall test form, need careful preparation. Each item must be clear and precise. These suggestions are given:

1. Word each item so the meaning is clear.
2. Construct items around the missing word.
3. Use one blank for one missing word.
4. Do not use more than two blanks within one item.
5. Provide "a," "an," and "the" within the item.
6. Use complete sentences with the missing word as the single blank.
7. Have the student place the word used to complete the blank to the left of the item for ease of grading.
8. Provide synonyms and terms used for each blank on the scoring key.
9. Score by counting correct answers.

PART III: Completion. In the following statements, a blank represents a missing word. Place the missing word in the column to the left.
Example:
ovaries    The human egg cell is produced in the female _____ .

1. _____ The period of a woman's life when the ovaries normally cease to produce and expel ova is the _____ .

*Problem-to-be-solved*

The problem-to-be-solved type of test form states a series of incidents presenting a problem. In order to solve the problem, the student must carefully read each incident, compile all given facts within a series of incidents, analyze the compilation, decide the steps to be taken in solving the problem, organize the steps in a logical manner, and state the solution to the problem. These suggestions are given:

1. Word the problem simply.
2. Avoid too many incidents within a problem.
3. Provide incidents to test whether the student can analyze the problem, decide the steps to be taken, and organize the solution in a logical manner.

4. Be aware of all possibilities in the solution of the problem.
5. Score the problem by giving credit to each part of the solved problem.

PART IV: Problem-to-be-solved. Read the problem carefully. Consider all given facts. State what you would do first, second, third, and so forth.
Example:
A housewife preparing a vegetable salad accidentally slices her left index finger between the palm and the second joint. The knife has cut deep and exposes muscles, tendons, and the bone of the finger.
Solution: Apply direct pressure over the wound with sterile gauze. If bleeding continues, apply pressure over the left brachial artery in the upper arm. Treat for shock. When bleeding is controlled, apply fresh sterile gauze over wound. Place a figure eight of the hand and wrist bandage over the gauze to hold it in place and prevent further injury to muscles and tendons. Seek immediate medical care.

_____

Problem 1. A man has fallen from a ladder. He is unconscious. There is bleeding from the right lower leg. The ends of the right lower leg bones have torn through flesh and clothes. There is bleeding at the right cheek.
Solution:

========

*True-False*

The true-false test form gives a complete statement which is either "true" or "false." It can be highly discriminating and useful. A true-false test is easy to construct, helpful in discovering misconceptions, suitable for situations involving just two alternatives, and easy to score. These suggestions are given:

1. Use straightforward statements.
2. Make the important part of the statement clear to the student.
3. Avoid any set pattern of answers, and avoid ambiguous statements.
4. Avoid the use of precise numbers in every statement.
5. Avoid statements that are too long.
6. Avoid the use of "only," "never," "always," "all," "usually," "frequently," "not," "none," and "almost always."

PART V: True-False. Determine if the following statements are True or False. Circle cor-

rect answer. If the statement is incorrect, reword it to make it correct in the space provided.
Example:
T (F) 1. Teeth should be brushed three times a day.
   Teeth should be brushed after eating.

_____

T F 1. Dentifrices are more important than tooth brushing.

========

When the test forms have been completed, the teacher should prepare a scoring key. For ease of use, the correct answers on the scoring key should line up directly with each test item on the students' test forms. In the completion test, synonyms should be listed on the scoring key.

When the test is completely constructed, pretesting takes place. During the pretesting, the teacher uses students familiar with the content to be tested but who will not be given the final test. Confusing or ambiguous items can be identified and eliminated with pretesting.

After the test has been given to the students for whom it was prepared, an item analysis takes place. The statistical tool used for this purpose is the "index of discrimination." In addition, the teacher may wish to determine the difficulty rating of a test item. Limits may be set to exclude those test items answered correctly by 25% or less of the group and those items answered correctly by 75% or more of the group, concentrating the difficulty rating around 50%.

*Evaluative Criteria in Health Education*

The teacher not only can evaluate health status, practices, attitudes, interests, and knowledge but also evaluate all phases of health education. Criteria for health education evaluation are found in the following:
Cauffman, J. G.: Appraisal of the health behavior of junior high school students. *Research Quarterly 34* (December, 1963): 425.
Cushman, W.: *School Health Instruction Survey Form.* Columbus, Ohio: The Author, Ohio State University, n.d.
Columbia Broadcasting System: *National Health Test.* New York: CBS, 1966.
Johns, E.: School health education evalua-

tive study, Los Angeles Area: an example of a modern evaluation plan. *J. School Health 32* (January, 1962):5.

Kilander, H. F.: A guide for the evaluation of the health instruction program. In *School Health Education.* 2nd ed. New York: The Macmillan Company, 1968, p. 514.

National Commission on Safety Education: *School Safety Education Checklist.* Washington, D.C.: National Education Association, 1967.

School Health Education Study: *Summary Report of a Nationwide Study of Health Instruction in the Public Schools.* Washington, D.C.: The Study, 1964, Appendix.

## TOTAL SCHOOL HEALTH PROGRAM

In this chapter, evaluative criteria for school health services, healthful school living, and health education have been discussed. Further evaluative criteria for the total school health program are discussed in these publications:

Anderson, C. L.: School health program evaluation scale. (Developed by Oregon State University, Corvallis, Ore.) In *School Health Practice.* 4th ed. St. Louis: The C. V. Mosby Company, 1968, p. 434.

California State Department of Education: *Criteria for Evaluating the Elementary School Health Program* (1962); and *Criteria for Evaluating the High School Health Program* (1962). Sacramento, Calif.: The Department.

*Evaluation of the Health Program in the Los Angeles City Schools.* #673. Los Angeles, Calif.: Division of Educational Services, 1962.

The results of evaluation of the total school health program can reveal whether the program does or does not influence the pupil's physical and mental health status and the pupil's health practices, attitudes, interests, and knowledge. The results can show the strengths and weaknesses of school health services, healthful school living, and health education. The results can disclose the effectiveness of the organization and administration of the pro-

gram. Finally, the results of evaluation can reveal whether school and community personnel work together well in the development of the school health program.

## References for Further Study

Anderson, C. L.: *School Health Practice.* 5th ed. St. Louis: The C. V. Mosby Company, 1972.

Beyrer, M., Nolte, A. E., and Solleder, M. K.: *A Directory of Selected References and Resources for Health Instruction.* 2nd ed. Minneapolis: Burgess Publishing Company, 1969.

Byrd, O. E.: *School Health Administration.* Philadelphia: W. B. Saunders Company, 1964.

Cornacchia, H., Staton, W. M., and Irwin, L. W.: *Health in the Elementary Schools.* 3rd ed. St. Louis: The C. V. Mosby Company, 1970.

Clark, H.: *Application of Measurement to Health and Physical Education.* 4th ed. Englewood Cliffs, N.J.: Prentice-Hall, Inc., 1967.

Joint Committee on Health Problems in Education of the National Education Association and the American Medical Association: *Healthful School Environment.* Washington, D.C.: National Education Association, 1969.

Kilander, H.: *School Health Education.* 2nd ed. New York: The Macmillan Company, 1968.

Latchaw, M., and Brown, C.: *The Evaluation Process in Health Education.* Englewood Cliffs, N.J.: Prentice-Hall, Inc., 1962.

Mayshark, C., and Shaw, D. D.: *Administration of School Health Programs.* St. Louis: The C. V. Mosby Company, 1967.

Mayshark, C., and Irwin, L. W.: *Health Education in Secondary Schools.* St. Louis: The C. V. Mosby Company, 1968.

Nemir, A.: *The School Health Program.* 3rd ed. Philadelphia: W. B. Saunders Company, 1970.

Oberteuffer, D., Harrelson, O., and Pollock, M.: *School Health Education.* 5th ed. New York: Harper & Row, 1972.

School Health Education Study: *Synthesis of Research in Selected Areas of Health Instruction.* Washington, D.C.: The Study, 1963.

Solleder, M. K.: *Evaluation Instruments in Health Education.* rev. ed. Washington, D.C.: American Association for Health, Physical Education and Recreation, 1969.

Turner, C. E., Randall, H. B., and Smith, S. L.: *School Health and Health Education.* 6th ed. St. Louis: The C. V. Mosby Company, 1970.

Willgoose, C. E.: *Health Education in the Elementary School.* 3rd ed. Philadelphia: W. B. Saunders Company, 1969.

# Appendix A

---
PUBLIC SCHOOLS
---

STATE

## HEALTH  RECORD

(Medical and dental examinations; screening for hearing, vision, and nutritional status;
posture screening; follow-through; teachers' observations)

THE INFORMATION CONTAINED IN EACH PART OF THIS HEALTH RECORD
IS TO REMAIN *CONFIDENTIAL*  AND IS A CUMULATIVE RECORD OF

| Last Name | First Name | Middle Name |
|---|---|---|
| Street Address | Town | County |
| Street Address | Town | County |
| Street Address | Town | County |

| PHYSICIAN TO BE CALLED IN EMERGENCY | TELEPHONE |
|---|---|
| | ,M.D. |
| | ,M.D. |
| | ,M.D. |

| DENTIST TO BE CALLED IN EMERGENCY | TELEPHONE |
|---|---|
| | ,D.D.S. |
| | ,D.D.S. |
| | ,D.D.S. |

HOME OR BUSINESS ADDRESSES AND TELEPHONE

| FATHER | TELEPHONE |
|---|---|

| MOTHER | TELEPHONE |
|---|---|

| NEXT OF KIN | TELEPHONE |
|---|---|

NAME

SEX

Last

DATE OF BIRTH

First

Initial

## TEACHER OBSERVATIONS OF PHYSICAL AND EMOTIONAL HEALTH PROBLEMS

Date                                                         Date

Date                                                         Date

Date                                                         Date

Date                                                         Date

Date                                                         Date

Date                                                         Date

Date                                                         Date

Date                                                         Date

Date                                                         Date

_____
PUBLIC SCHOOLS

_____
STATE

# PUPIL HEALTH HISTORY

*(to be filled out by the parent, nurse, student, or teacher*
*previous to the medical and dental examinations)*

NAME _____ DATE OF BIRTH _____ SEX _____

**RECORD OF ILLNESS** *(Check those which occurred at any time;*
*star (\*) significant illness within the past five years):*

| | | | | | |
|---|---|---|---|---|---|
| ALLERGY | _____ | EAR INFECTION | _____ | MONONUCLEOSIS | _____ |
| ANEMIA | _____ | FREQUENT COLDS | _____ | MUMPS | _____ |
| APPENDICITIS | _____ | HAY FEVER | _____ | PNEUMONIA | _____ |
| ASTHMA | _____ | HEART DISEASE | _____ | RHEUMATIC FEVER | _____ |
| BRONCHITIS | _____ | HERNIA | _____ | SCARLET FEVER | _____ |
| CHICKEN POX | _____ | HIVES | _____ | SINUSITIS | _____ |
| CHOREA | _____ | INFECTIOUS HEPATITIS | _____ | TETANUS | _____ |
| DIABETES | _____ | MEASLES | _____ | WHOOPING COUGH | _____ |
| DIPHTHERIA | _____ | | | | |

OTHER: (SPECIFY) _____

**TUBERCULOSIS CONTROL** *(physician or nurse fills in)*

TUBERCULIN
POSITIVE _____ NEGATIVE _____ DATE _____
POSITIVE _____ NEGATIVE _____ DATE _____
TEST
POSITIVE _____ NEGATIVE _____ DATE _____

**IMMUNIZATION RECORD** (record year) *(physician or nurse fills in)*

SMALLPOX_____ WHOOPING COUGH _____ TYPHOID_____
POLIO_____ DIPHTHERIA _____ TETANUS _____
MUMPS _____ RUBEOLA_____ RUBELLA _____

**RECORD OF SERIOUS INJURIES AND OPERATIONS** (record year)

INJURIES_____ OPERATIONS _____

**MENSTRUATION**

REGULAR _____ IRREGULAR _____
DURATION _____ SEVERE _____

DO ANY OF THE FOLLOWING OCCUR FREQUENTLY? *(Yes___No___Doubtful___Date___)*

| | | |
|---|---|---|
| ACHING EYES_____ | HOARSENESS_____ | HEART AND LUNGS_____ |
| BLINDNESS_____ | NASAL DISCHARGE___ | CHEST PAIN_____ |
| BLURRED VISION_____ | NOSEBLEED_____ | PALPITATIONS_____ |
| INFLAMED EYELIDS____ | SORE THROAT_____ | SHORTNESS OF BREATH___ |
| RECURRING HEADACHE_ | ABDOMINAL PAIN____ | PAINFUL URINATION_____ |
| STYS_____ | DIARRHEA_____ | FREQUENT URINATION_____ |
| COLOR BLIND_____ | NAUSEA_____ | WEIGHT—SUDDEN GAIN____ |
| DEAFNESS_____ | JAUNDICE_____ | —SUDDEN LOSS_____ |
| TOOTHACHE_____ | CONSTIPATION_____ | NIGHT SWEATS_____ |
| COUGH (PROLONGED)___ | VOMITING_____ | FAINTING_____ |

## SOCIAL AND EMOTIONAL HEALTH

*(Check which of the following have been observed and date)*

**ELEMENTARY SCHOOL**

| | |
|---|---|
| SELFISH | EASILY DISCOURAGED |
| EXCITABLE | SHY |
| ANGERS EASILY | NAIL BITING |
| VERY EASY TO MANAGE | THUMB SUCKING |
| RESENTFUL | HAPPY DISPOSITION |
| IS GENEROUS TO OTHERS | ORDERLY |
| JEALOUS | HELPFUL AROUND THE HOUSE |
| DEPENDABLE | HAS MANY FRIENDS |
| LIKES TO PLAY WITH OTHERS | SELF-RELIANT |
| HAS MANY FEARS | PREFERS TO BE ALONE |
| WORRIES A GREAT DEAL | |

**SECONDARY SCHOOL**

| | |
|---|---|
| HAPPY DISPOSITION | HAS MANY FEARS |
| ORDERLY | JEALOUS |
| HAS MANY FRIENDS | DEPENDABLE |
| IS A LEADER | SELFISH |
| IS A FOLLOWER | EXCITABLE |
| HAS FEW FRIENDS | SUSPICIOUS |
| PREFERS TO BE ALONE | AWKWARD |
| EASILY DISCOURAGED | DAYDREAMING |
| WORRIES A GREAT DEAL | EASILY EMBARRASSED |
| SELF-RELIANT | LOSES TEMPER |
| RESENTFUL | TOLERANT |

DATE OF LAST DENTAL EXAMINATION OR TREATMENT

DATE LAST ATTENDED BY FAMILY PHYSICIAN AND REASON

---
PUBLIC SCHOOLS
---

---
STATE
---

# MEDICAL EXAMINATION

*(to be filled out by the physician and may be mailed to the*
*principal of the school or may be kept in the physician's office)*

NAME_____ DATE OF BIRTH_____ SEX_____

PARENTS' NAMES_____

**FILL IN EACH SPACE; USE SPACE AT BOTTOM FOR REMARKS**

| | | | | | | |
|---|---|---|---|---|---|---|
| **DATE** | | | | | | |
| GENERAL APPEARANCE | | | | | | |
| GENERAL NUTRITION | | | | | | |
| POSTURE | | | | | | |
| **SKIN** | | | | | | |
| SCALP | | | | | | |
| **EYES AND LIDS** | | | | | | |
| VISION WITHOUT GLASSES | R L | R L | R L | R L | R L | R L |
| VISION WITH GLASSES | R L | R L | R L | R L | R L | R L |
| OTHER | | | | | | |
| **EARS** | | | | | | |
| GENERAL CONDITION | R L | R L | R L | R L | R L | R L |
| DISCHARGE | R L | R L | R L | R L | R L | R L |
| **HEARING** | R L | R L | R L | R L | R L | R L |
| **NASOPHARYNX** | | | | | | |
| TONSILS | | | | | | |
| NASAL OBSTRUCTION | | | | | | |
| | | | | | | |
| **MOUTH** | | | | | | |
| | | | | | | |
| TEETH | | | | | | |
| SOFT TISSUES | | | | | | |
| **THYROID** | | | | | | |
| **LYMPH GLANDS** | | | | | | |
| CERVICAL | | | | | | |
| OTHER | | | | | | |
| **LUNGS** | | | | | | |

| | | | | | | |
|---|---|---|---|---|---|---|
| **HEART** | | | | | | |
| MURMURS | | | | | | |
| ENLARGEMENT | | | | | | |
| | | | | | | |
| | | | | | | |
| **PULSE RATE** | | | | | | |
| | | | | | | |
| **ABDOMEN** | | | | | | |
| GENERAL | | | | | | |
| SCARS | | | | | | |
| HERNIA | | | | | | |
| **BONES AND MUSCLES** | | | | | | |
| CHEST | | | | | | |
| SPINE | | | | | | |
| UPPER EXTREMITIES | | | | | | |
| LOWER EXTREMITIES | | | | | | |
| | | | | | | |
| | | | | | | |
| | | | | | | |
| | | | | | | |
| **NERVOUS SYSTEM REFLEXES** | | | | | | |
| | | | | | | |
| **EMOTIONAL PROBLEMS** | | | | | | |

PHYSICIAN'S SIGNATURE: _____

REMARKS: _____

_____

_____

_____

_____

_____

_____

_____

_____

_____

PUBLIC SCHOOL

STATE

**PHYSICIAN'S REPORT TO THE SCHOOL ON SIGNIFICANT
FINDINGS OF THE MEDICAL EXAMINATION**

*(to be filled out by the physician and mailed to the school principal)*

NAME_____ DATE OF BIRTH_____

PARENTS' NAMES_____

**RECOMMENDATIONS FOR CORRECTION**

DATE_____

DATE_____

DATE_____

DATE_____

**RECOMMENDATIONS TO THE TEACHER**

IS PUPIL CAPABLE OF CARRYING A FULL PROGRAM OF     Yes_____ No_____
SCHOOL WORK?     Yes_____ No_____

    Yes_____ No_____

SHOULD THERE BE RESTRICTIONS ON UP-AND-DOWN     Yes_____ No_____
STAIRS TRAVEL?     Yes_____ No_____

    Yes_____ No_____

IS SPECIAL SEATING PLACEMENT RECOMMENDED?     Yes_____ No_____

    Yes_____ No_____

    Yes_____ No_____

DO YOU ADVISE SUPPLEMENTARY IN-BETWEEN-MEAL     Yes_____ No_____
FEEDING?     Yes_____ No_____

    Yes_____ No_____

DOES PUPIL HAVE ANY CHRONIC HEALTH CONDITIONS?     Yes_____ No_____

    Yes_____ No_____

    Yes_____ No_____

IS THERE EVIDENCE OF UNUSUAL EMOTIONAL     Yes_____ No_____
TENDENCIES?     Yes_____ No_____

    Yes_____ No_____

*(DETACHABLE)*

**REMARKS TO AID TEACHER**

DATE_____

DATE_____

DATE_____

DATE_____

**CLASSIFICATION FOR PHYSICAL EDUCATION** *(Check the one best suited to student)*

| | DATE | DATE | DATE | DATE |
|---|---|---|---|---|
| A. Unlimited physical education activity, including interscholastic and intramural sports. | | | | |
| B. Moderate physical activity: Limited to physical education classes and excluding interscholastic sports and more strenuous activities. | | | | |
| C. Adapted physical education or physical education for the handicapped. | | | | |

**RECOMMENDED ACTIVITIES FOR "B" AND "C" CLASSIFICATIONS**

DATE _____

DATE _____

DATE _____

DATE _____

**PLEASE INDICATE ANY SPECIAL NEED FOR DENTAL, PSYCHIATRIC, MEDICAL, OR SURGICAL CARE.**

DATE_____ SIGNATURE OF EXAMINING PHYSICIAN _____M.D.

DATE_____ SIGNATURE OF EXAMINING PHYSICIAN _____M.D.

DATE_____ SIGNATURE OF EXAMINING PHYSICIAN _____M.D.

DATE_____ SIGNATURE OF EXAMINING PHYSICIAN _____M.D.

DETACHABLE

_____
PUBLIC SCHOOLS

_____
STATE

## FOLLOW-THROUGH

*(to be filled out by the school nurse)*

NAME_____ DATE OF BIRTH_____

PARENTS' NAMES_____

| NOTIFICATION OF PHYSICIAN OF SCREENING RESULTS | FOLLOW-THROUGH OF MEDICAL RECOMMENDATIONS | FOLLOW-THROUGH OF DENTAL RECOMMENDATIONS |
|---|---|---|
| DATE | DATE | DATE |
| DATE | DATE | DATE |
| DATE | DATE | DATE |
| DATE | DATE | DATE |
| DATE | DATE | DATE |
| DATE | DATE | DATE |
| DATE | DATE | DATE |

PUBLIC SCHOOLS

STATE

## HEARING AND VISION SCREENING

NAME_____DATE OF BIRTH_____

PARENTS' NAMES_____

### AUDIOGRAM

Date_____ By_____ Grade_____

| | 500 | 1000 | 2000 | 4000 | 6000 |
|---|---|---|---|---|---|
| 10 | | | | | |
| 0 | | | | | |
| 10 | | | | | |
| 20 | | | | | |
| 30 | | | | | |
| 40 | | | | | |
| 50 | | | | | |
| 60 | | | | | |
| 70 | | | | | |
| 80 | | | | | |
| 90 | | | | | |
| 100 | | | | | |

Loss in Decibles

Left Ear—X          Right Ear—O

### AUDIOGRAM

Date_____ By_____ Grade_____

| | 500 | 1000 | 2000 | 4000 | 6000 |
|---|---|---|---|---|---|
| 10 | | | | | |
| 0 | | | | | |
| 10 | | | | | |
| 20 | | | | | |
| 30 | | | | | |
| 40 | | | | | |
| 50 | | | | | |
| 60 | | | | | |
| 70 | | | | | |
| 80 | | | | | |
| 90 | | | | | |
| 100 | | | | | |

Left Ear—X          Right Ear—O

## MASSACHUSETTS VISION TEST

| DATE | EXAMINER | GLASSES | TESTS | | | | | | RETEST | RECOMMENDATIONS |
|---|---|---|---|---|---|---|---|---|---|---|
| | | | I | | II | | III | | | |
| | | | L | R | L | R | a | b | c | |
| | | | | | | | | | | |
| | | | | | | | | | | |
| | | | | | | | | | | |
| | | | | | | | | | | |
| | | | | | | | | | | |
| | | | | | | | | | | |

PUBLIC SCHOOL

STATE

# DENTAL RECORD

*(to be filled out by dentist; may be mailed to principal or kept in dentist's office)*

NAME_____DATE OF BIRTH_____

PARENTS' NAMES_____

### TOOTH CHART

*Record on the Tooth Chart conditions of each tooth. Permanent teeth are referred to in numbers. Deciduous teeth are referred to in letters.*

| | **RIGHT SIDE OF PATIENT** | **LEFT SIDE OF PATIENT** |
|---|---|---|
| | 8  7  6  5  4  3  2  1 | 1  2  3  4  5  6  7  8 |
| | E  D  C  B  A | A  B  C  D  E |

DETACHABLE

**1ST DENTAL EXAM**
  UPPER
  LOWER

**2D DENTAL EXAM**
  UPPER
  LOWER

**3D DENTAL EXAM**
  UPPER
  LOWER

**4TH DENTAL EXAM**
  UPPER
  LOWER

**5TH DENTAL EXAM**
  UPPER
  LOWER

**6TH DENTAL EXAM**
  UPPER
  LOWER

**7TH DENTAL EXAM**
  UPPER
  LOWER

**8TH DENTAL EXAM**
  UPPER
  LOWER

— — — — — — — — — — — — — — — — — — — — — — — —

PUBLIC SCHOOLS_____ STATE_____

NAME_____ PARENTS' NAMES_____

**DENTAL RECOMMENDATIONS**

**6TH DENTAL EXAM**
DATE_____
                                                      D.D.S

**5TH DENTAL EXAM**
DATE_____
                                                      D.D.S

*Note below any abnormal or pathological conditions and special examinations requested, such as x-rays.*

1ST DENTAL EXAM

2D DENTAL EXAM

3D DENTAL EXAM

4TH DENTAL EXAM

5TH DENTAL EXAM

6TH DENTAL EXAM

7TH DENTAL EXAM

8TH DENTAL EXAM

REMARKS:

- - - - - - - - - - - - - - - - - - - - - - - - - - - - - - - - - - - - - - -

4TH DENTAL EXAM
DATE                                                                    D.D.S.
3D DENTAL EXAM
DATE                                                                    D.D.S.
2D DENTAL EXAM
DATE                                                                    D.D.S.
1ST DENTAL EXAM
DATE                                                                    D.D.S.

PUBLIC SCHOOLS

STATE

NAME _____ SEX _____

PARENTS' NAMES _____ DATE OF BIRTH _____

### HEIGHT WEIGHT INTERPRETATION FOR BOYS

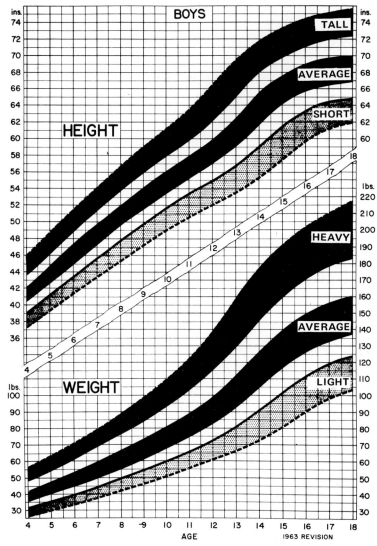

Reprinted with the permission of the Joint Committee on Health Problems in Education of the National Education Association and the American Medical Association.

*Section 7, back cover*

PUBLIC SCHOOLS

STATE

NAME _____ SEX _____

PARENTS' NAMES _____ DATE OF BIRTH _____

## HEIGHT WEIGHT INTERPRETATION FOR GIRLS

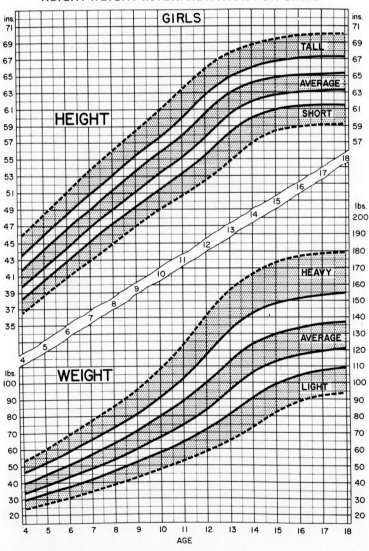

Reprinted with the permission of the Joint Committee on Health Problems in Education of the National Education Association and the American Medical Association.

DETACHABLE

_____
PUBLIC SCHOOL

_____
STATE

## POSTURE SCREENING

NAME _____ SEX _____

PARENTS' NAMES _____ DATE OF BIRTH _____

HEIGHT _____ WEIGHT _____

| | SCORE | | | | | | SCORE | | | |
|---|---|---|---|---|---|---|---|---|---|---|
| STANDING AP POSTURE | | | | | LEG IMBALANCE | | | | |
| SHOULDER OVERHANG | | | | | FOOT IMBALANCE | | | | |
| FORWARD HEAD | | | | | MECHANICS OF SITTING | | | | |
| ROUND BACK | | | | | DOWN | | | | |
| HOLLOW BACK | | | | | UP | | | | |
| HYPER KNEES | | | | | WALKING AP POSTURE | | | | |
| PRONATED FEET | | | | | LATERAL BALANCE | | | | |
| LATERAL BALANCE | | | | | PELVIC CONTROL | | | | |
| SHOULDER HEIGHT<br>L | | | | | FOOT POSITION<br>HEEL-BALL-TOE | | | | |
| R | | | | | REACHING MECHANICS | | | | |
| HIP PROMINENCE<br>L | | | | | STAIR CLIMBING<br>UP | | | | |
| R | | | | | DOWN | | | | |
| RIB PROMINENCE<br>L | | | | | LIFTING MECHANICS<br>LOWERING WEIGHT | | | | |
| R | | | | | RAISING WEIGHT | | | | |
| | | | | | ROPE SKIPPING | | | | |

RATING SCALE:
1-EXCELLENT  3-FAIR
2-GOOD  4-POOR*

_____
Name of examiner                                    Date

_____
Name of examiner                                    Date

_____
Name of examiner                                    Date

_____
Name of examiner                                    Date

*Mathews, D. K.: *Measurement in Physical Education*, 3rd ed. Philadelphia: W. B. Saunders Co., 1968, p. 271.

_____
PUBLIC SCHOOLS
_____
STATE

## SUMMARY OF ALL HEALTH DATA TO BE USED BY TEACHER
## IN INSTRUCTIONAL PROGRAM

_____

DATE _____

_____

DATE _____

_____

DATE _____

_____

DATE _____

_____

DATE _____

_____

DATE _____

_____

DATE _____

_____

DATE _____

_____

DATE _____

_____

DATE _____

_____

# SOURCES OF FREE OR INEXPENSIVE PRINTED MATERIALS OF INSTRUCTION FOR HEALTH EDUCATION

1. Aetna Life Affiliated Companies
   Education Department
   151 Farmington Avenue
   Hartford, Conn. 10015
2. American Academy of Pediatrics, Inc.,
   1801 Hinmon Avenue
   Evanston, Ill. 60204
3. American Association for Health, Physical Education and Recreation
   1201 16th Street, N.W.
   Washington, D.C. 20036
4. American Cancer Society
   219 East 42nd Street
   New York, N.Y. 10017
5. American Diabetes Association
   18 East 48th Street
   New York, N.Y. 10017
6. American Dietetic Association
   620 North Michigan Avenue
   Chicago, Ill. 60611
7. American Dental Association
   Bureau of Dental Health Education
   211 East Chicago Avenue
   Chicago, Ill. 60611
8. American Dental Hygienists' Association
   211 East Chicago Avenue
   Chicago, Ill. 60611
9. American Heart Association
   44 East 23rd Street
   New York, N.Y. 10010
10. American Home Economics Association
    1600 20th Street, N.W.
    Washington, D.C. 20036
11. American Institute of Baking
    400 East Ontario Street
    Chicago, Ill. 60611
12. American Medical Association
    Department of Health Education
    535 North Dearborn Street
    Chicago, Ill. 60610
13. American National Red Cross
    Office of Publications
    17th and D Streets, N.W.
    Washington, D.C. 20006
14. American Nurses' Association
    10 Columbus Circle
    New York, N.Y. 10019
15. American Optometric Association
    7000 Chippewa
    St. Louis, Mo. 63119
16. American Pharmaceutical Association
    2215 Constitution Avenue, N.W.
    Washington, D.C. 20037
17. American Public Health Association, Inc.
    1015 18th St., N.W.
    Washington, D.C. 20036
18. American School Health Association
    107 South Depeyster
    Kent, Ohio 44240
19. American Social Health Association
    1740 Broadway
    New York, N.Y. 10019
20. Arthritis Foundation
    1212 Avenue of the Americas
    New York, N.Y. 10036
21. Association for Family Living
    6 North Michigan Avenue
    Chicago, Ill. 60602
22. Borden Company
    Consumer's Service
    350 Madison Avenue
    New York, N.Y. 10017
23. Carnation Milk Company
    Home Service Department
    5045 Wilshire Boulevard
    Los Angeles, Calif. 90036
24. Cereal Institute, Inc.
    Educational Director
    135 South LaSalle Street
    Chicago, Ill. 60603

25. Consumers Union of the U.S., Inc.
    Mount Vernon, N.Y. 10550
26. Eli Lilly Company
    Educational Division
    740 South Alabama Street
    Indianapolis, Ind. 46206
27. Employers Mutual of Wausau
    407 Grant Street
    Wausau, Wisc. 55402
28. Epilepsy Foundation of America
    733 15th Street, N.W.
    Washington, D.C. 20005
29. Equitable Life Assurance Society of the
    United States
    1285 Avenue of the Americas
    New York, N.Y. 10019
30. Evaporated Milk Association
    910 17th Street, N.W.
    Washington, D.C. 20036
31. Florida Citrus Commission
    Lakeland, Fla. 33802
32. General Mills, Inc.
    Education Section
    9200 Wayzata Boulevard
    Minneapolis, Minn. 55426
33. Good Housekeeping Institute
    8th Avenue and 57th Street
    New York, N.Y. 10019
34. H. J. Heinz Company
    P.O. Box 57
    Pittsburgh, Pa. 15230
35. Hogg Foundation for Mental Health
    Will C. Hogg Building
    The University of Texas at Austin
    Austin, Texas 78712
36. John Hancock Mutual Life Insurance
    Company
    Health Education Service
    200 Berkeley Street
    Boston, Mass. 02117
37. Johnson & Johnson
    New Brunswick, N.J. 08903
38. Kellogg Company
    Department of Home Economics
    Services
    Battle Creek, Mich. 49016
39. Kimberly-Clark Corporation
    The Life Cycle Center
    Neenah, Wisc. 54956
40. Kraft Cheese Company
    500 Peshtigo Court
    Chicago, Ill. 60690
41. Lederle Laboratories
    Pearl River, N.Y. 10965

42. Lever Brothers
    Educational Department
    390 Park Avenue
    New York, N.Y. 10022
43. Licensed Beverage Industries, Inc.
    155 East 44th Street
    New York, N.Y. 10017
44. Maternity Center Association
    48 East 92nd Street
    New York, N.Y. 10028
45. Mental Health Materials Center
    419 Park Avenue South
    New York, N.Y. 10016
46. Metropolitan Life Insurance Company
    School Health Bureau
    Health and Welfare Division
    One Madison Avenue
    New York, N.Y. 10010
47. Muscular Dystrophy Associations of
    America, Inc.
    1740 Broadway
    New York, N.Y. 10019
48. National Association for Mental Health, Inc.
    180 North Kent Street
    Rosslyn, Va. 22209
49. National Association of Hearing and
    Speech Agencies
    919 18th Street, N.W.
    Washington, D.C. 20006
50. National Better Business Bureau, Inc.
    230 Park Avenue
    New York, N.Y. 10017
51. National Board of Fire Underwriters
    85 John Street
    New York, N.Y. 10038
52. National Clearinghouse for
    Drug Abuse Information
    5600 Fisher Lane
    Rockville, Md. 20852
53. National Clearinghouse for Smoking
    and Health
    5600 Fishers Lane
    Rockville, Md. 20852
54. National Congress of Parents
    and Teachers
    700 North Rush Street
    Chicago, Ill. 60611
55. National Council on Alcoholism
    2 East 103rd Street
    New York, N.Y. 10029
56. National Dairy Council
    Program Service Department
    111 North Canal Street
    Chicago, Ill. 60606

57. National Easter Seal Society for
Crippled Children and Adults
2023 West Ogden Avenue
Chicago, Ill. 60612
58. National Education Association
1201 16th St., N.W.
Washington, D.C. 20036
59. National Foundation—March of Dimes
1275 Mamaroneck Avenue
White Plains, N.Y. 10605
60. National Health Council
1740 Broadway
New York, N.Y. 10019
61. National League for Nursing, Inc.
10 Columbus Circle
New York, N.Y. 10019
62. National Livestock and Meat Board
36 South Wabash Avenue
Chicago, Ill. 60603
63. National Kidney Foundation
315 Park Avenue South
New York, N.Y. 10010
64. National Multiple Sclerosis Society
257 Park Avenue South
New York, N.Y. 10010
65. National Safety Council
425 North Michigan Avenue
Chicago, Ill. 60611
66. National Society for the *Prevention*
of Blindness, Inc.
79 Madison Avenue
New York, N.Y. 10016
67. National Tuberculosis and Respiratory
Diseases Association
1740 Broadway
New York, N.Y. 10019
68. Nutrition Foundation, Inc.
99 Park Avenue
New York, N.Y. 10016
69. Personal Products Company
Education Department
Milltown, N.J. 08850
70. Pharmaceutical Manufacturers
Association
1155 15th Street, N.W.
Washington, D.C. 20005

71. Planned Parenthood—World Population
810 Seventh Avenue
New York, N.Y. 10019
72. Proctor and Gamble Company
P.O. Box 171
Cincinnati, Ohio 45201
73. Public Affairs Committee, Inc.,
381 Park Avenue South
New York, N.Y. 10016
74. Rutgers Center of Alcohol Studies
Rutgers—The State University
Box 560
New Brunswick, N.J. 08903
75. School Health Education Study
3M Education Press
3M Center
St. Paul, Minn. 55101
76. Science Research Associates, Inc.
259 East Erie Street
Chicago, Ill. 60611
77. Scott Paper Company
Industrial Highway—Tinicum
Island Road
Philadelphia, Pa. 19153
78. Sex Information and Education Council
of the United States (SIECUS)
1855 Broadway
New York, N.Y. 10023
79. Smith, Kline & French Laboratories
1500 Spring Garden Street
Philadelphia, Pa. 19101
80. Society of Public Health Educators
81 Hillside Road
Rye, N.Y. 10580
81. Tampax, Inc.
Educational Director
5 Dakota Drive
Lake Success, N.Y. 11040
82. United Cerebral Palsy Associations, Inc.
321 West 44th Street
New York, N.Y. 10036
83. Wheat Flour Institute
14 East Jackson Boulevard
Chicago, Ill. 60604

# Appendix C

## PUBLISHERS OF ELEMENTARY AND SECONDARY SCHOOL, COLLEGE FRESHMAN, AND PROFESSIONAL SCHOOL HEALTH EDUCATION TEXTBOOKS AND PAPERBACKS

Allyn & Bacon, Inc., 470 Atlantic Ave., Boston, Mass. 02210

American Association for Health, Physical Education and Recreation, 1201 16th St., N.W., Washington, D.C. 20036

American Book Company, 450 West 33rd St., New York, N.Y. 10001

Appleton-Century-Crofts, 440 Park Avenue South, New York, N.Y. 10016

Bobbs-Merrill Company, Inc., 4300 West 62nd Street, Indianapolis, Ind. 46268

W. C. Brown Company, 135 South Locust St., Dubuque, Iowa 52001

Burgess Publishing Company, 426 South 6th St., Minneapolis, Minn. 55415

The John Day Company, 257 Park Avenue South, New York, N.Y. 10010

Doubleday & Company, 277 Park Ave., New York, N.Y. 10017

Ginn and Company, Statler Office Building, Back Bay, P.O. Box 191, Boston, Mass. 02117

Glencoe Press, 8701 Wilshire Blvd., Beverly Hills, Calif. 90211

Harcourt, Brace and Jovanovich, Inc., 757 Third Ave., New York, N.Y. 10017

Harper & Row, 49 East 33rd St., New York, N.Y. 10016

D. C. Heath & Company, 125 Spring St., Lexington, Mass. 02173

Holbrook Press, Inc., 470 Atlantic Ave., Boston, Mass. 02210

Holt, Rinehart and Winston, Inc., 383 Madison Ave., New York, N.Y. 10017

Houghton Mifflin Company, 2 Park St., Boston, Mass. 02107

Joint Committee on Health Problems in Education of the National Education Association and the American Medical Association, 1201 16th St., Washington, D.C. 20036

Laidlaw Brothers, Thatcher and Madison Sts., River Forest, Ill. 60305

Lea & Febiger, 600 Washington Square, Philadelphia, Pa. 19106

J. B. Lippincott Company, East Washington Square, Philadelphia, Pa. 19105

Lyons and Carnahan, 407 East 25th St., Chicago, Ill. 60616

McGraw-Hill Book Company, 330 West 42nd St., New York, N.Y. 10036

The Macmillan Company, 866 Third Ave., New York, N.Y. 10022

Charles E. Merrill Publishing Company, 1300 Alum Creek Drive, Columbus, Ohio 43216

The C. V. Mosby Company, 11830 Westline Industrial Drive, St. Louis, Mo. 63141

Prentice-Hall, Inc., Englewood Cliffs, N.J. 07632

Ronald Press Company, 79 Madison Ave., New York, N.Y. 10016

W. B. Saunders Company, West Washington Square, Philadelphia, Pa. 19105

School Health Education Study, 3M Education Press, 3M Center, St. Paul, Minn. 55101

Scott, Foresman and Company, 1900 East Lake Ave., Glenview, Ill. 60025

The Steck-Vaughn Company, P.O. Box 2028, Austin, Texas 78767

Charles C Thomas, Publisher, 301-327 East Lawrence Ave., Springfield, Ill. 62703

Van Nostrand Reinhold Company, 300 Pike St., Cincinnati, Ohio 45202

Wadsworth Publishing Company, Inc., 10 Davis Drive, Belmont, Calif. 94002

John Wiley & Sons, 605 Third Ave., New York, N.Y. 10016

# Index

Strep throat, 54
Sty, 18
Superintendent of schools, 11-274, 211-218
  administrative control, 212
  approval, policies and procedures, 212
  cooperation, local health department, 217
  elementary school health education, 215
  equipment and supplies, 213
  evaluation, 217-218
  facilities, 213
  funds, 213
  in-service health education, 216-217
  legal regulations, 214-215
  liaison agent, 216
  noonday school meals, 215
  public relations, 216
  school health council, 217
  secondary school health education, 215
  supervision of health education, 212-213, 221-222
Supervision, 221-222
  health education, 212-213
  methods, 136-137
  school day, 136-137
Supervisor of health education, 141-230, 212-213, 221-222, 247-253
Supplementary feeding, 127
Survey, 195
Sweep Test, 29
Syphilis, 60, 185-187

**T**

Tacoma Public Schools, 29
Tachycardia, 30
Tapeworms, 48
Tartar, 65
Teacher, of health education, 149, 152, 219-221
  certification, 97, 154, 220
  content, 161-189
  lessons, 177-189
  methods and materials, 190-198
  preparation, 219-221
  school day, 130-137
    change of class activities, 136-137
    characteristics, 133-134
    organization, 135-136
    placement of classroom activities, 136
    preparation of instruction, 134-135
    pupil rest and relaxation, 136
    units, 162-176
Teacher-made knowledge tests, 249-253
  objective, 250-252
    completion, 251
    matching, 250-251
    multiple choice, 250
    problem-to-be-solved, 251-252
    true-false, 252
  subjective, 249-250
Teacher-pupil relations, 133
*Teach Us What We Want To Know*, 160
Teeth, 63-65
  crown, 65
  deciduous, 63
  permanent, 64
  root, 65
  See also Dental Health
Temperature, classroom, gymnasium, 109

Tenure, 103
Tetanus, 56-57
  effects, 57
  signs, 57
  toxoid, 57
Threadbare skin, 19
Threshold Test, 29
Tonometer, 83
Tonsillitis, 17
Toothache, 68
Tooth brushing, 70-72
  demonstration, 71
  effectiveness, 70
Tooth brushing after eating, 72, 177-178
Topical fluoride application, 66
Tornado, 118, 164-165
Tort liability, 86-87
Trachoma, 18
Treponemas, 60
Trichinae, 48
True-false questions, 252
Tuberculin tests, 35, 58, 98-99
  Heaf, 58
  jet injection, 58
  Mantoux, 58
  negative reaction, 58
  positive reaction, 58
  purposes, 58
  school personnel, 98-99
  Tine, 58
Tuberculosis, 57-59
  bacilli, 57
  chemoprophlaxis, 59
  chemotherapy, 59
  control, 59
  detection, 58
    tuberculin tests, 35, 58, 98-99
  effect on lung tissue, 57
  miliary, 57
  prevention, 58-59
  signs, 58
  reinfection, 57-58
  treatment, 59
  tubercle, 57
Type "A" lunch, 124-126
Typhoid fever, 107

**U**

Unconsciousness, 90
Unit, 161-176
  Alcoholic-beverages—their use, abuse, and misuse, 165-166
  Cancers, 167-169
  defined, 163
  Dental health, 163-164
  Eye infections, injuries, and defects, 164
  Hallucinogens, 165
  lessons, 177-189
  Menstrual hygiene, 170-172
  objectives, 177-189
  Quackery, 166-167
  Rabies, 169-170
  reasons, 161
  Self-preservation in the event of tornado, 164-165
United Cerebral Palsy Associations, Inc., 80
United States Department of Agriculture, 4, 124, 246
United States Department of Labor, 4